The Atlas of

Aesthetic Facial Surgery

Comprehensive Surgical Atlases in Otolaryngology and Head and Neck Surgery

Editor-in-Chief

K. J. Lee, M.D., F.A.C.S.

Director, Ear Research and Educational Center
Chairman, Education and Research Committee
Coordinator, Laser Surgery Center
President, Hospital of St. Raphael Medical Staff
Chairman, Medical Board
Hospital of St. Raphael
New Haven, Connecticut
Attending, Hospital of St. Raphael, Yale–New Haven Hospital, and Milford Hospital
New Haven and Milford, Connecticut
Consultant, Backus Hospital and Windham Community Hospital
Norwich and Willimantic, Connecticut
Assistant Clinical Professor, Department of Surgery
Yale University School of Medicine
New Haven, Connecticut

The Surgical Atlas of Otology and Neuro-otology
Eiji Yanagisawa, M.D., F.A.C.S., and Gale Gardner, M.D., F.A.C.S.

The Atlas of Head and Neck Surgery
Bruce W. Jafek, M.D., F.A.C.S., and Clarence T. Sasaki, M.D., F.A.C.S.

The Atlas of Aesthetic Facial Surgery
Douglas D. Dedo, M.D., F.A.C.S.

The Surgical Atlas of Airway and Facial Trauma
Robert H. Miller, M.D., F.A.C.S.

The Atlas of Cleft Lip and Cleft Palate Surgery
Howard W. Smith, M.D., D.M.D., F.A.C.S.

Foreword

In the five volumes in this series, the editors, contributors, and I have attempted to illustrate succinctly the current acceptable techniques in otolaryngology and head and neck surgery. When possible and appropriate, we have included alternative techniques for comparison.

I am greatly indebted to the editorial staff of Grune & Stratton, Inc., for their support and patience. I also thank the volume editors, contributors, and illustrators for enduring my numerous phone calls and letters. As usual, my wife and family have been most supportive.

In recognition of our teachers, the volume editors have dedicated these texts to their mentors.

K. J. Lee, M.D., F.A.C.S.
Editor-in-Chief

The Atlas of
Aesthetic Facial Surgery

Douglas D. Dedo, M.D., F.A.C.S.

Clinical Assistant Professor
Department of Otolaryngology
University of Miami School of Medicine
Miami, Florida
Attending, Good Samaritan and St. Mary's Hospital
West Palm Beach, Florida
Attending, Palm Beach Gardens Hospital
Palm Beach Gardens, Florida
Director, Biennial Palm Beach Aesthetic Surgery Symposium
Palm Beach, Florida

Illustrated by

Marcelino Obaya
Carl Gulledge
Francine Mehler

G&S

GRUNE & STRATTON
A Subsidiary of Harcourt Brace Jovanovich, Publishers
New York London Paris San Diego San Francisco São Paulo Sydney Tokyo Toronto

Figure 6-1 is reprinted with permission from Norwood, O'T.: Hair Transplant Surgery, Charles C. Thomas, Springfield Ill., 1973, p. 6.

Figure 6-15 is reprinted with permission from Unger, W.P.: Hair Transplantation, Marcel Dekker, New York, 1979, p. 90.

Library of Congress Cataloging in Publication Data

Main entry under title:

The Atlas of aesthetic facial surgery.

(Comprehensive surgical atlases in otolaryngology and head and neck surgery)
Includes bibliographies and index.
1. Face—Surgery. 2. Surgery, Plastic. I. Dedo, Douglas D. II. Obaya, Marcelino. III. Gulledge, Carl. IV. Mehler, Francine. V. Series. [DNLM: 1. Face—Surgery—Atlases. 2. Surgery, Plastic—Atlases. WE 17 A877]
RD119.5.F33A75 1983 617'.520592 83-22610
ISBN 0-8089-1616-5

Grune & Stratton, Inc.
Orlando, Florida

Distributed in the United Kingdom by
Grune & Stratton, Inc. (London) Ltd.
24/28 Oval Road, London NW 1

Library of Congress Catalog Number 83-22610
International Standard Book Number 0-8089-1616-5
Printed in the United States of America

To

The late Joseph H. Ogura, M.D.

Lindbergh Professor and Chairman
Department of Otolaryngology–Head and Neck Surgery
Washington University Medical School
St. Louis, Missouri

For providing a foundation in
head and neck and facial plastic surgery.

Richard Webster, M.D.

Chief, Plastic Surgical Service
Melrose–Wakefield Hospital
Melrose, Massachusetts
Associate Surgeon, Plastic and Reconstructive Surgery
Massachusetts Eye and Ear Infirmary
Boston, Massachusetts
Lecturer, Department of Otolaryngology
Harvard Medical School
Boston, Massachusetts

For developing, teaching, and heading
the subspecialty of facial plastic and reconstructive surgery.

Contents

Preface

When performed to improve the appearance of the face, aesthetic surgery reaches its pinnacle. At no time is the postoperative result of any surgery more open to scrutiny than it is when it involves the alteration of facial lines and defects. Although skillfully applied makeup surely can modify or even camouflage minor flaws, it obviously cannot change the numerous imperfections that affect the face.

It is hoped that this book will provide a concise and completely illustrated description of the common procedures used in cosmetic surgery of the head and neck. The format of the text should enable the reader to understand easily the steps used in each procedure. Elaboration and discussion of the indications for surgery and postoperative evaluation have been kept to a minimum since the surgeon trained in plastic surgery will have a firm foundation in the basic techniques of patient evaluation. At the end of each chapter, the author discusses his rationale for preferring one technique to another.

The contributing authors, each of whom specializes in the topic he covers, are all relatively young surgeons whose instructors were established clinicians. The reader therefore can learn the basic procedures that have been proven by time as well as the latest techniques and modifications that the authors have either developed or found worthwhile on the basis of their own clinical experience.

I would like to thank Drs. Bruce B. Chrisman, Charles E. Clark, III, Jeffrey N. Hausfeld, K. J. Lee, John A. McCurdy, and Michael Patipa for their contributions to this volume. While it is impossible to compensate them adequately for their time and energy, I hope that they will feel rewarded when they see residents and other surgeons using this atlas as a guide.

Thanks are also due to the illustrators, Marcelino Obaya, Carl Gulledge, and Francine Mehler, whose outstanding illustrations complement the text. Excellent diagrams are the key to a surgical atlas since they enable the reader to understand and interpret each procedure.

Contributors

Bruce B. Chrisman, M.D.
Assistant Clinical Professor
Department of Medicine, (Dermatology)
John A. Burns School of Medicine
University of Hawaii
Attending, Kapiolani Children's Medical Center and Queen's Medical Center
Honolulu, Hawaii

Charles E. Clark, III, M.D., F.A.C.S.
Assistant Clinical Professor
Department of Otolaryngology
Duke University Medical School
Attending, Head and Neck Surgery, McPherson Hospital
Durham, North Carolina

Jeffrey N. Hausfeld, M.D.
Clinical Instructor
Department of Otolaryngology
George Washington University Medical Center
Attending, Otorhinolaryngology and Facial Plastic and Reconstructive Surgery, Shady Grove Adventist Hospital, Rockville, Maryland, and George Washington University Medical Center, Washington Hospital Center, Children's Hospital National Medical Center, and Sibley Memorial Hospital
Washington, D.C.

John A. McCurdy, Jr., M.D., F.A.C.S.
Assistant Clinical Professor
Department of Surgery
John A. Burns School of Medicine
University of Hawaii
Honolulu, Hawaii
Attending, Maui Memorial Hospital, Wailuku, Maui, Hawaii, and Castle Memorial Hospital
Honolulu, Hawaii

Michael Patipa, M.D.
Attending Oculoplastic Surgeon
Good Samaritan Hospital and St. Mary's Hospital
West Palm Beach, Florida

1
Cervicofacial Rhytidectomy

Rejuvenation of the lower one-third of the face and upper neck is achieved primarily by means of the myeloplasty, rhytidectomy, or facelift operation. Since the first description in the early 1900s of localized skin and muscle excision to correct wrinkling, the facelift operation has developed into a procedure that involves wide undermining of the skin with subsequent rotation, advancement, and trimming. Present controversy now centers around the extent of undermining and the appropriate method for manipulation of the deeper subcutaneous layers. As new instrumentation and techniques are developed, the postoperative cosmetic result and its duration will continue to improve.

ANATOMY

The topographic anatomy allows identification of key landmarks to plan incisions, the extent of undermining, high-risk zones, and the precise diagnosis of the pathologic anatomy causing the cosmetic deformity.

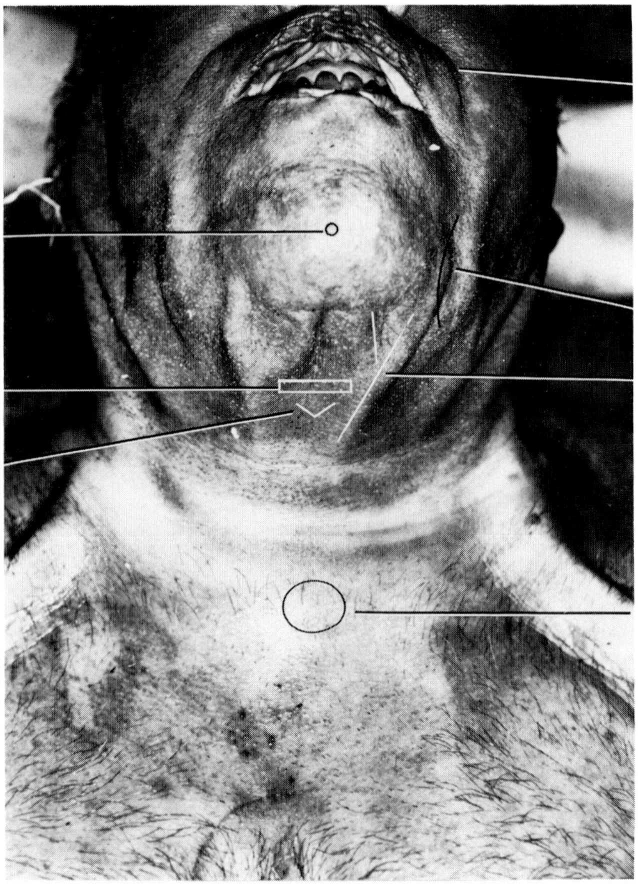

Figure 1-1

The topography is illustrated in Figure 1-1 on the anterior views of the cadaver. The nasolabial fold that entends inferiorly to the jowl, the pogonion, the hyoid bone, the thyroid cartilage notch, the sternal notch, and the anterior folds of the platysma are identified.

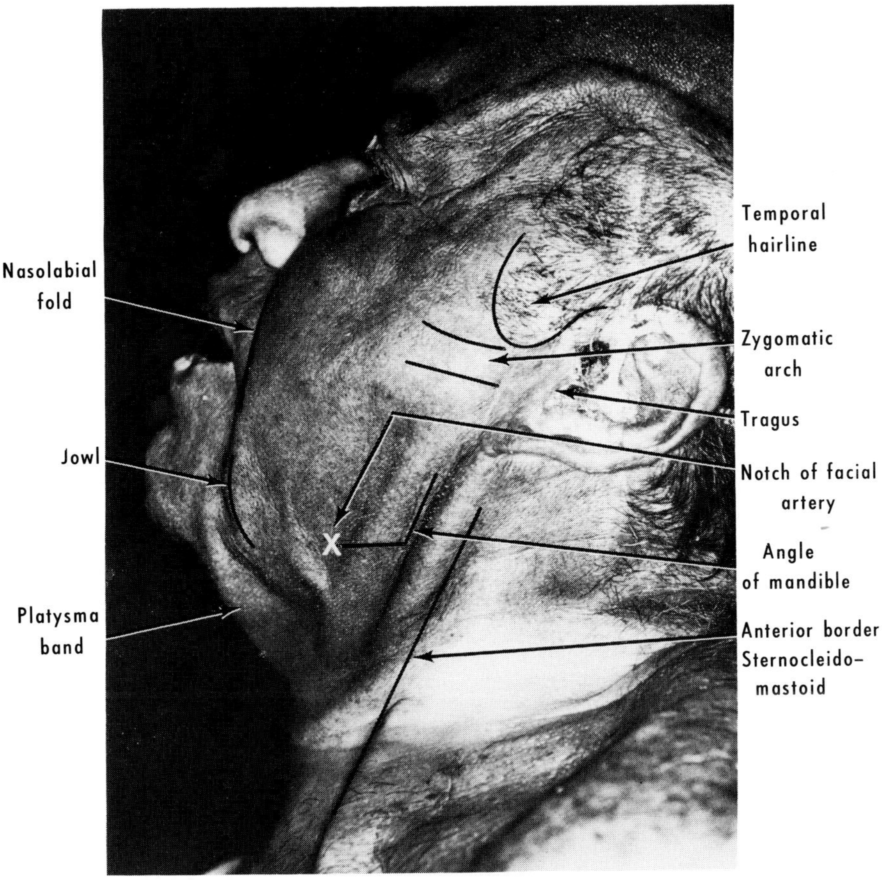

Figure 1-2

On the lateral view (Figure 1-2), the temporal hairline, the zygomatic arch, the tragus, the notch of the facial artery, the mandibular angle, and the anterior border of the sternocleidomastoid muscle and the intimate relationship of the nasolabial fold, jowl, and platysma banding are shown.

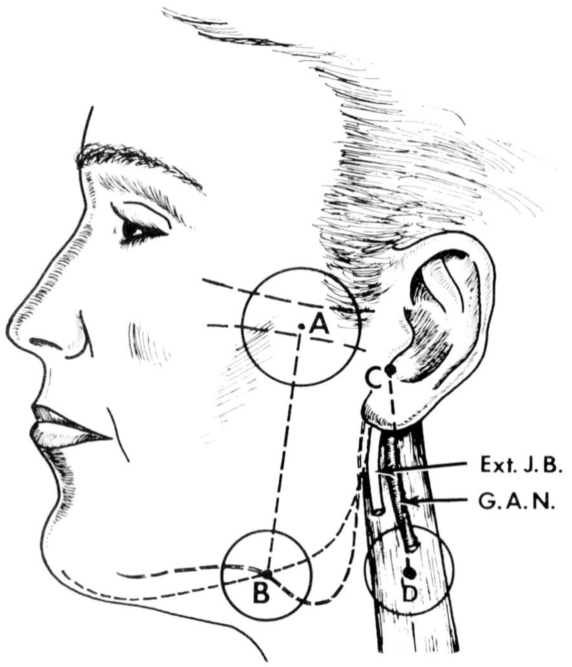

Figure 1-3

Figure 1-3 shows the high-risk zones of the face. Line AB runs from the anterior edge of the temporal hairline to the notch of the facial artery, and posterior to this line a relatively comfortable cushion of subcutaneous tissue protects the facial nerve. Anterior to this line the subcutaneous musculoaponeurotic system (SMAS) becomes thinner and the branches of the facial nerve course more superficially to enter the undersurface of the facial musculature. Anterior to point A in the circumscribed circle, the temporal branch enters a transition zone from a deeper to a more superficial plane as it subsequently enters the outer surface of the frontalis muscle. Note that this zone extends 1 cm below the zygomatic arch. Dissection over the zygomatic arch must be very superficial and lateral to the SMAS. Dissection superior to the zygomatic arch and anterior to the temporal hairline toward the eyebrow must be deep and in the supraperiosteal layer. Anterior to the notch of the facial artery (point B) the mandibular branch of the facial nerve begins to ascend from its position in the fibrous capsule of the submaxillary gland to course over the horizontal ramus of the mandible and ennervate the corner of the mouth. If the SMAS is elevated in continuity with the platysma muscle, it can be safely carried to the anterior border of the parotid gland and the notch of the facial artery. Any SMAS undermining beyond these landmarks risks injury to the branches of the facial nerve. Dissection lateral to, or on top of, the platysma muscle in the neck will prevent injury to the nerve. A line dropped 6.5 cm from the external auditory canal (point C) to the midportion of the sternocleidomastoid muscle, with the head turned 45° (point D), identifies the precise location of the greater auricular nerve (G.A.N. in Figure 1-3). Also in Figure 1-3, the external jugular vein (Ext J. B.) runs parallel and 0.5 cm anterior to the nerve at point D. The greater auricular nerve lies under the SMAS, which itself is intimately connected to the dermis and the fascia overlying the mastoid and sternocleidomastoid muscle, respectively. Preservation of this sensory nerve is achieved by elevating a thin flap in the occipital and subauricular regions once the hairline has been passed. By identifying the location of the nerve (line CD), platysma muscle and SMAS plication sutures are placed to avoid damaging the nerve.

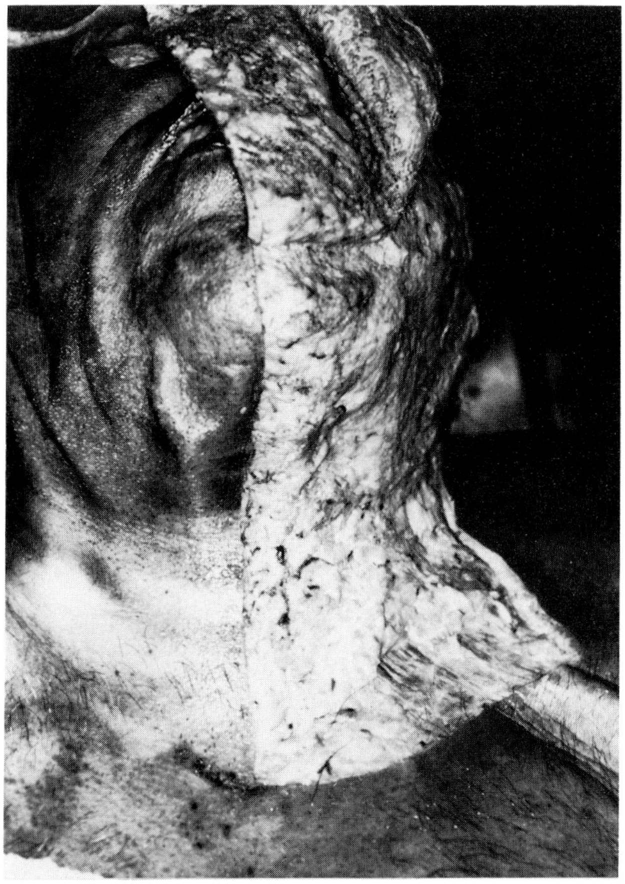

Figure 1-4A

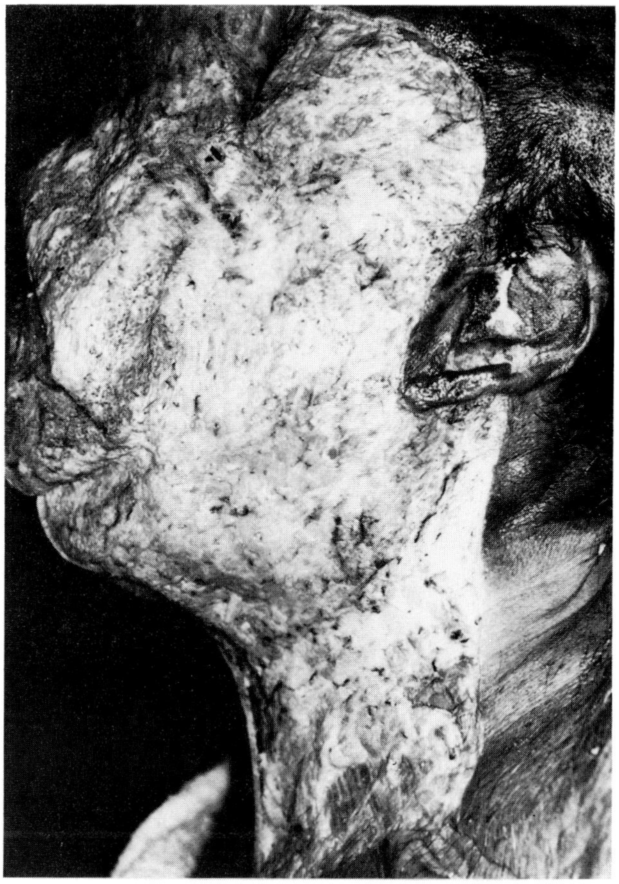

Figure 1-4B

The subcutaneous layer shown in Figure 1-4A (anterior view) and Figure 1-4B (lateral view) has been exposed by elevating the skin. There are no vital structures lateral to this layer. In effect, the SMAS has been exposed with a thin layer of fat. (*Note:* The skin flap also has a fine layer of fat.)

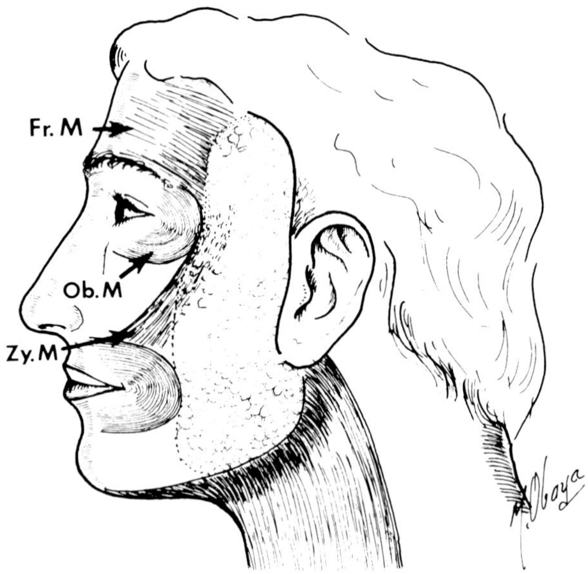

Figure 1-5A

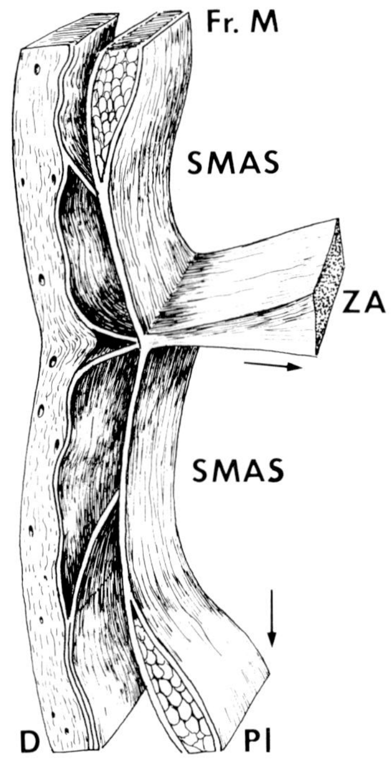

Figure 1-5B

Figure 1-5A and B is a schematic illustration of the SMAS layer, which is shown extending from the frontalis muscle (Fr. M) and obicularis oculi (Ob. M) to become intimately attached to the platysma muscle (P1). A coronal cut depicts the fibrous attachments to the zygomatic arch (ZA). Cadaver dissections more clearly define the extent of this important anatomic layer.

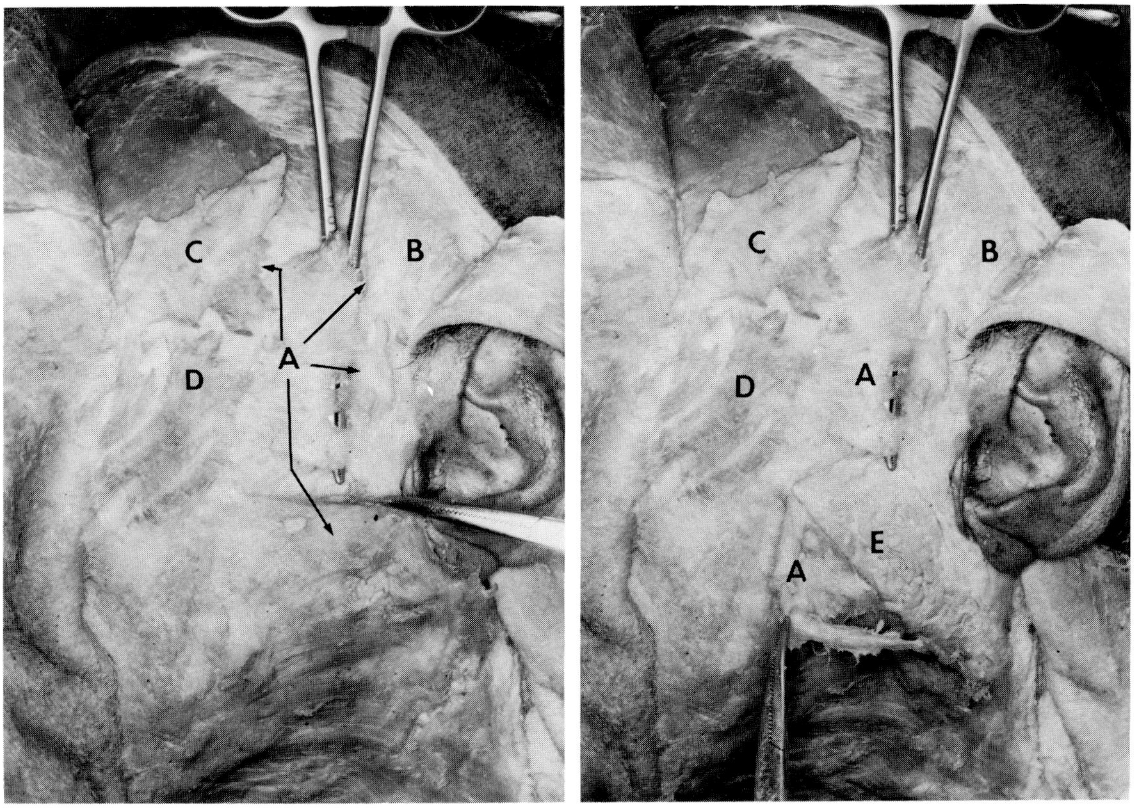

Figure 1-6

In Figure 1-6, in the temporal area the SMAS (A) is lateral to the temporalis fascia (B) and is continuous with the frontalis muscle (C) and orbicularis oculi (D). The hemostat lies on top of the temporalis fascia and under the SMAS. When the SMAS is split, the parotid gland (E) is exposed.

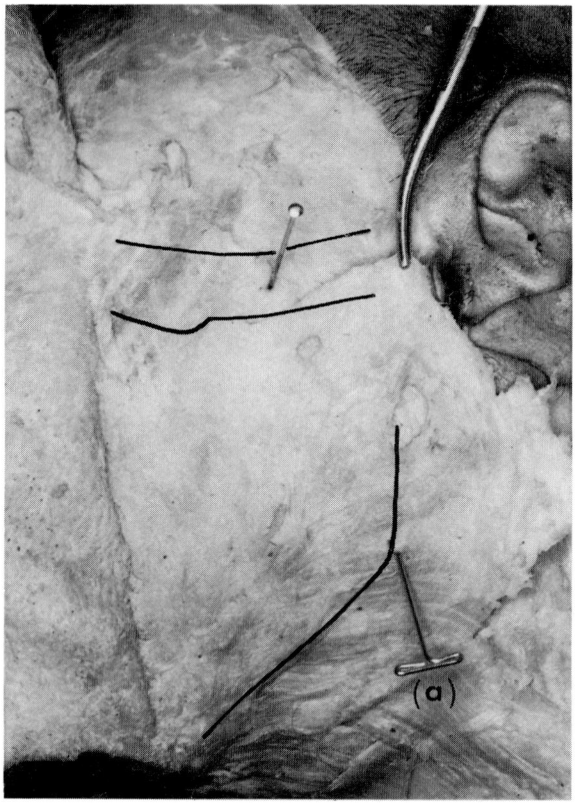

Figure 1-7

As shown in Figure 1-7, the preauricular SMAS from the zygoma (superior pin) to the angle of the mandible (a) is densely adherent to the parotid fascia. Note the insertion of the platysma fibers into the SMAS just above the horizontal ramus of the mandible.

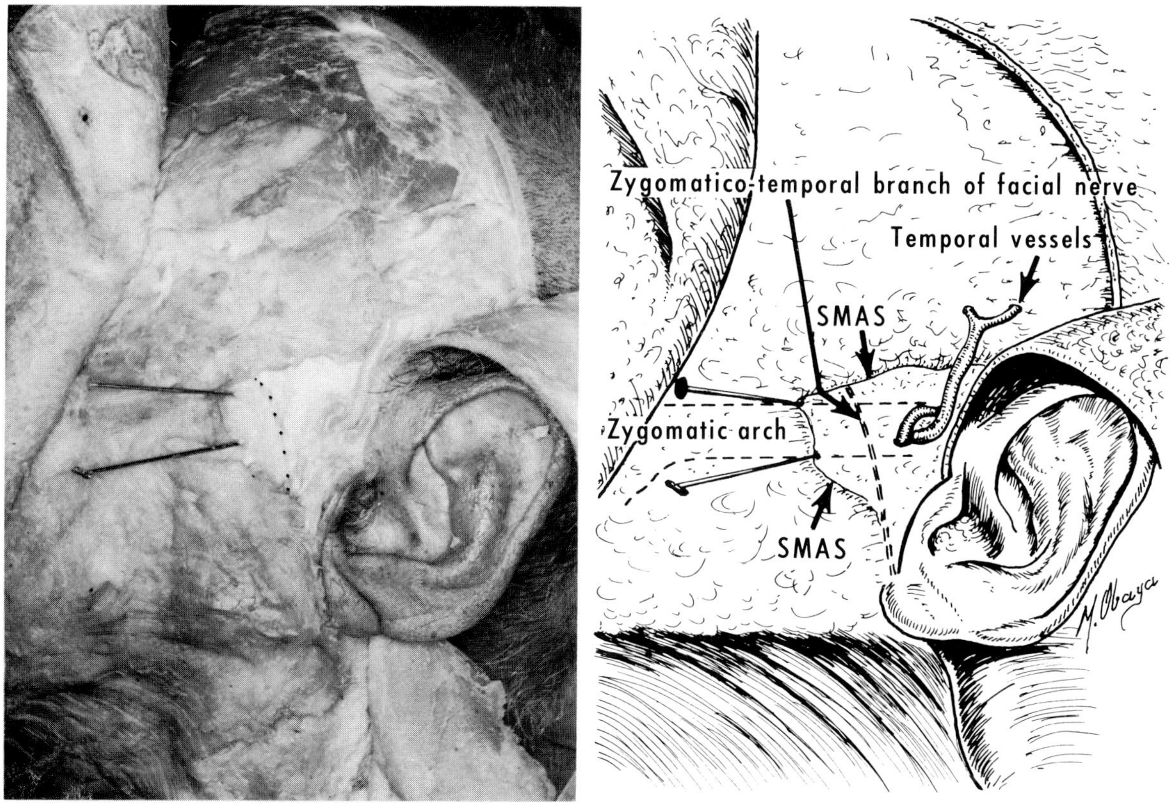

Figure 1-8

When dissection extends beneath the SMAS over the zygomatic arch as well as 1 cm below it (Figure 1-8), the temporal branch of the facial nerve is exposed, thereby making this level of dissection inappropriate for facelift surgery.

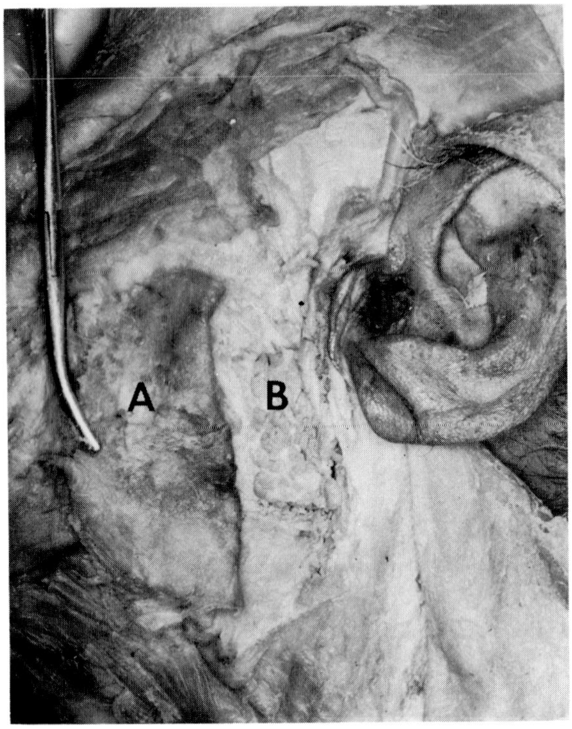

Figure 1-9

As the SMAS (point A in Figure 1-9) is elevated over the parotid gland beginning 1 cm below the zygoma, the facial nerve is protected by the superficial lobe of the parotid gland (point B in Figure 1-9).

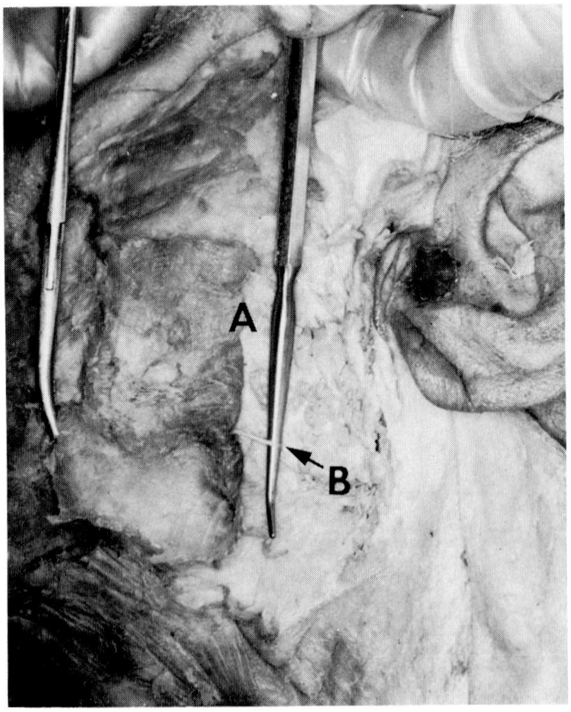

Figure 1-10

In Figure 1-10, at the anterior border of the parotid (A) the various facial nerve branches begin to surface, thereby increasing the risk of nerve injury when dissection of this layer extends beyond the anterior border of the parotid. The probe is retracting a buccal branch (B). Safe undermining of the cheek area, anterior to the parotid gland, may thus be done only in a superficial plane, lateral to the SMAS.

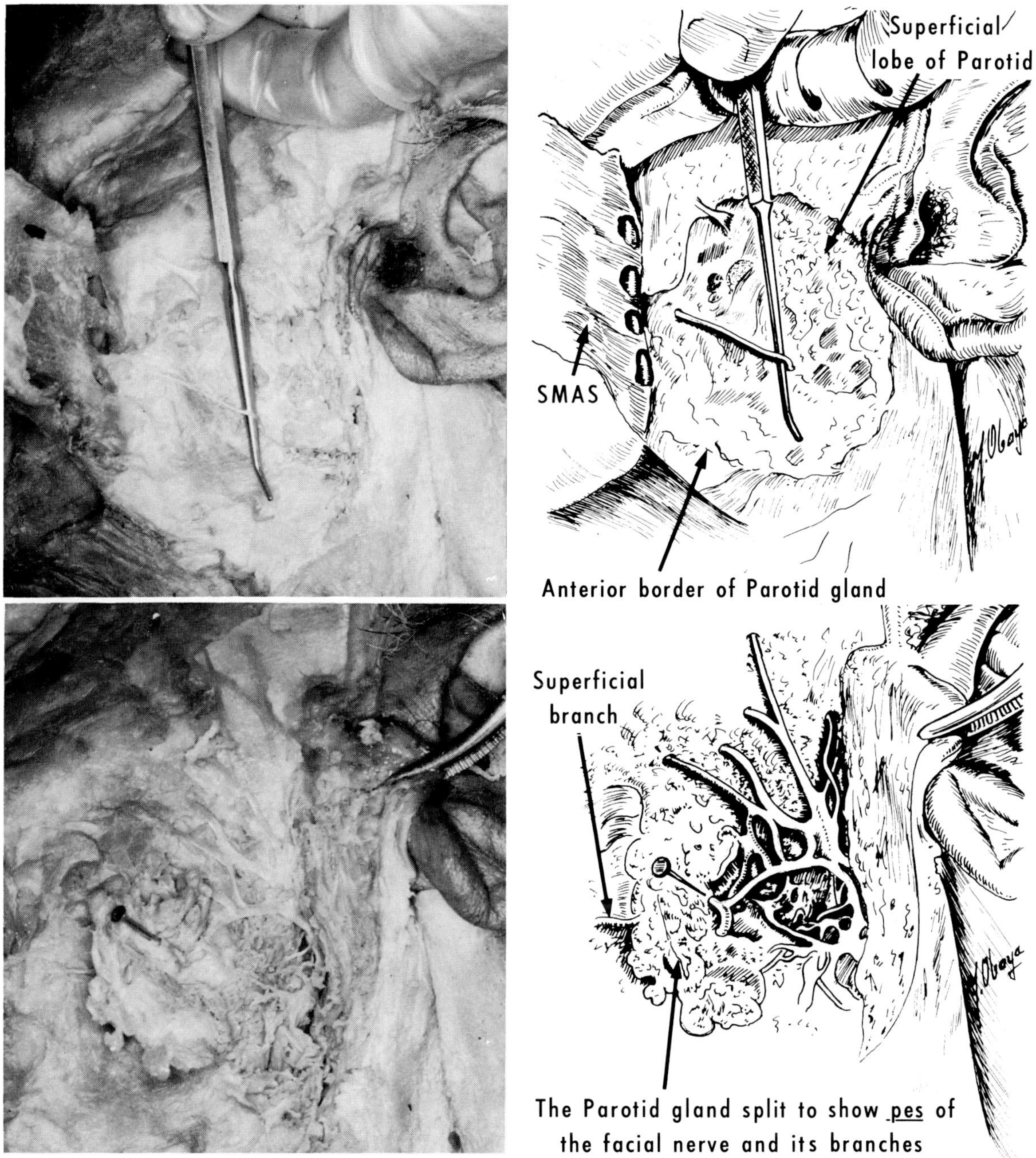

Figure 1-11

As shown in Figure 1-11, the SMAS becomes thinner and more difficult to delineate as dissection extends anteriorly over the parotid. When the superficial lobe is split, the pes of the facial nerve and its branches are identified.

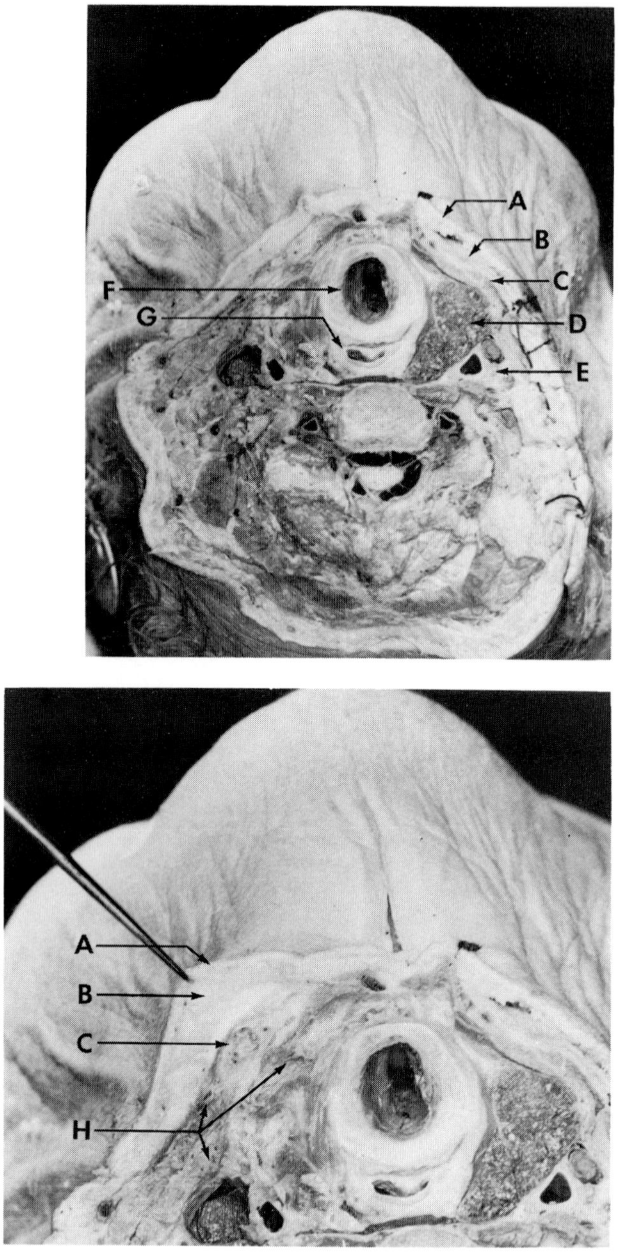

Figure 1-12

A superficial layer of fat lies lateral to the platysma muscle in the submandibular and submental areas. Figure 1-12 shows a cross section of the neck at the level of the cricoid cartilage. This layer of insulating fat is shown at point B. The skin (A), fat (B), platysma muscle (C), sternocleidomastoid muscle (D), carotid sheath (E), trachea (F), esophagus (G), and strap muscles (H) are identified.

In Figure 1-13, the fat (A) has been removed from the left half of the specimen to expose the platysma muscle (B).

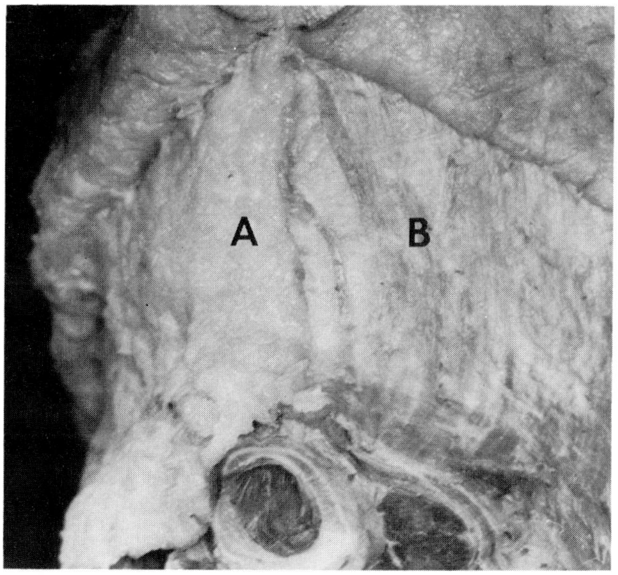

Figure 1-13

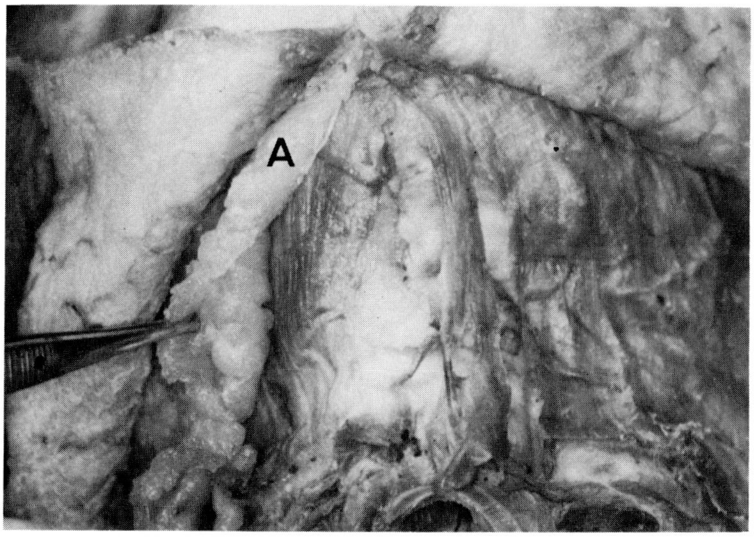

Figure 1-14

Figure 1-14 shows how the fat may be elevated as a single layer (A) from the platysma.

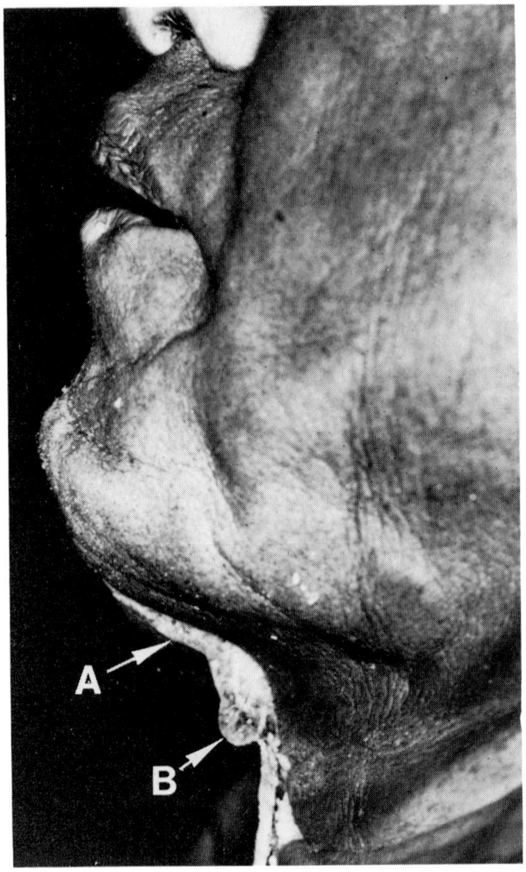

Figure 1-15

As shown in Figure 1-15, after the skin flap (A) is redraped following excision of the subcutaneous fat, the submental contour has been improved while the persistent fold of skin and fat (B) is well demonstrated on the untreated side. This gives credibility to those who advocate sculpturing the neck in facelift surgery.

In Figure 1-16, the superficial layer of fat in the neck is continuous with the jowl (A) and nasolabial fold (B) areas. Since it lies lateral to the SMAS and platysma, it could conceivably be removed to effectively sculpture the jowl area without injuring the facial nerve. Unfortunately, the vasculature and bleeding makes fat excision in this area difficult clinically.

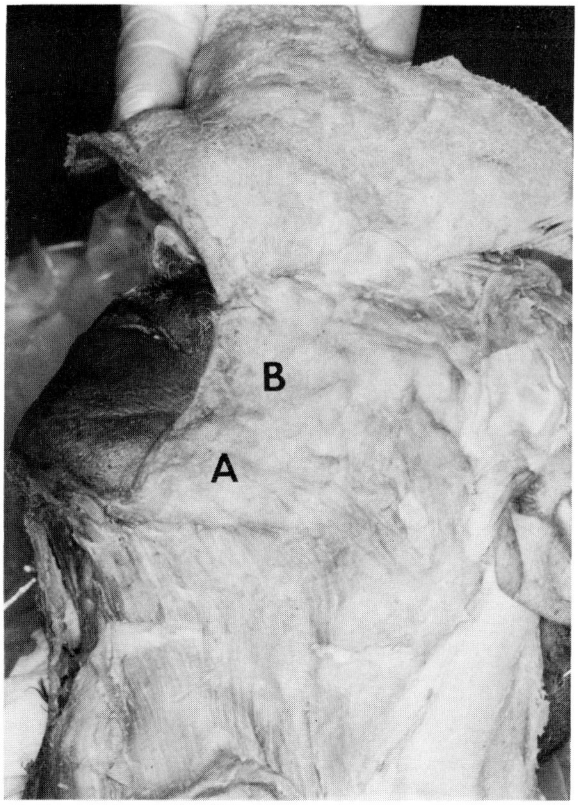

Figure 1-16

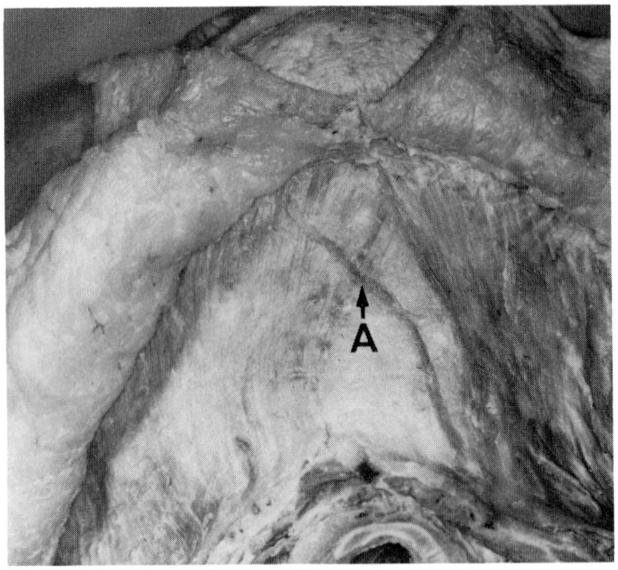

Figure 1-17

The platysmal muscle shown in Figure 1-17 is similar to the other 17 paired facial muscles because of its intimate relationship with the skin, fat, and fascia of the subcutaneous layers. The platysma arises from the deltoid and pectoral areas of the chest. It inserts into the lower one-third of the face between the quadratus labi inferioris (depressor of the lip) and SMAS of the inferior and posterior cheek. Frequently the anterior border (A) of this muscle bifurcates one or more times to form a band of muscle fibers that either cross the midline to interdigitate with the opposite side or run parallel to the main body of the muscle. This accounts for the wide or occasional multiple folds in the submental area.

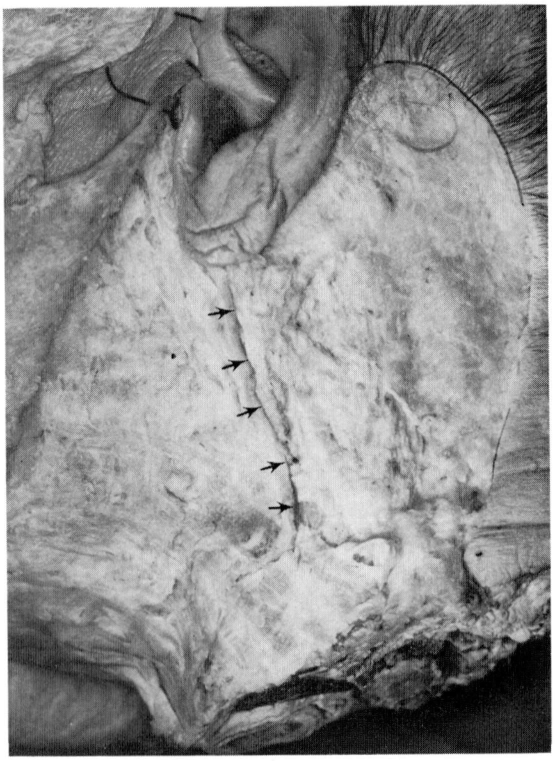

Figure 1-18

As seen in Figure 1-18, the posterior border of the platysma is continuous with the SMAS and may be identified inferior to the lobule of the ear, along the anterior border of the sternocleidomastoid muscle (arrows).

When the posterior border of the platysma (A) is elevated and subsequently raised superiorly, the submaxillary gland (B) is identified (Figure 1-19).

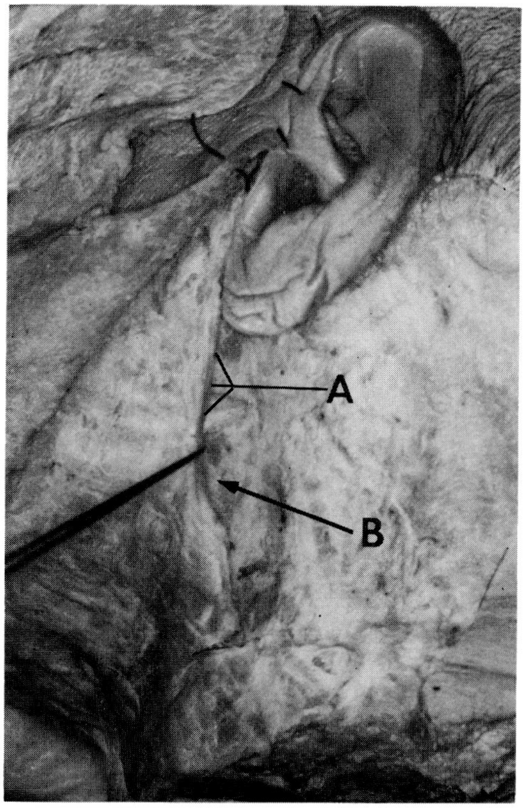

Figure 1-19

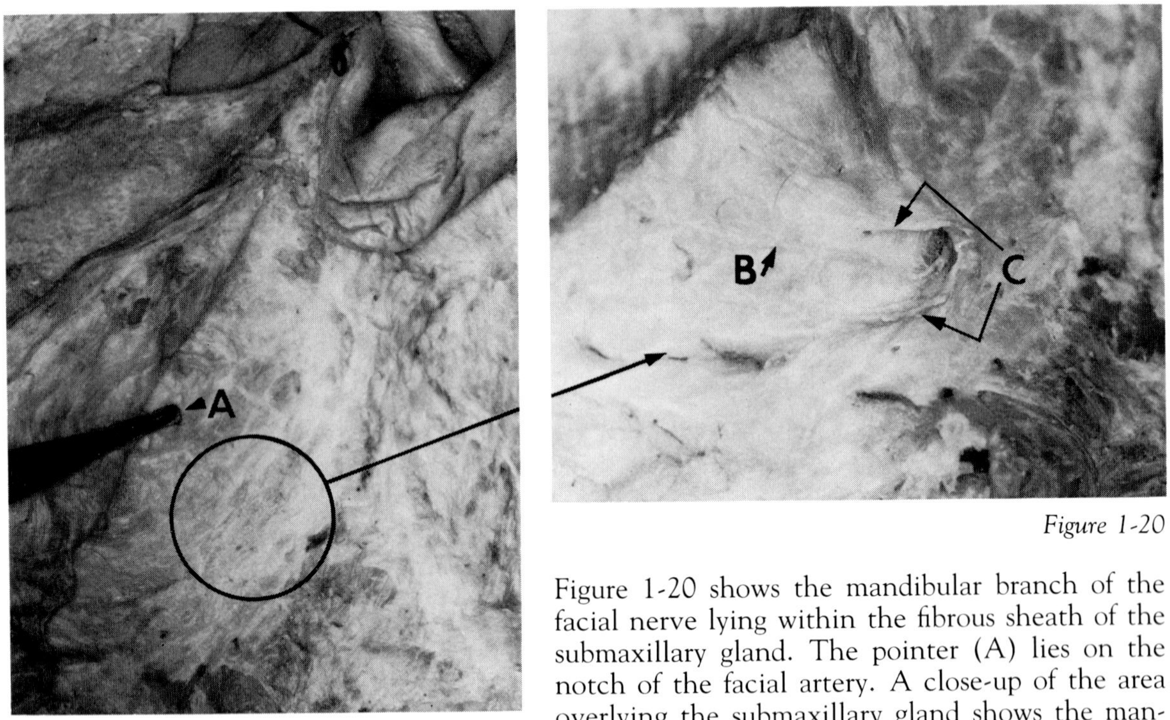

Figure 1-20

Figure 1-20 shows the mandibular branch of the facial nerve lying within the fibrous sheath of the submaxillary gland. The pointer (A) lies on the notch of the facial artery. A close-up of the area overlying the submaxillary gland shows the mandibular branch (B) encased by the fibrous capsule (C) of the submaxillary gland. By hugging the undersurface of the platysma muscle and staying at least two finger breadths below the ramus of the mandible (Figure 1-20), the platysma may be mobilized without damage to the mandibular branch of the facial nerve. Posterior to the notch of the facial artery, the nerve may be vulnerable to injury if dissection of the SMAS-platysma complex is carried too deeply. Anterior to the notch, the nerve begins to run superiorly and even more superficially, thus making elevation of this musculofascial layer very dangerous anterior to the artery notch.

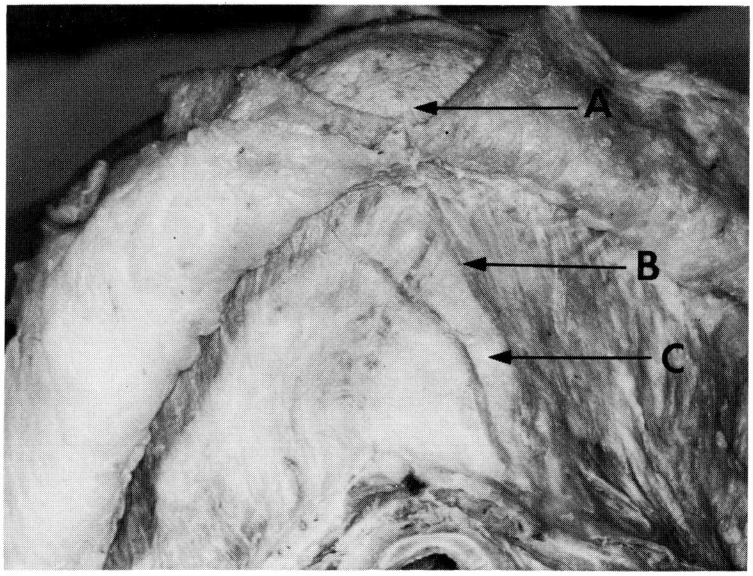

Figure 1-21

As shown in Figure 1-21, the submental fat pad (C) lies in the submental triangle deep to the platysma muscle (B). The pogonion (A) provides a reference point.

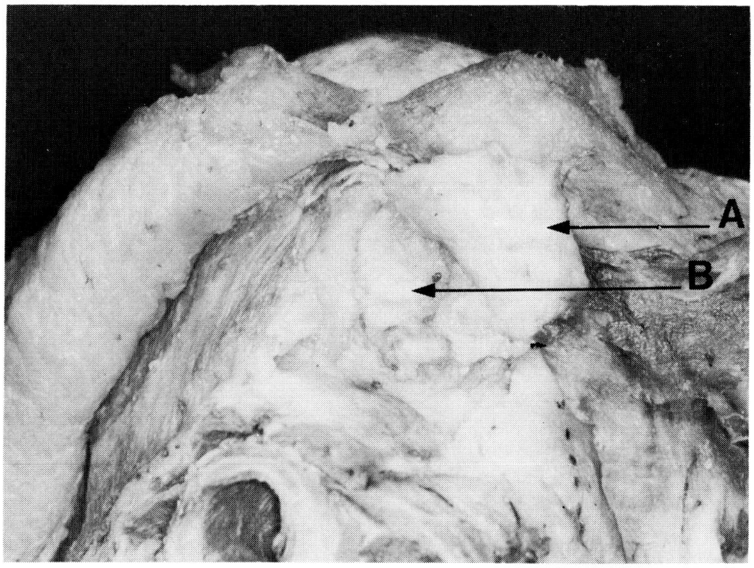

Figure 1-22

In Figure 1-22, after elevation of the fibrofatty tissue (A) that attaches to the hyoid, a deeper, slightly whiter collection of adipose tissue (B) is identified.

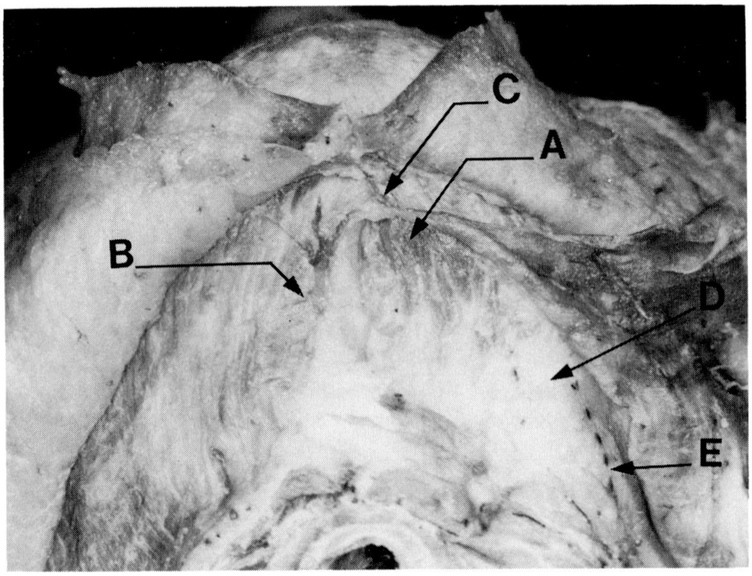

Figure 1-23

Figure 1-23 shows that the fat has been removed only from the left half of the submental triangle to expose the mylohyoid muscle (A), which forms the floor of the triangle. The right half of the submental fat pad (B) is in place, and the platysma (C), anterior border of the submaxillary gland (D), and marginal mandibular branch of the seventh facial nerve (E) are labeled. Attempts at removal of submental fat lateral to the mylohyoid in the region of the submaxillary gland may endanger the mandibular nerve.

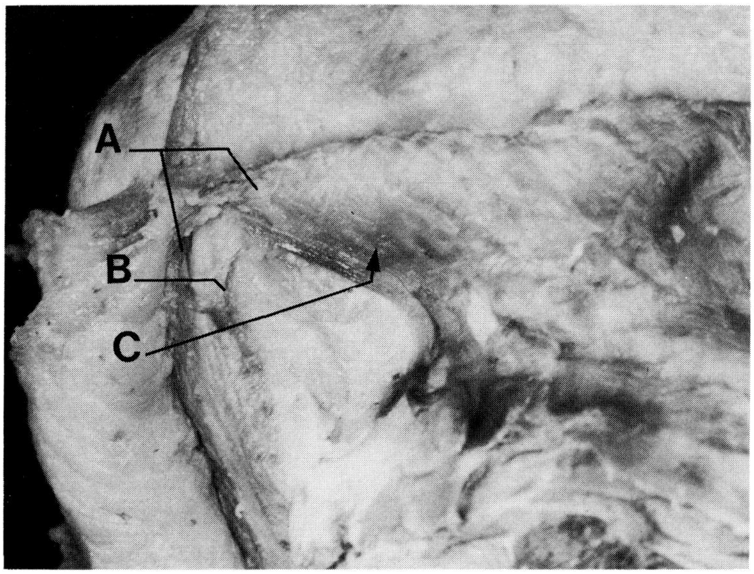

Figure 1-24

The oblique view of the submental triangle shown in Figure 1-24 clearly defines two layers: platysma muscle (A) and submental fat (B). When the left half of the platysma muscle is redraped after fat excision on this side, a depression is apparent (C).

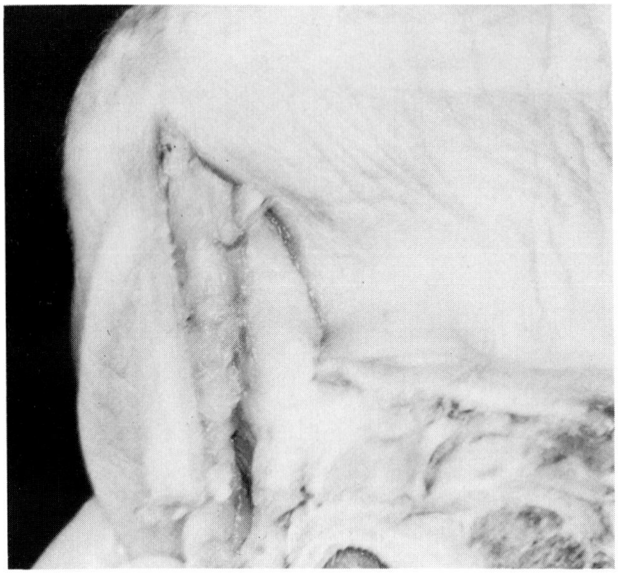

Figure 1-25

As shown in Figure 1-25, injudicious removal of the submental fat pad will produce an unnatural depression. When the skin flap is replaced, it will adhere to the mylohyoid muscle and create what has been called the "cobra" deformity.

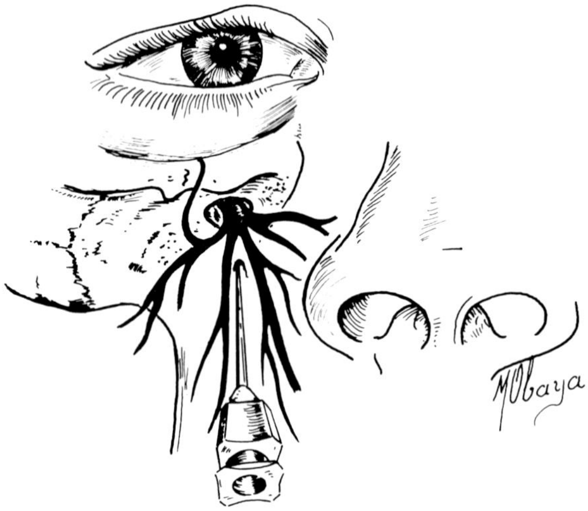

Figure 1-26

TECHNIQUE

ANESTHESIA

As shown in Figure 1-26, the infraorbital nerve is located 1–2 cm below the infraorbital margin in a line dropped from the pupil, perpendicular to the interpupillary plane; 1–2 ml of 0.5% Marcaine (bupivacaine hydrochloride; see Discussion section at end of chapter for reasons for its use in this procedure) with 1 : 200,000 Adrenalin is injected around the nerve as it leaves the foramen.

The third branch of the trigeminal nerve (mandibular) is blocked through the mandibular notch with a 25-gauge spinal needle (Figure 1-27). As the needle meets the pterygoid plate, it is "marched" posteriorly until bone is no longer contacted. After the syringe is preaspirated to prevent intravascular injection, 2–4 ml of 0.5% Marcaine with 1 : 200,000 Adrenalin is infiltrated.

The superficial cervical plexus shown in Figure 1-28A is blocked with a similar bolus of anesthetic along the midportion of the posterior margin of the sternocleidomastoid muscle. The area of skin anesthesia thus achieved is mapped out (shaded) in Figure 1-28B.

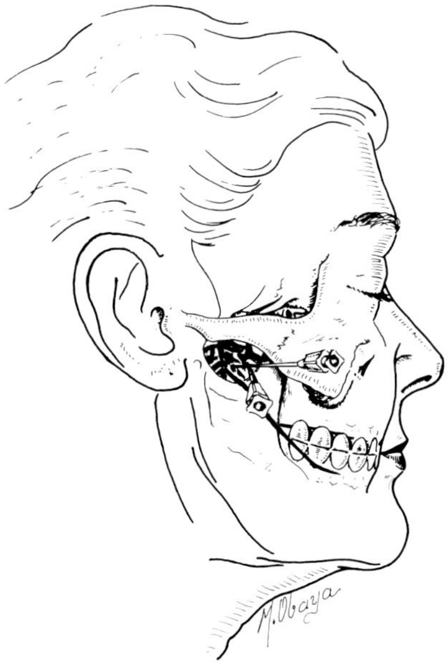

Figure 1-27

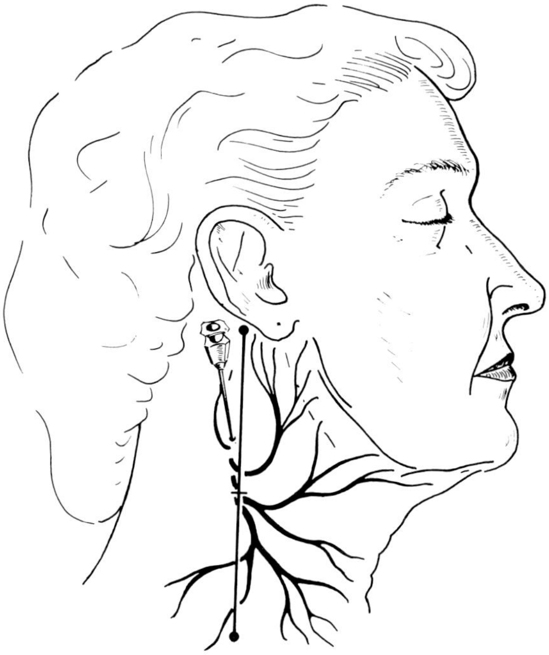

Figure 1-28A

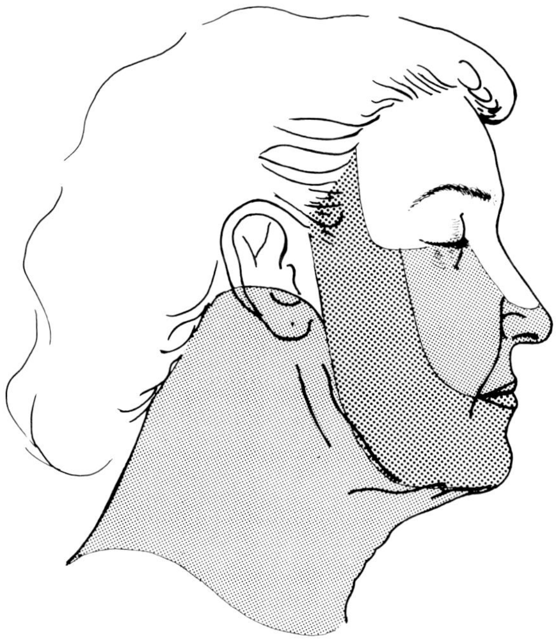

Figure 1-28B

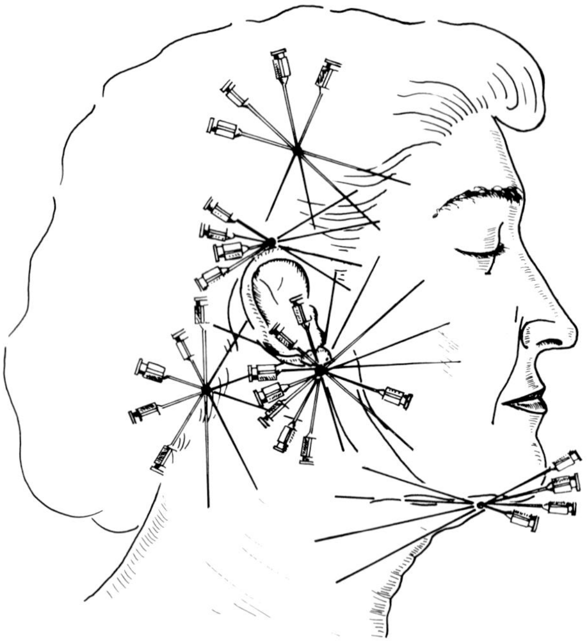

Figure 1-29

Figure 1-29 shows the injection of a local infiltrative anesthesia: 0.25% Marcaine with 1 : 200,000 Adrenalin is infiltrated with a 22-gauge spinal needle under the area of proposed undermining. The incision lines are supplemented with 1% Xylocaine with 1 : 200,000 Adrenalin.

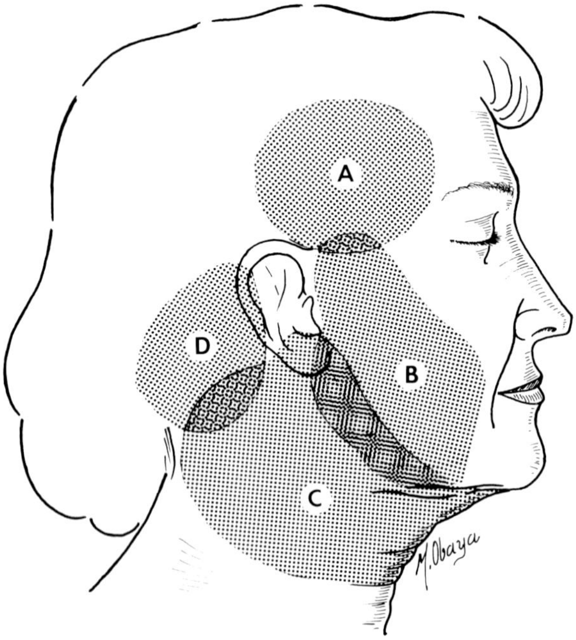

Figure 1-30

CLASSIC FACELIFT

The "classic facelift" operation shown in Figure 1-30 involved undermining the integument of the scalp and face to create four flaps of skin. The temporal (A) and occipital (D) flaps are elevated in a deeper plane to preserve the hair follicles. The preauricular (B) and cervical skin flaps (C) are much thinner and lateral to the SMAS to prevent injury to the facial nerve.

The extent of undermining varied considerably and absorbable or permanent plication sutures were considered by some to be efficacious (Figure 1-31).

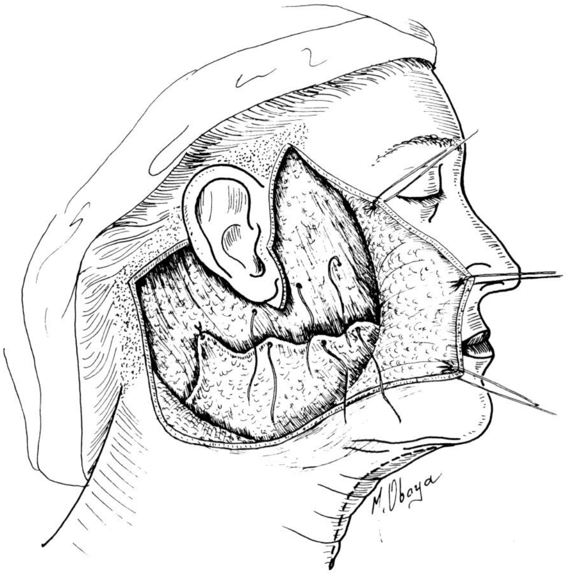

Figure 1-31

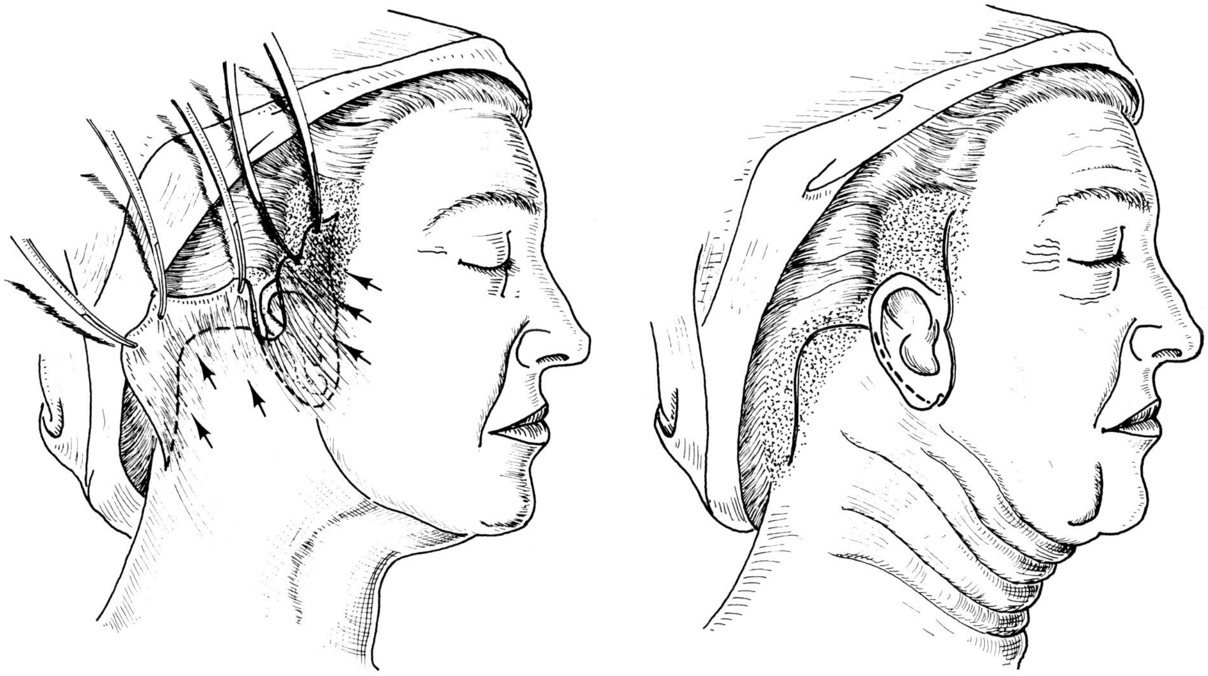

Figure 1-32

By rotating the skin posterosuperiorly, the cheek and cervical areas were lifted (Figure 1-32).

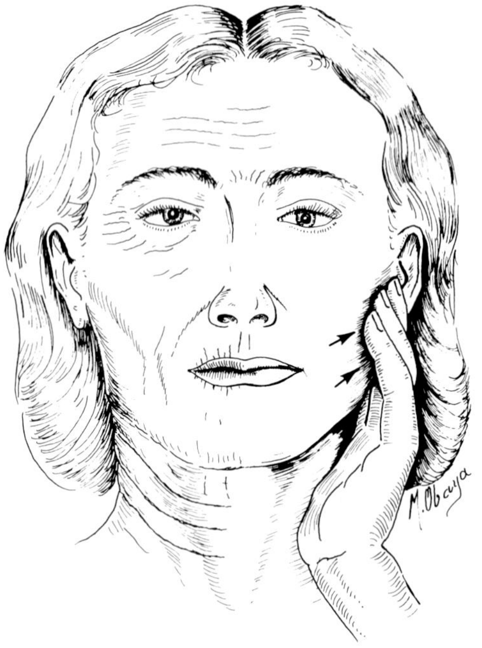

Figure 1-33

To effect a change in one area, dissection and undermining must extend a few millimeters beyond the area to be corrected. This partially explains the failure to improve the nasolabial folds (despite what most patients expect) (Figure 1-33) and the "turkey wattle" deformity.

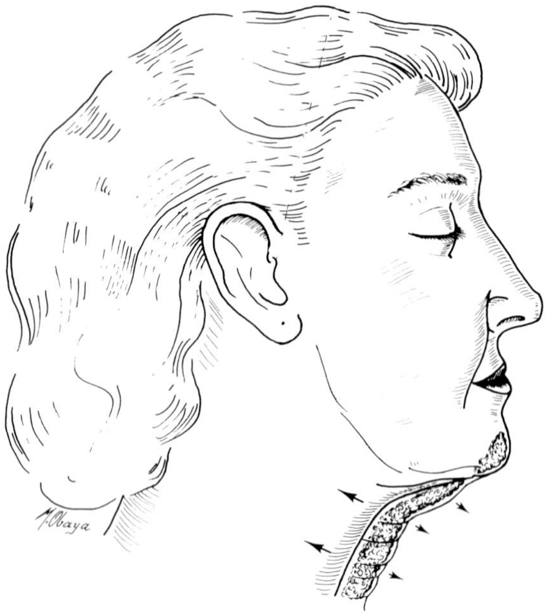

Figure 1-34

As shown in Figure 1-34, simple advancement of skin over a mound of fat produces a temporary improvement. The foundation (adipose tissue) will gradually produce recurrent bulging and fullness as the edema subsides. This is particularly evident in the cervicomental contour, which will gradually return over 8–12 months to its preoperative position if no fat is removed.

Short flaps to rotate and advance skin (Figure 1-35) will not affect distant musculodermal attachments, and hence the cosmetic deformity. The posterior and superior rotation on the mastoid and preauricular skin will *not* correct anterior platysma banding nor the rhytids of the lateral canthal area. The points of tension and support are too far removed from the area to be improved.

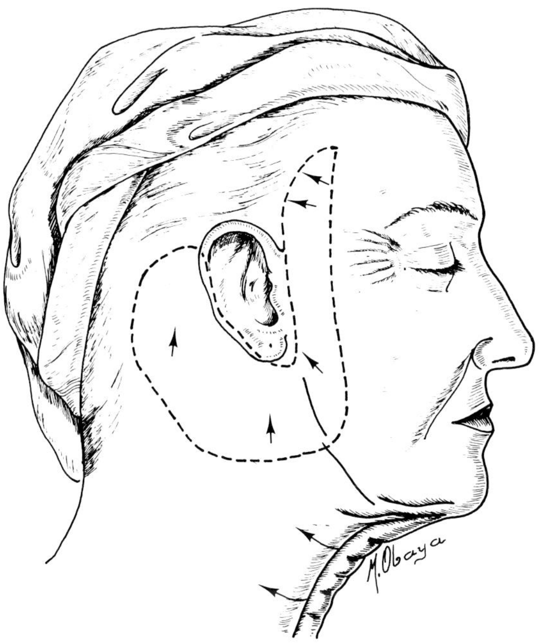

Figure 1-35

Modification of the Classic Facelift

With the development of more extensive techniques, it is now possible to tailor the classic facelift operation for each patient. The key factor is an accurate diagnosis of the pathologic anatomy causing the particular cosmetic deformity. By classifying the cervical region of each patient, the anatomy is carefully evaluated and the patient informed as to the proposed incisions, extent of undermining and risks, necessity of muscle excision and/or plication, and the need for implants.

Table 1-1 presents six classes of the cervical region based on the specific pathology of the anatomic layers of the neck. During the preoperative evaluation, the patient is placed in the class with the deepest layer involved. A Class I patient may be advised to delay surgery for a few years. Learning when not to operate on someone is as important as being able to operate well. If the patient is psychiatrically stable and realizes that the postoperative result will not be startling, a "prophylactic" skin flap procedure (Figure 1-30) may be indicated to help the patient maintain the present visage.

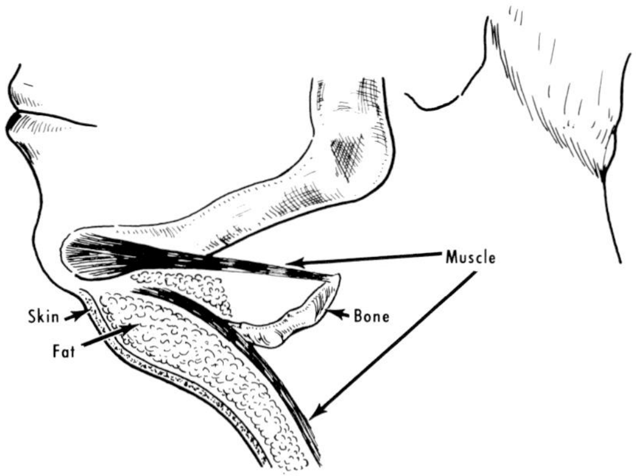

Table 1-1
Classification of Cervical Abnormalities

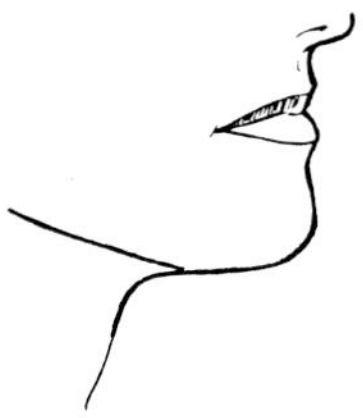

Class I: Minimal Deformity—Well-Defined Cervical Mental Angle, Good Platysma Tone, No Accumulation of Fat (Younger Patient)

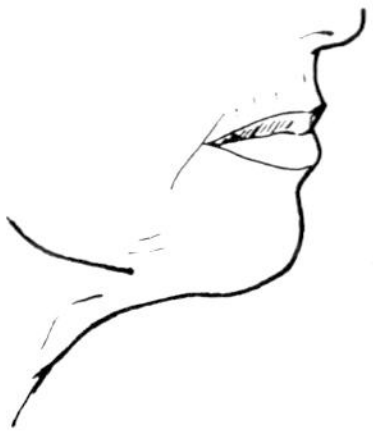

Class II: Laxity of the Cervical Skin—Begins to Hang Like a Curtain; No Fat Accumulation, No Platysma Weakness

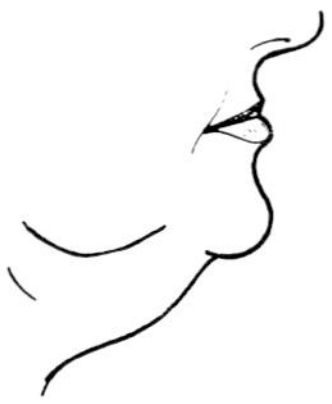

Class III: Fat Accumulation

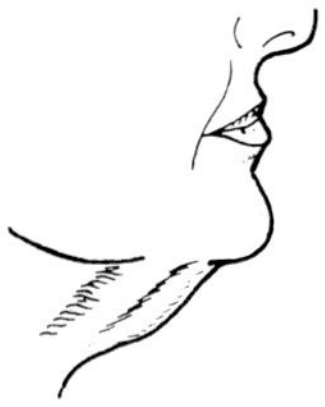

Class IV: Muscle Accentuation (Banding Present in Repose or on Contraction)

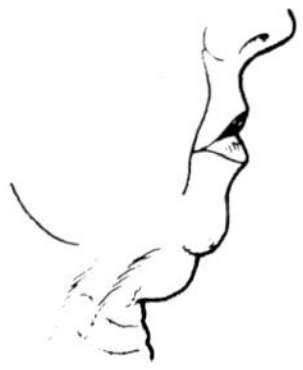

Class V: Congenital or Acquired Retrognathia

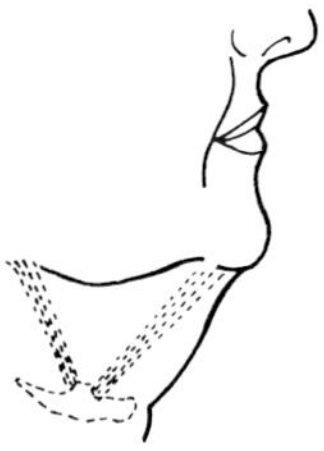

Class VI: Low Hyoid

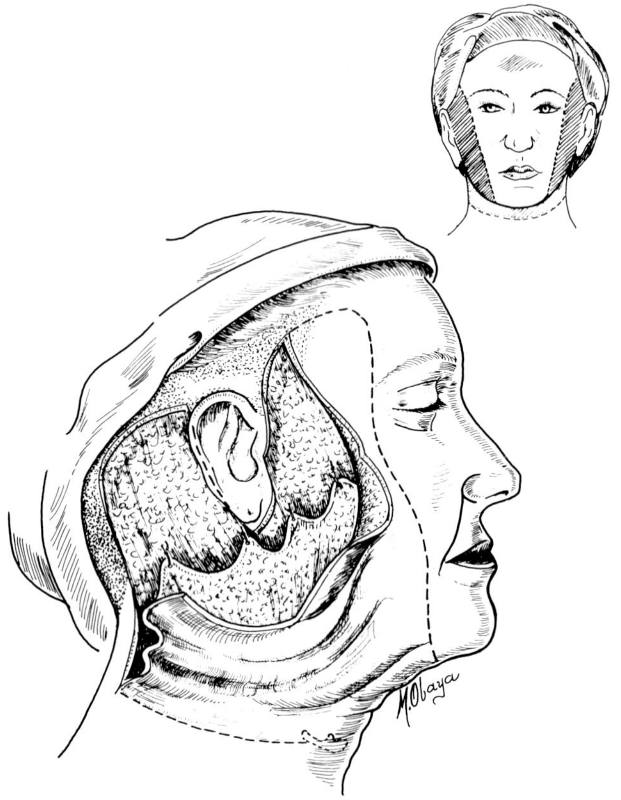

To correct skin laxity in Class II patients, the procedure shown in Figure 1-36 will allow redraping of the skin with maximum rotation and excision. Years later as a tuck-up becomes necessary, the layer of scar between the skin and subcutaneous tissue may be excised and plicated to obtain a result as satisfactory as the original facelift. Plication of the SMAS and posterior border of the platysma muscle will firm the foundation of the cervicofacial unit to prolong the cosmetic result.

Figure 1-36

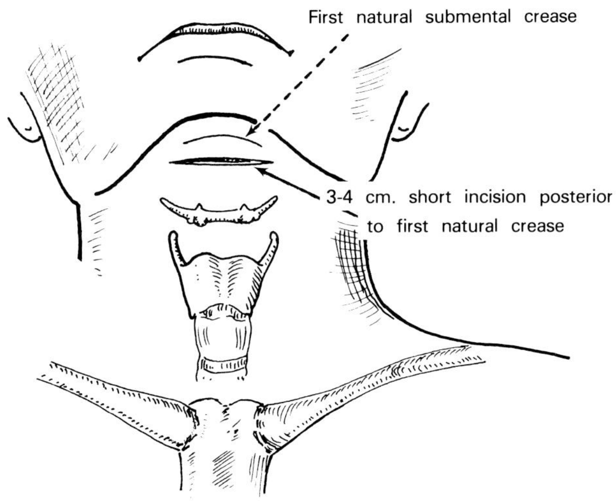

Figure 1-37A

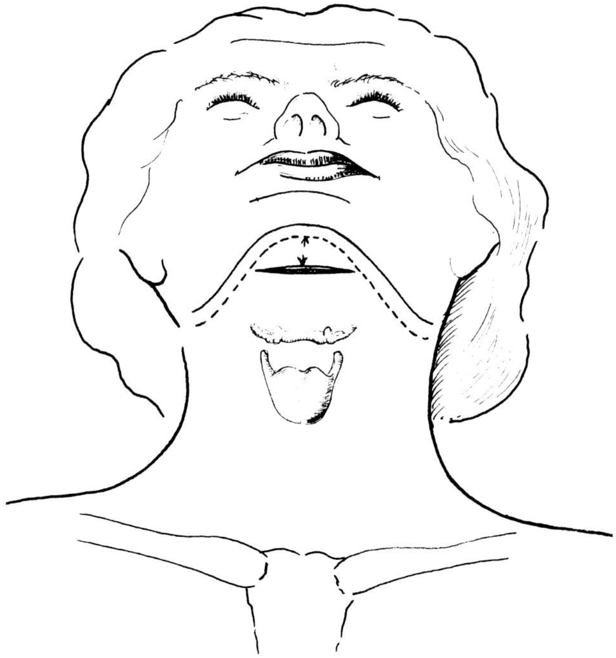

Figure 1-37B

In Class III patients with fat accumulation, the obtuse cervicomental contour is due to an excess of fat in the submandibular and/or submental areas.

To facilitate undermining of the cervical flaps and excision of fat, a 3–4 cm submental incision is made at or posterior to the first submental crease (Figure 1-37A). The precise location of the submental incision will vary with the angle of the pogonion (Figure 1-37B and C). The more obtuse the angle (Figure 1-37B), the closer the incision is placed to the first submental crease and the chin. When the angle of the horizontal ramus at the pogonion is acute, the incision must be placed further from the chin to prevent the incision from extending up on the borders of the mandible.

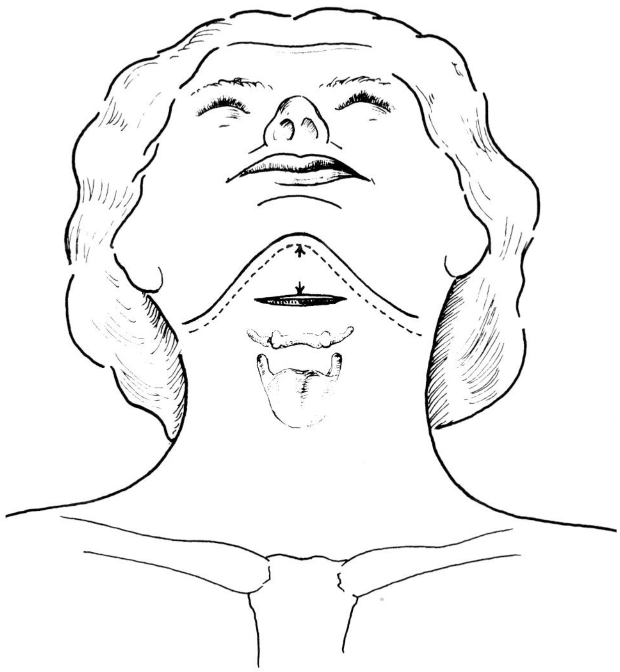

Figure 1-37C

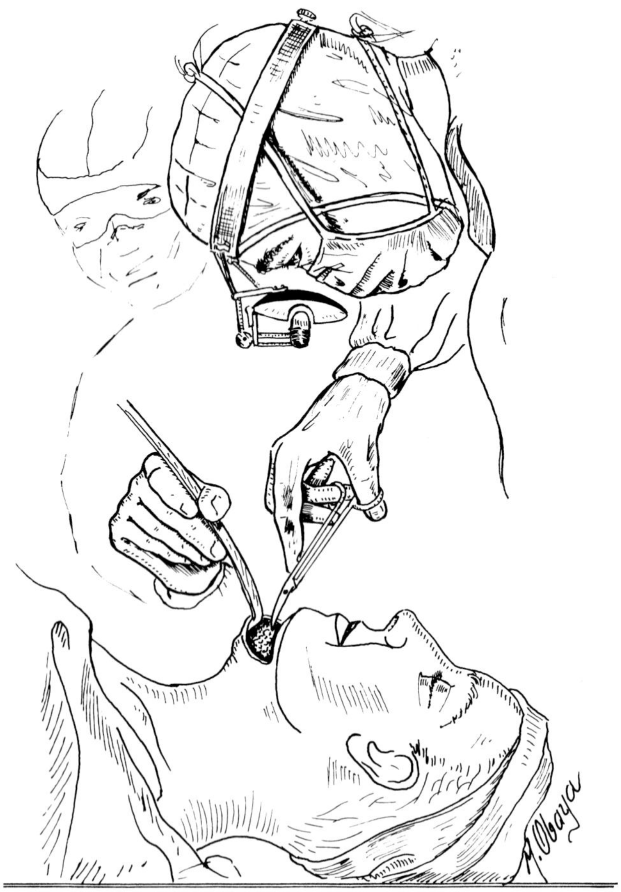

Figure 1-38A

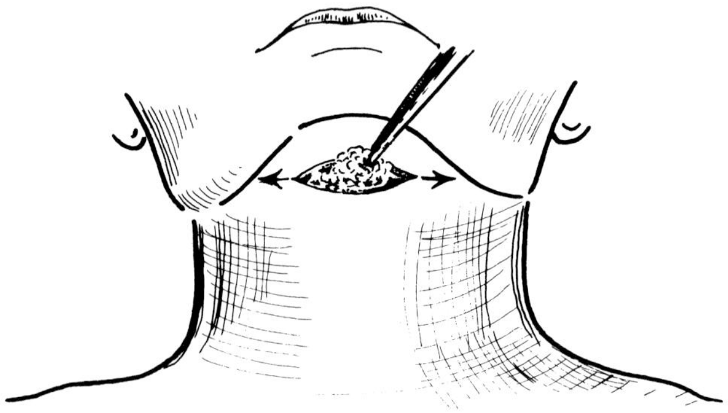

Figure 1-38B

The cervical area may be sculptured by removing fat from angle to angle lateral to the platysma muscle (see anatomy in Figures 1-13 and 1-14). As shown in Figure 1-38A, a headlight, slender Metzenbaum scissors, and an Aufricht retractor facilitate skin elevation to the thyrohyoid membrane in the midline and laterally to the angle of the mandible. The major area of submental fat excision is between and superficial to the medial bands of the platysma muscle. Lateral traction on the flaps (Figure 1-38B) will also guide fat removal as it bulges through the incision.

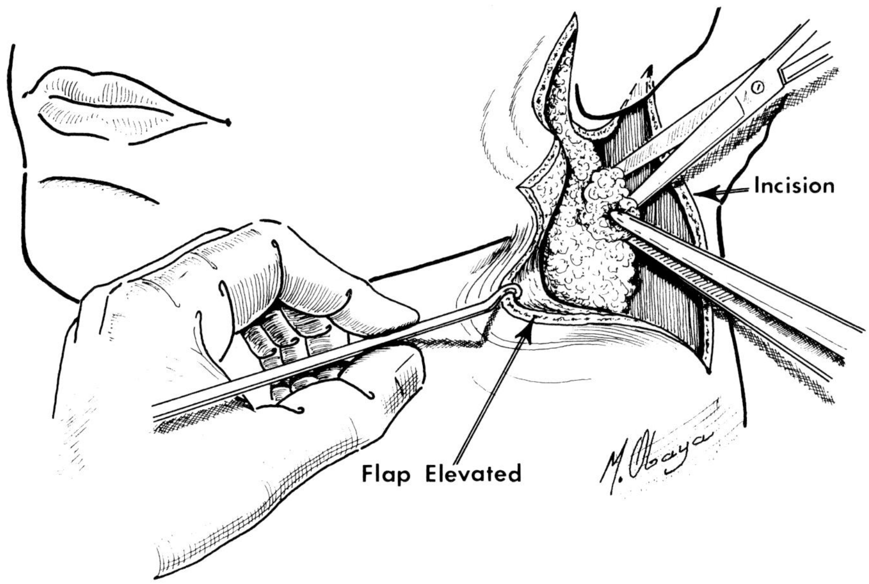

Figure 1-39

Figure 1-39 shows lateral removal of the fat superficial to the platysma from the inferior border of the mandible to approximately the level of the hyoid bone. Extreme care must be taken not to penetrate the fibers of the platysma muscle nor to tent the platysma muscle up when dissecting this layer of fat, in order to avoid injuring the marginal mandibular branch of the facial nerve.

In extremely obese individuals, the edges of the adipose layer are tapered to prevent a sharp line of demarcation postoperatively (Figure 1-40). By reducing this layer of insulating fat, the inferior border of the mandible now becomes apparent and creates a more youthful neck.

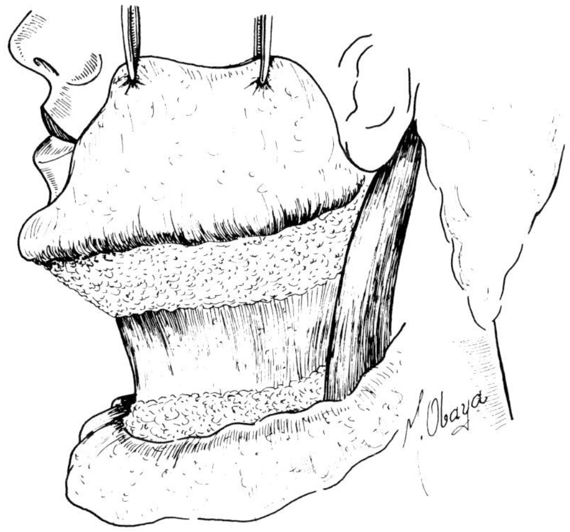

Figure 1-40

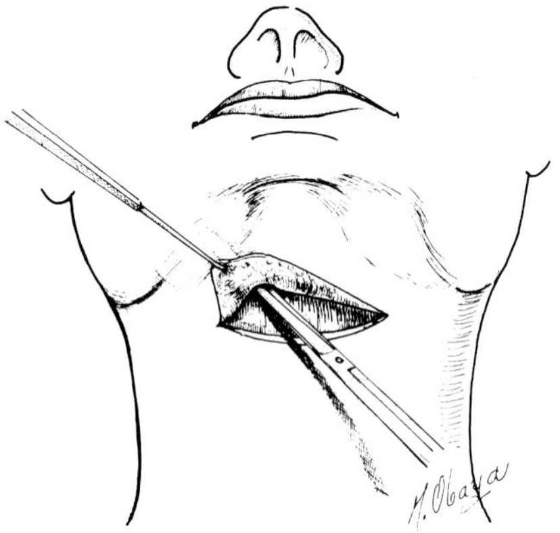

Figure 1-41A

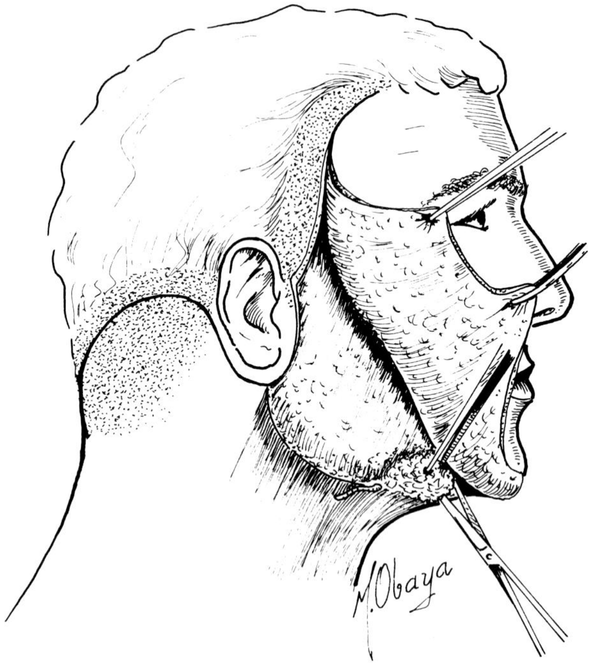

Figure 1-41B

As shown in Figure 1-41A and B, meticulous removal of fat 1 cm above the horizontal ramus of the mandible may also be done through the submental incision and laterally under direct vision. Bleeding is frequently a problem in the jowl area and is controlled with cautery and suture.

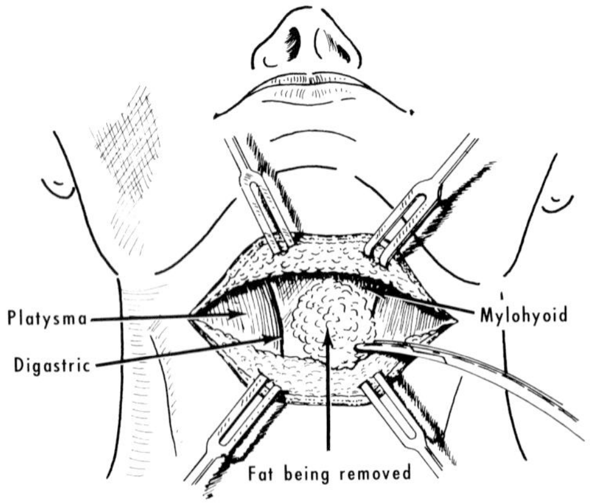

Figure 1-42

The classic submental lipectomy is rarely used to sculpture the submental contour, as injudicious fat removal may lead to a postoperative depression (Figure 1-42).

In Class IV patients with muscle accentuation, the platysma muscle may be prominent in repose or accentuated by voluntary contraction. Frequently there will be an excess of adipose tissue as previously described and these patients would be classified as Class IV with fat. After the fat is removed, the vertical fibers of the platysma are well visualized.

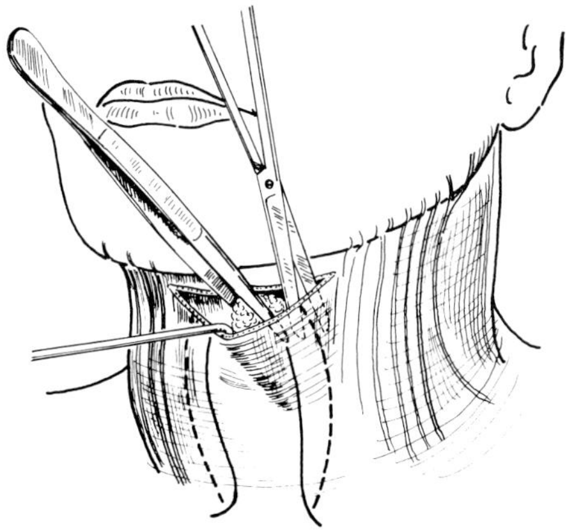

Figure 1-43

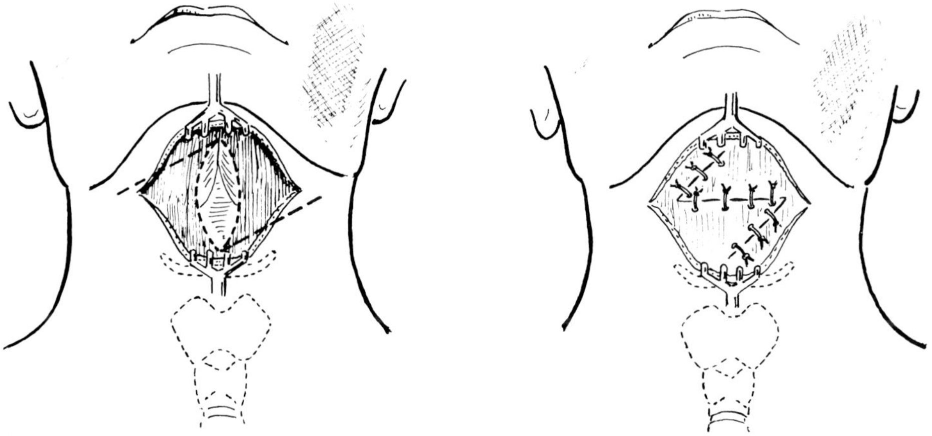

Figure 1-44

The anterior borders of the platysma muscle may be manipulated in a variety of ways. Figure 1-43 shows an excision made as deep in the neck as possible. Figure 1-44 illustrates the creation of interdigitating flaps with Z-plasty of the free border.

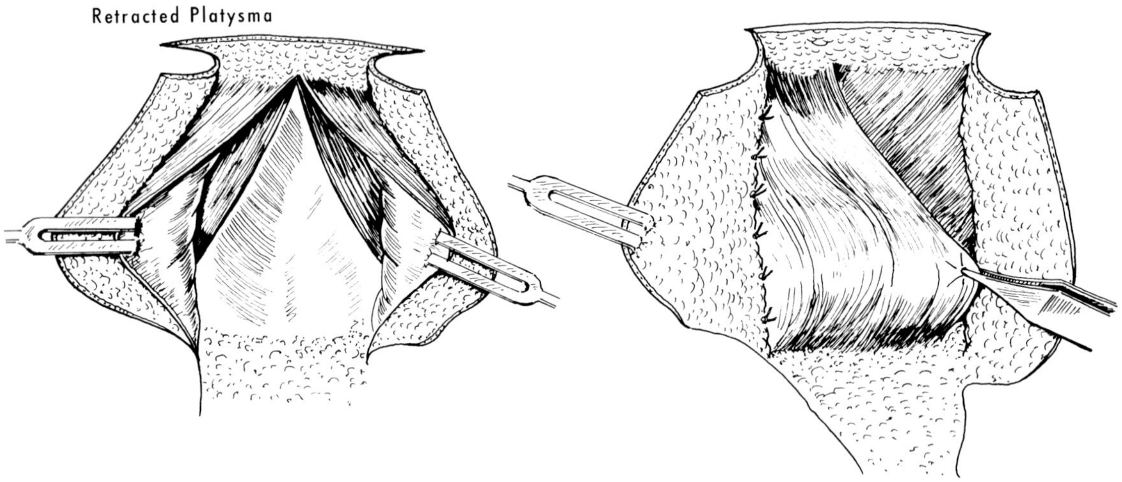

Figure 1-45

Plication of the medial borders is shown in Figure 1-45. Figure 1-46 shows the creation of laterally based flaps with sutures in the midline using permanent buried sutures to form a muscle sling.

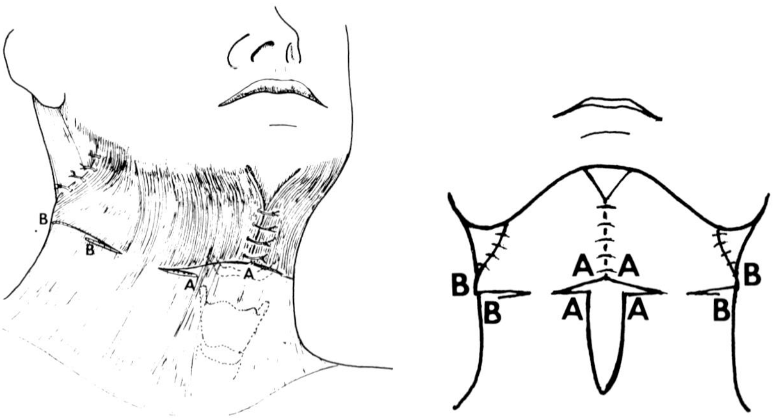

Figure 1-46

Selection of the proper techniques to correct "stringiness about the neck" depends on the patient's particular anatomy and degree of laxity of the muscle's medial borders. In patients who have wide anterior banding in repose, resection and suturing in the midline will create a satisfactory result. If the anterior folds are present only on voluntary contraction, then creation of laterally based flaps sutured or plicated in the midline without resection will prevent overcorrection and puckering of the cervical skin (Figure 1-47).

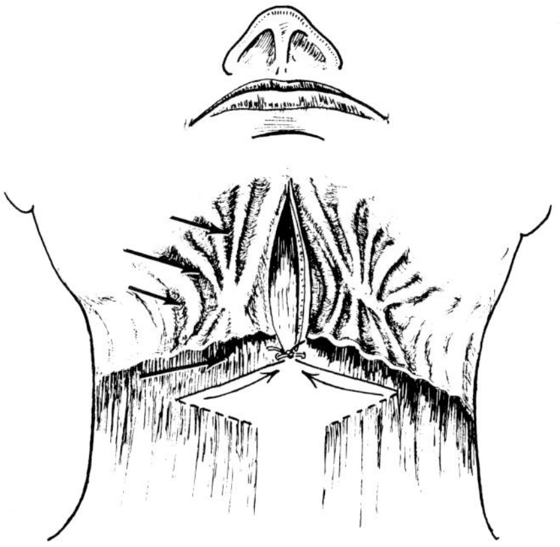

Figure 1-47

Once the submental area is completed, the posterior border of the platysma and SMAS are identified. The shaded area in Figure 1-48 outlines the proposed extent of SMAS undermining. Note that it begins 1 cm below the zygomatic arch and 1 cm in front of the tragus. As the dissection extends inferiorly along the anterior border of the sternocleidomastoid muscle, the posterior border of the platysma is separated from the investing layer of superficial cervical fascia that covers the sternocleidomastoid muscle.

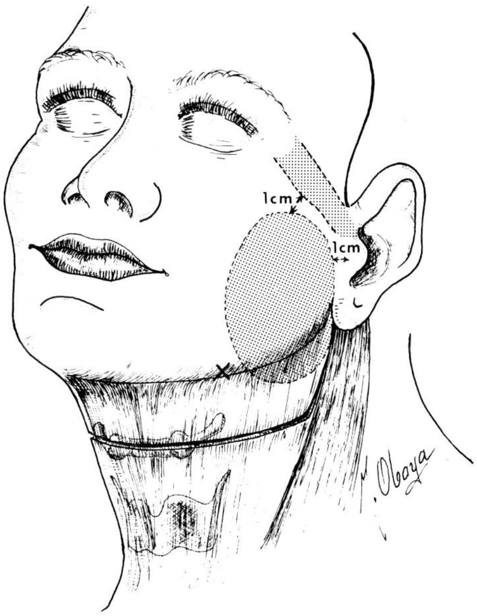

Figure 1-48

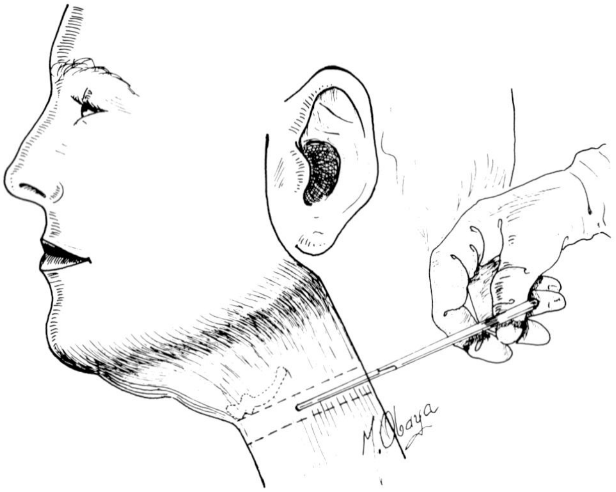

Figure 1-49

Complete or partial horizontal sectioning of the platysma muscle at the level of the hyoid bone may be safely done to further define the youthful neck. As shown in Figure 1-49, elevation and horizontal sectioning of the platysma is done with the tips of the scissors hugging the undersurface of the muscle at or below the level of the hyoid. Once a small tract is created, a hemostat is gently squeezed on the muscle, prior to clamp closure. If the corner of the mouth does not move, the clamp is closed and the muscle sectioned *below* the clamp. If the corner of the mouth moves, the clamp is positioned lower until a level is found that does not cause facial movement. This clamp-squeeze technique is used whenever concern exists about sectioning vital structures.

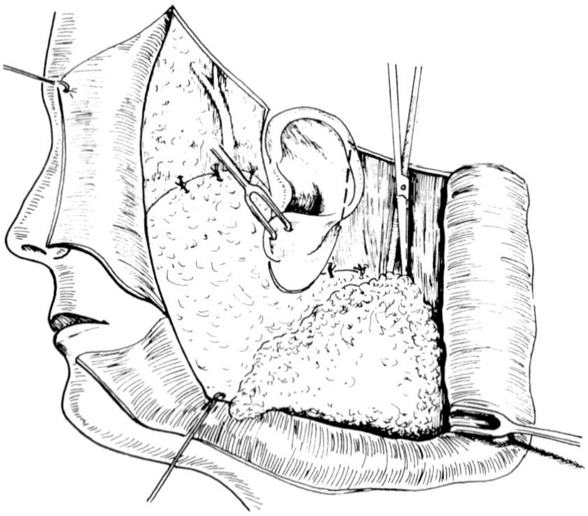

Figure 1-50

Once the SMAS-platysma unit has been mobilized, it is rotated posterosuperiorly (arrow) to tighten the foundation of the face (Figure 1-50). The edge of the SMAS is anchored in key points with a buried permanent suture. The edge is further supported with 3-0 Dexon sutures. The posterior border of the platysma is manipulated in a variety of techniques and sutured to the fascia of the sternocleidomastoid muscle with vertical sutures to reduce the likelihood of injury to the greater auricular nerve.

The posterior border of the platysma may be simply advanced posteriorly and sutured (Figure 1-51).

The posterior border of the platysma may be created into a short flap that is advanced posteriorly to support the cervical region and reduce posterior platysma banding (see Figure 1-46).

As shown in Figure 1-49, the platysma may be completely sectioned horizontally across the neck and rotated posterosuperiorly as a muscle sling for submental and submandibular support. Incomplete horizontal sectioning of the platysma muscle may leave residual vertical banding that is evident immediately after surgery. Occasionally these bands have developed as late as 2 years after surgery and are thought to be due to scarring and fibrosis between the cut ends of the muscle.

Congenital microgenia or relative retrognathia from atrophy of the soft tissues and bone absorbtion is corrected with chin augmentation (Figure 1-52). A submental incision through which undermining, fat sculpturing, or muscle work was done is used to approach the pogonion. A pocket is created superficial to the periosteum, and a Snyder gel-filled implant is placed. Two or three 4-0 clear nylon sutures are placed to close the soft-tissue pocket inferiorly and prevent implant migration.

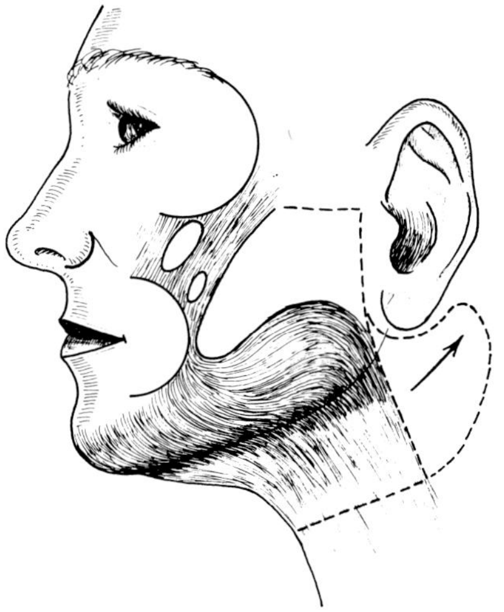

Figure 1-51

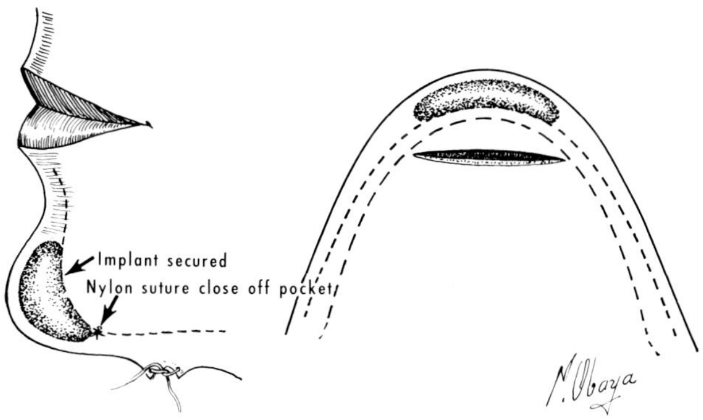

Figure 1-52

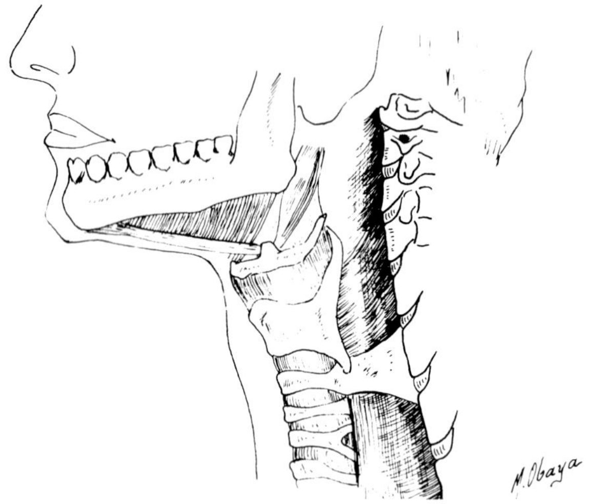

Level of the hyoid bone at 4th. cervical vertebra.

Figure 1-53

Ideally, the hyoid bone should lie at or above the fourth cervical vertebra (Figure 1-53). In the Class VI patient, the hyoid bone lies below the fourth cervical vertebra, limiting the postoperative result.

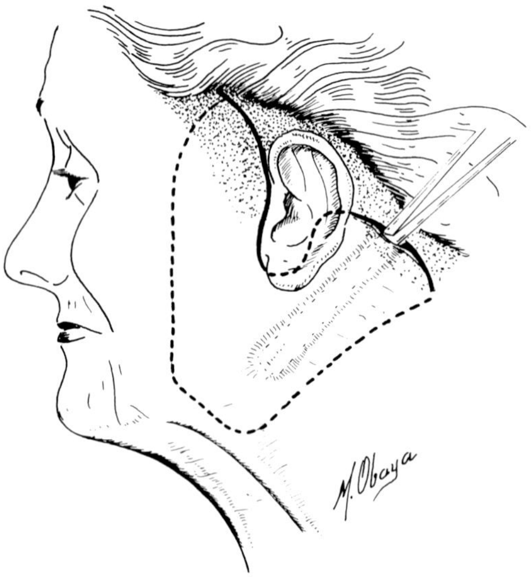

Figure 1-54

SEGMENTAL EXCISION LIFE

An alternative to the wide undermining described previously is the minimal or conservative facelift. It could actually be called a segmental excision lift. Undermining is carried forward approximately 2.5–3.5 cm as illustrated in Figure 1-54.

Buried plication sutures of 2-0 braided permanent material (Figure 1-55) tighten the SMAS and posterior border of the platysma to the perochindrium of the tragus and mastoid periosteum, respectively.

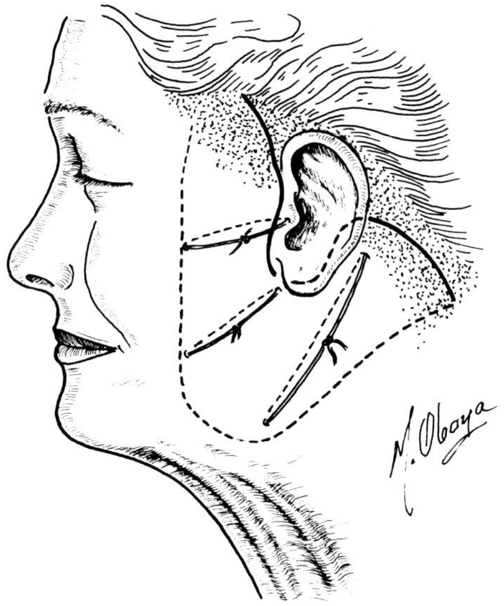

Figure 1-55

FINESSE

INCISIONS

Temporal

If the incision follows the temporal hairline, the superior displacement of the sideburn tuft of hair that occurs with other incisions is reduced. However, scarring, hair loss, and a receding hairline make this a less frequently used incision.

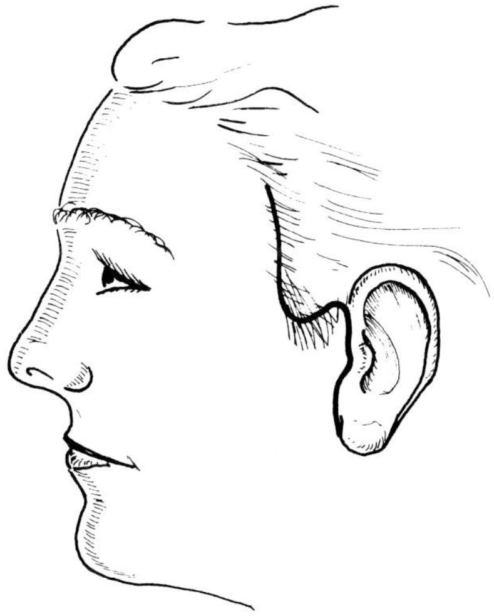

Figure 1-56

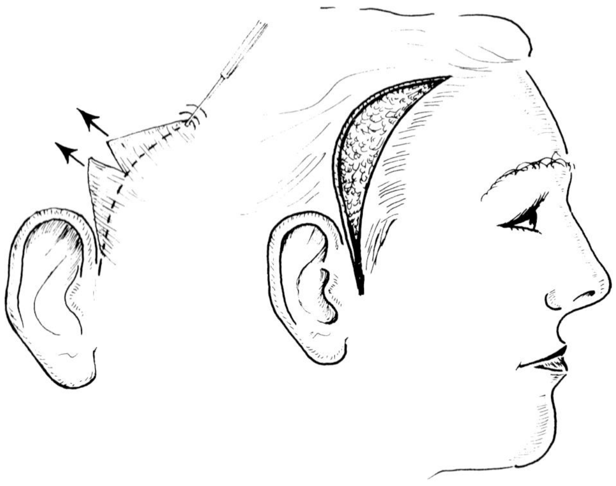

A gentle curving incision placed inside the hairline of the temporal area is most frequently used (Figure 1-57). It allows excision of the advanced flap without "dog-ear" formation (Figure 1-57 inset).

Figure 1-57

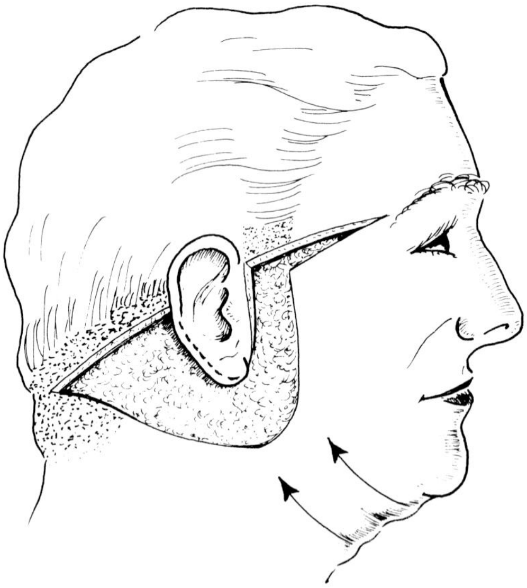

Another approach to elevation of the cheek flap is an incision that runs from the eyebrow posteriorly to the hairline and then inferiorly in front of the ear (see Figure 1-58). Makeup and other ancillary procedures will be necessary to adequately camouflage this incision. If the patient will accept the scar, it provides the maximum direction of pull for the cheek and jowl areas.

Figure 1-58

An alternative to the eyebrow-to-hairline incision is one that allows a horizontal triangle of skin to be excised in the preauricular area with a W-plasty to reduce dog-ear formation (Figure 1-59).

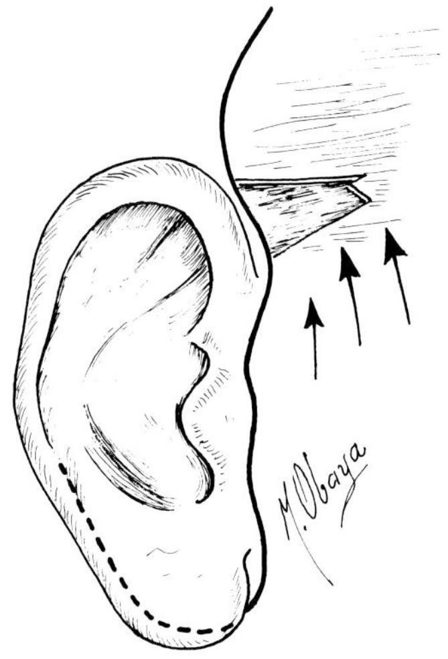

Figure 1-59

Preauricular

The incision shown in Figure 1-60 follows the root of the auricle to dip into the superior tragal crease, run anterior to the tragus, and dip into the inferior tragal crease before running inferiorly and under the lobule. This is excellent for patients with a thin, prominent tragal cartilage.

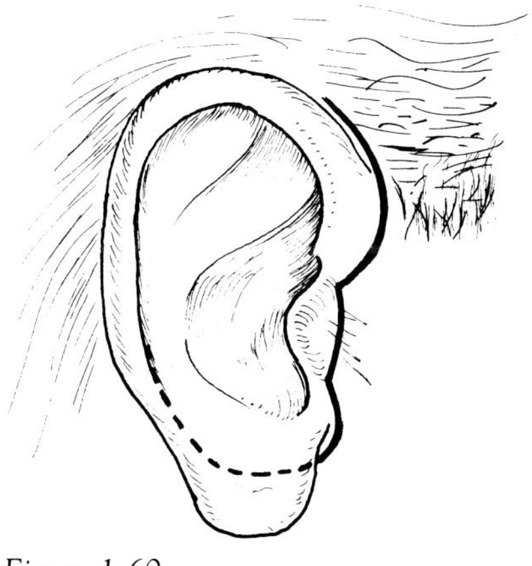

Figure 1-60

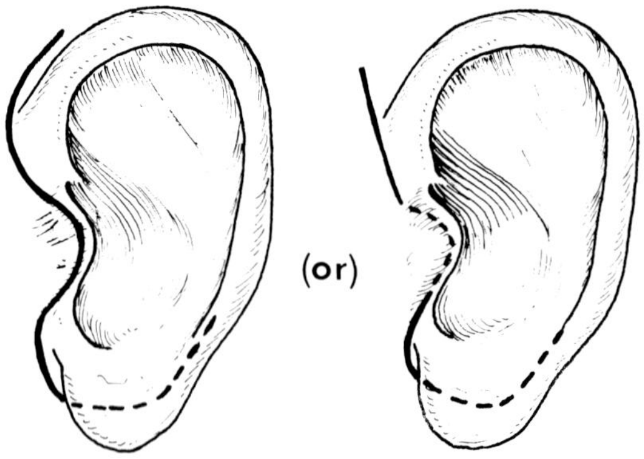

Figure 1-61

The incision shown in Figure 1-61 goes on top of or just posterior to the tragal cartilage. This is excellent in camouflaging the incision but may cause distortion of the tragus postoperatively if the skin is not trimmed and thinned correctly. In patients with thick squatty traguses, this is the incision of choice.

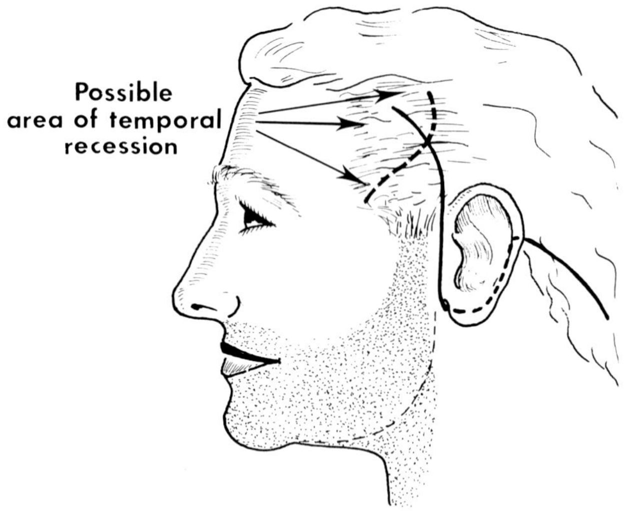

Figure 1-62

The incision in the male patient shown in Figure 1-62 must be made with consideration of the possibility of subsequent temporal hair recession and balding as well as rotating hair-bearing skin into the ear. Therefore, the temporal aspect must curve posteriorly behind the root of the ear. In front of the ear, the non-hair-bearing skin is divided approximately in half with the incision. Because hair-bearing skin is rotated posteriorly behind the ear, the patients are told that they will have to shave this area.

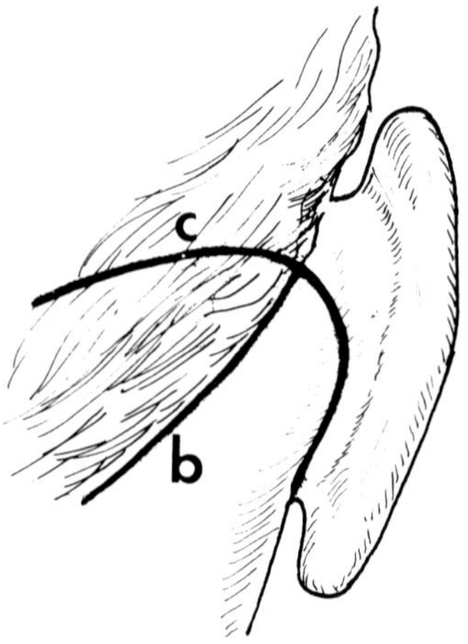

Figure 1-63

Postauricular

The classic incision was one that extended a short distance up onto the conchal cartilage to prevent subsequent migration of the scar inferiorly out of the sulcus (Figure 1-63). At the level of the external meatus it ran posteriorly into or along the hairline.

The incision that follows the hairline (line b in Figure 1-63) allows a more direct posterior pull on the cervical skin (Figure 1-64).

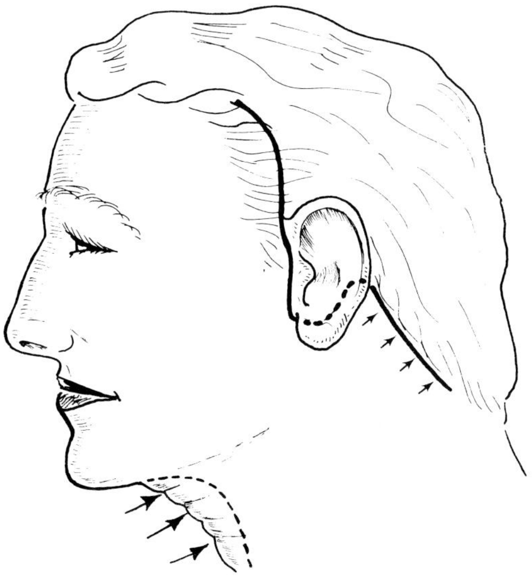

Figure 1-64

Figure 1-65 shows a step deformity in the posterior hairline that usually poses no problems (Figure 1-65).

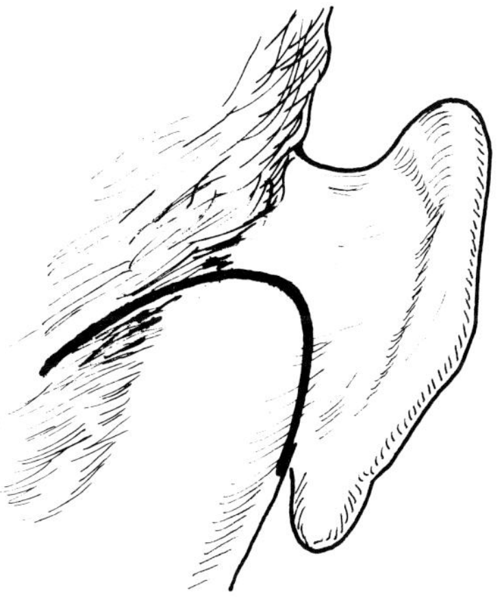

Figure 1-65

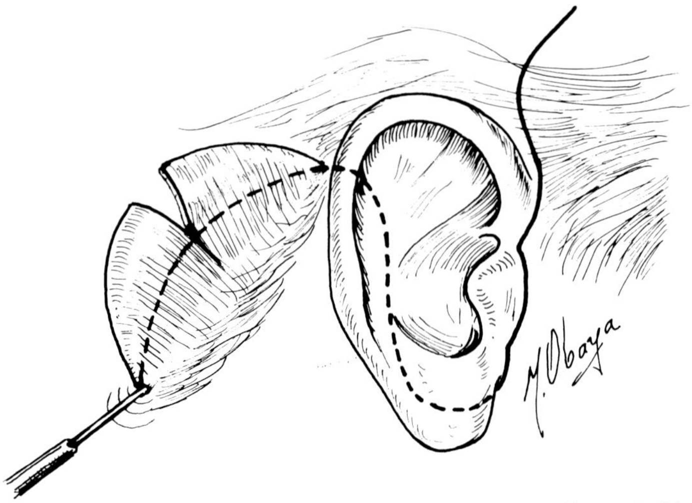

Figure 1-66

An incision that curves superiorly into the hairline from the conchal cartilage allows rotation and advancement of the flaps with no dog-ear formation. Any step deformity in the hairline is superior and hidden behind the auricle. The "triangles" of skin to be excised are in reality an ellipse of skin.

SCULPTURING A LOBULE

Frequently the incision around the auricle ignores the shape, size, or even the presence of a lobule. By identifying preoperatively a large lobule, or the absence of one, the incision is altered as it circumscribes the auricle to permit sculpturing a new earlobe.

In patients who desire a small lobule and have none, the earlobe is grasped and pulled anteriorly and laterally to produce a verticle fold that is incised with straight scissors (Figure 1-67).

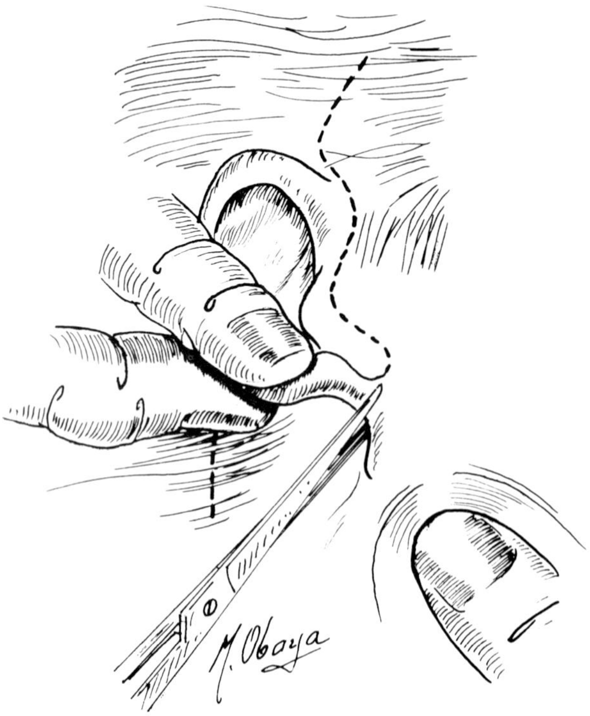

Figure 1-67

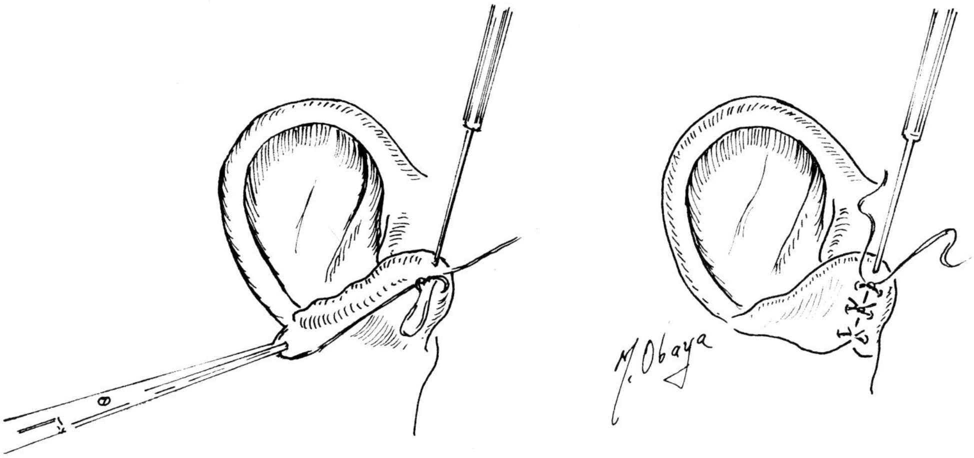

Figure 1-68

Closure with 5-0 nylon sutures with a hook placed in the apex of the "V" will create a small lobule (Figure 1-68).

The pre- and postauricular incisions are subsequently carried into the incision thus made.

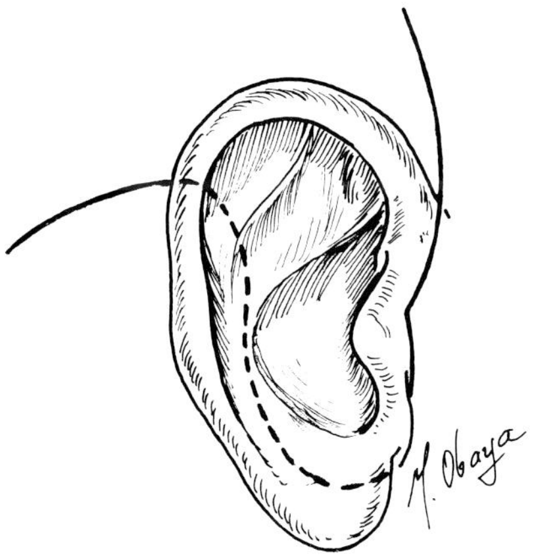

Figure 1-69

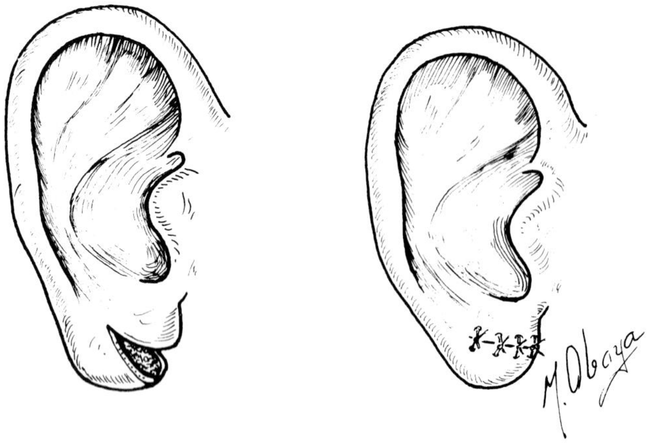

Figure 1-70

As shown in Figure 1-70, reduction of a large lobule may be accomplished by carrying the incision into the lobule and excising a wedge of tissue. Meticulous closure with 5-0 clear nylon subcutaneously and 5-0 black nylon interrupted will minimize the scar.

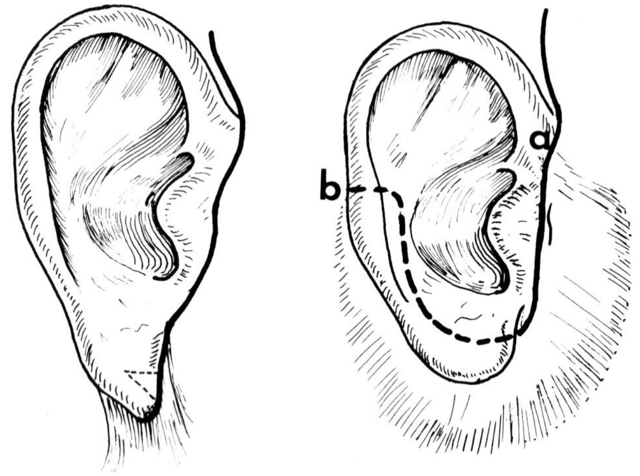

Figure 1-71A

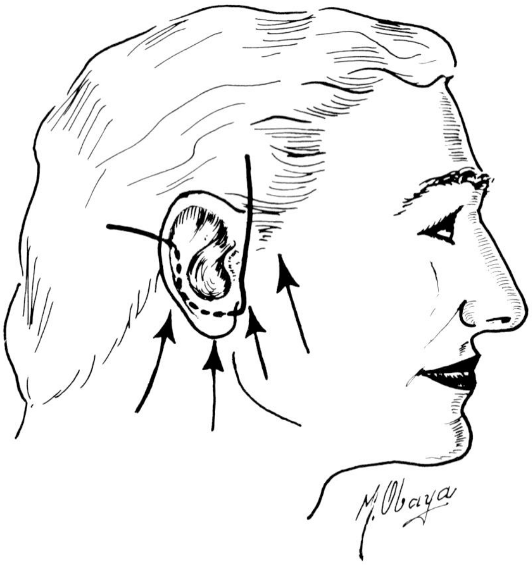

Figure 1-71B

If the ear lobule becomes floppy and more noticeable after a facelift, an office procedure using one of the above techniques can be used. Prevention of the pulled-down lobule or "pixie ear" (Figure 1-71A) is dependent on the tension on the lobule at closure. The lobule must hang freely from the side of the face with the flaps tucked up under it. If a pixie ear develops postoperatively, wide exposure (shaded area in Figure 1-71A) and support of the skin flaps in front of (curve a in Figure 1-71A) and behind (curve b) the ear are necessary to take tension from the earlobe and allow it to hang freely (Figure 1-71B). Occasionally a wedge of tissue must be excised to reduce the size of the lobe.

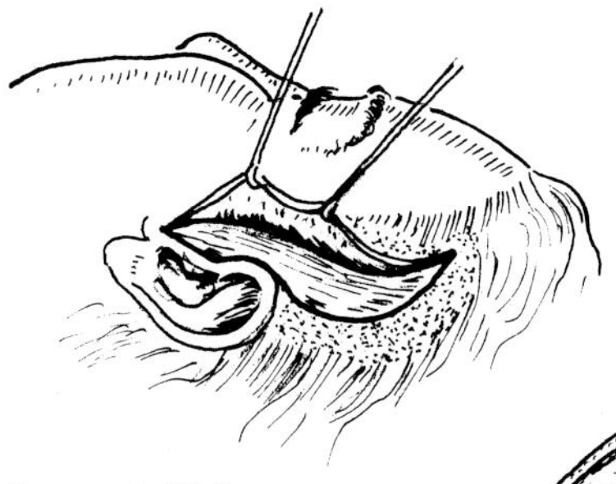

Figure 1-72A

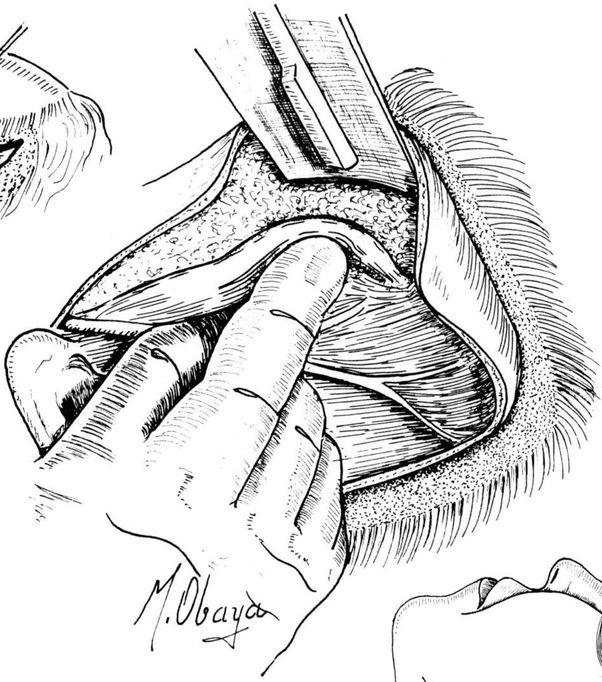

Figure 1-72B

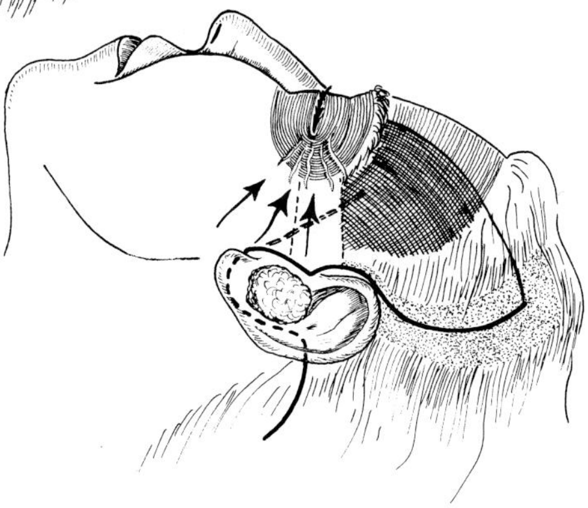

Figure 1-72C

UNDERMINING

The temporal flap is readily elevated at the level of the temporalis fascia. Once the incision is carried to but not through the fascia (Figure 1-72A), a finger on a sponge will readily peel the temporal flap from the temporalis fascia and vessels (Figure 1-72B). If dissection is to extend anterior to the temporal hairline (shaded area in Figure 1-72C) blunt dissection in a deeper plane on top of the periosteum is done to prevent injury to the temporal branch of the facial nerve.

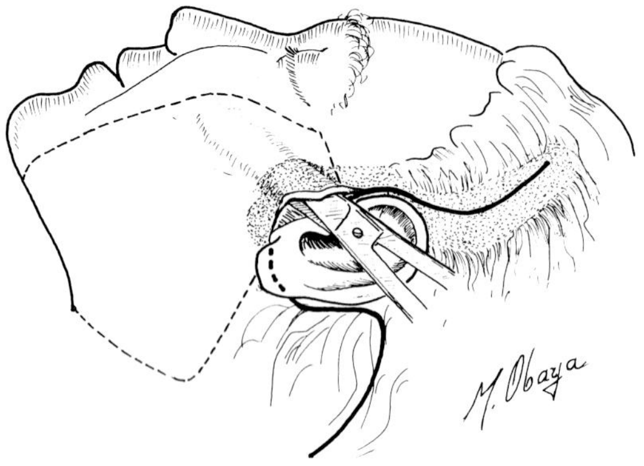

Figure 1-73

The preauricular flap is started with knife dissection (dotted area in Figure 1-73) and after 1–2 cm is continued with scissor tunneling, spreading, and connecting of the tunnels. A common problem is creation of flaps that are too thick. The thinner the flap, the less bleeding that will occur and less chance of injury to the facial nerve. A transition zone between the temporal and preauricular flap lies over the zygomatic arch. These two different levels of undermining are not to be connected anterior to the hairline. If dissection is to extend to the orbicularis oculi muscle, extremely blunt and superficial dissection is to be done. The occipital flap is thick to preserve the hair follicles and, once anterior to the hairline, becomes very superficial.

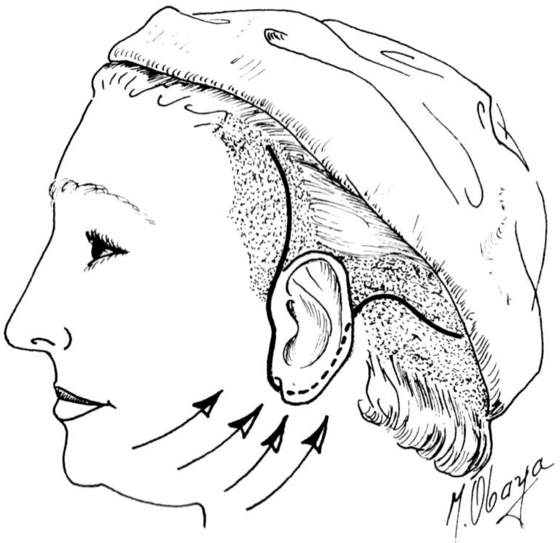

Figure 1-74

FLAP ADVANCEMENT: TRIMMING AND CLOSURE

Distribution of the facial and cervical skin is dependent on the cosmetic deformity being corrected (Figure 1-74).

As shown in Figure 1-75, excessive superior rotation of the cervical and temporal flaps will not only distort the hairline at the root of the auricle, but leave excess folds of skin in the neck below the lobule.

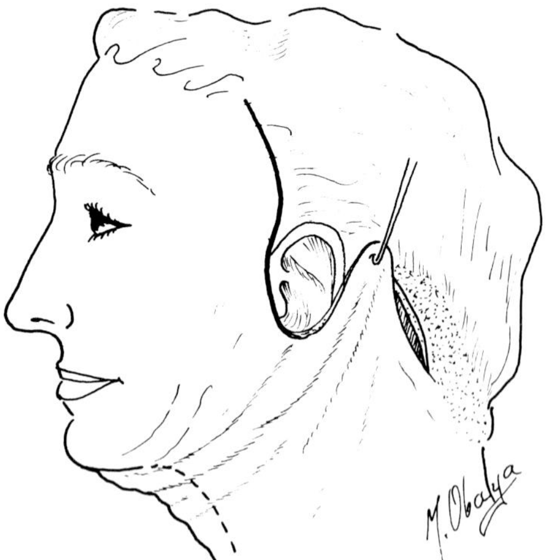

Figure 1-75

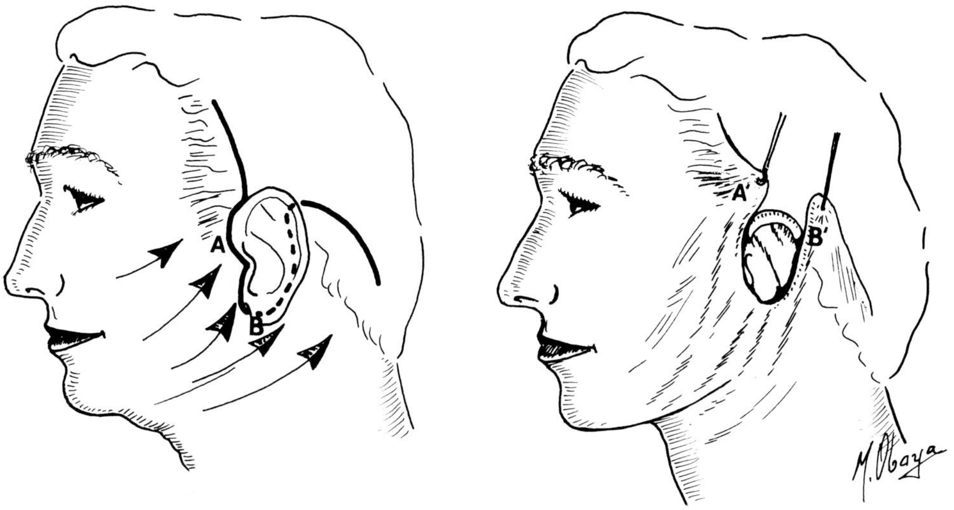

Figure 1-76

By advancing the flaps posterosuperiorly, the preauricular hairline of the temporal flap will be advanced superiorly to the root of the auricle (Figure 1-76A′). The cervical skin below the lobule will be rotated up toward the apex of the sulcus behind the ear (Figure 1-76B′). Excision of the redundant skin is begun in the temporal area after two tacking sutures are placed at points A′ and B′ (Figure 1-76).

The temporal flap is first split while a hook provides countertraction at the apex of the incision. The redundant flaps of hair-bearing skin are excised. Preservation of hair follicles is increased by beveling the cut edge of the flaps away from the hair roots.

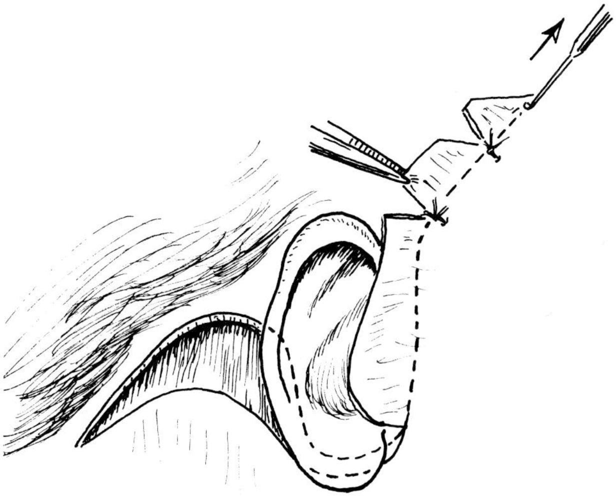

Figure 1-77

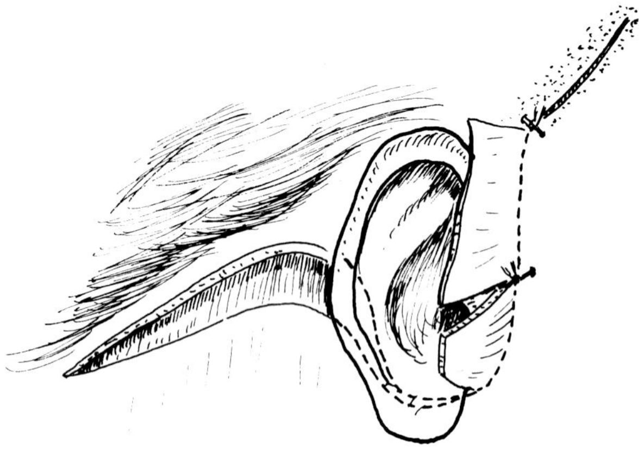

Figure 1-78

The preauricular incision is carefully trimmed and tailored to the tragus and lobule (Figure 1-78). If the incision extends behind the tragus, the subcutaneous fat must be removed from the flap to allow a snug, nondistorting fit as it drapes over the tragus.

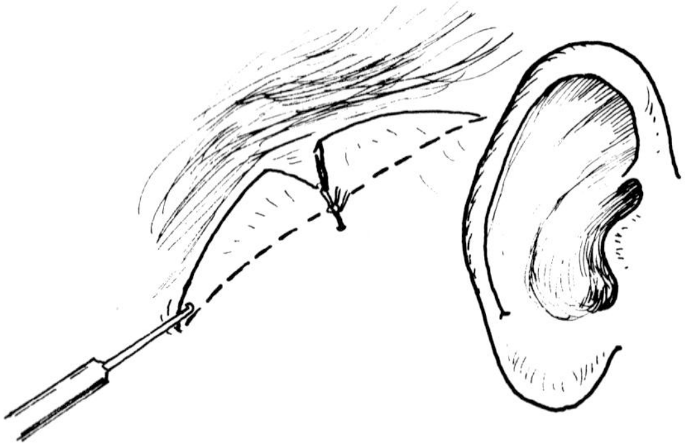

Figure 1-79

The occipital flap is trimmed next, again with a hook providing countertraction. The flap is split as before and sutured, and the excess hair-bearing skin is excised.

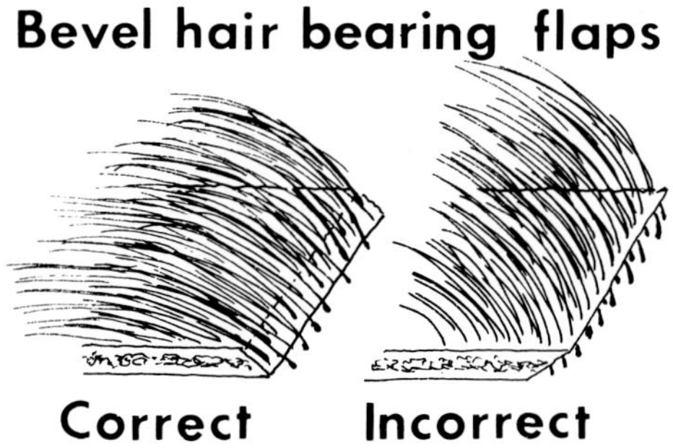

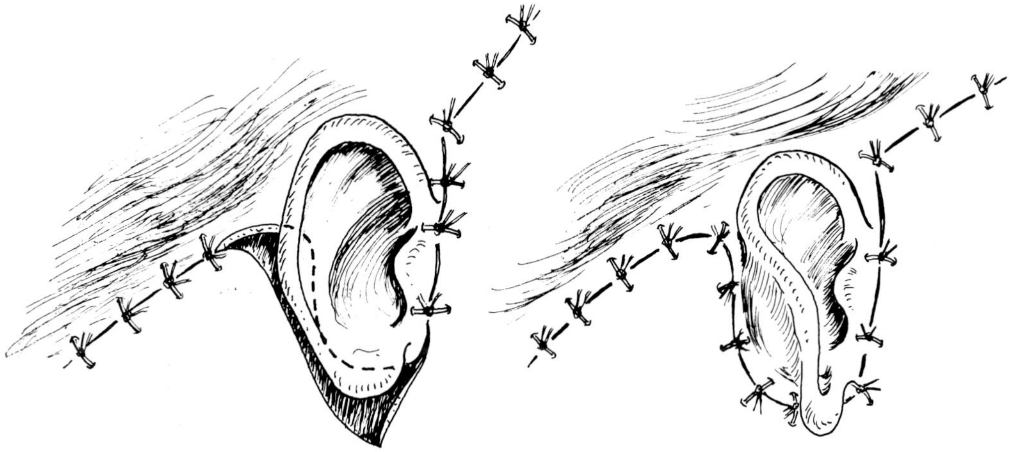

Figure 1-80

The infra-auricular skin is excised last (Figure 1-80).

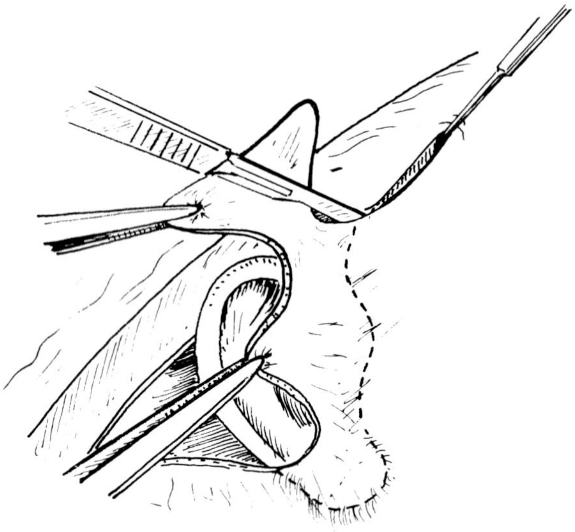

Figure 1-81

An alternative to the tacking suture method is the sequential excision of redundant skin as advocated by Kamer.[5] Instead of using using the anchor points of support, the temporal flap is rotated about a hook placed in the most superior extent of the incision. After beginning the excision near the hook, the excised portion of skin is used as a retractor to approximate the wound edges while the suture is placed.

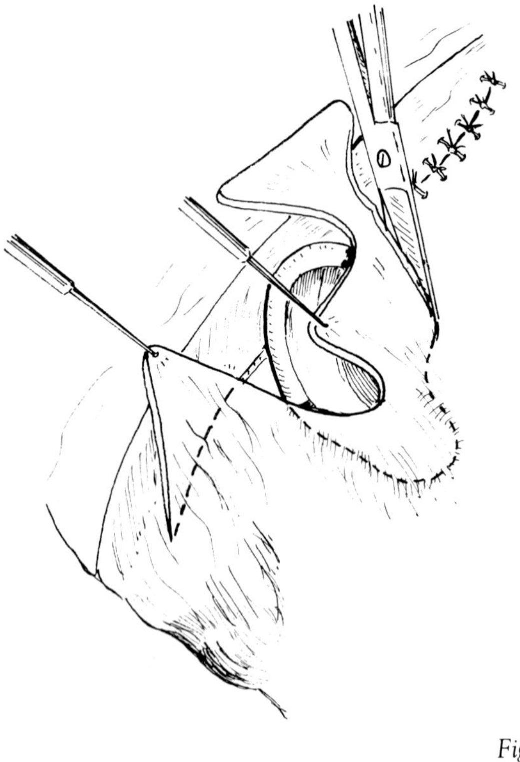

Figure 1-82

Excess skin in the preauricular area is excised in two steps (Figure 1-82). First, an incision is made from the last temporal suture down to the groove between the anterior helical rim and tragus. After this incision is sutured, the redundant skin is excised in a similar fashion between the tragus and the earlobe.

The cervical flap is excised by drawing the apex of the occipital flap cephalad and retracting the pinna anteriorly (Figure 1-83). With the skin held taut, the excess lying over the posterior sulcus is excised from the lobule to the apex of the incision.

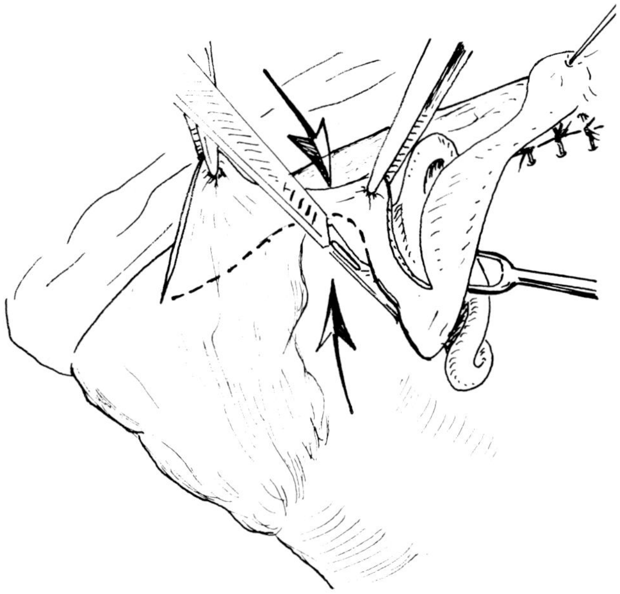

Figure 1-83

The occipitomastoid flap is trimmed by placing a hook at the end of the incision and pulling the flap in an anterosuperior direction. The excess skin is removed with a scalpel or scissors.

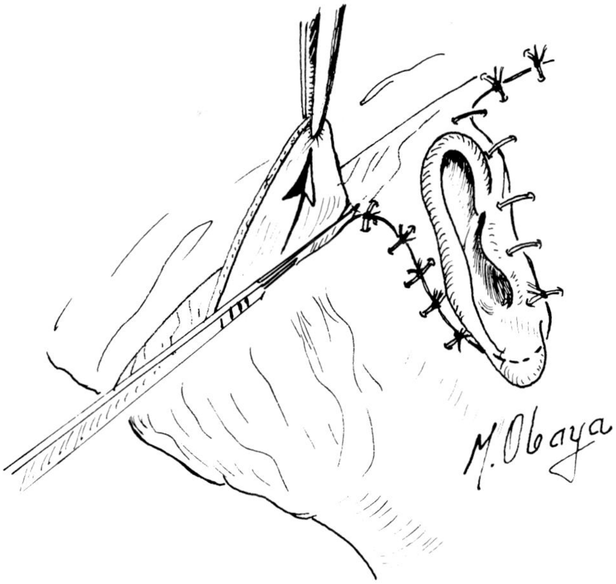

Figure 1-84

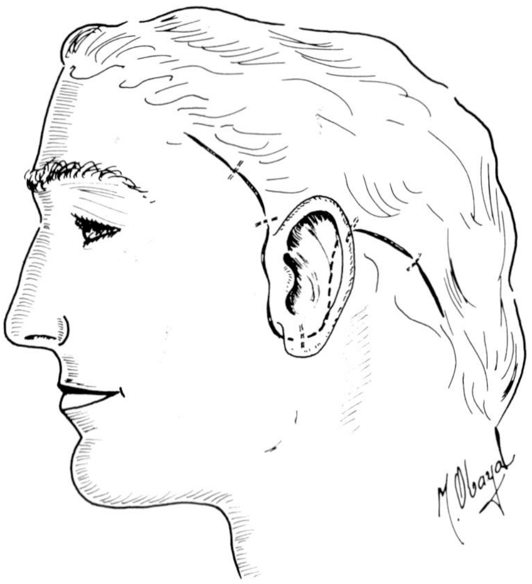

Figure 1-85

Careful approximation of the wound edges will not guarantee a satisfactory scar (Figure 1-85). If excessive tension on the wound edges exists, gradual separation with subsequent widening of the scar will occur. To prevent wide scars, subcutaneous 3-0 Dexon sutures are placed in strategic tension bearing areas to protect the incision. If there is any gaping of the incision in the preauricular area after the excess skin has been excised, the edges of the incision are approximated with buried 5-0 clear nylon sutures to prevent a wide scar. Closure of the temporal and occipital hair-bearing areas with skin staples saves time. They are also very inert and can be removed 10–14 days after surgery.

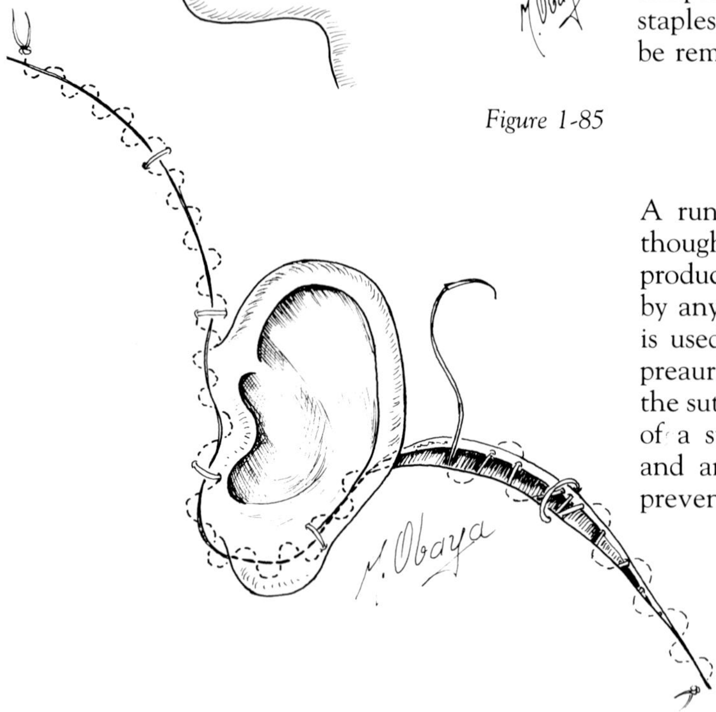

Figure 1-86

A running subcuticular suture (Figure 1-86), although slightly more time-consuming to place, will produce a scar that is far superior to that obtained by any other technique. A 4-0 black nylon suture is used in the hair-bearing skin and a 5-0 in the preauricular area. To correct any irregularities in the suture line, "twists" that constitute the first half of a surgeon's knot reapproximate the epidermis and are subsequently removed 2–3 days later to prevent suture scars.

DRESSINGS AND DRAINS

Because of the large raw surface area of these widely undermined flaps, tissue exudation and oozing can retard healing. Therefore, it is advisable to drain the cervical-cheek flap areas with a flat drain that exits from a separate stab incision (Figure 1-87). The drain runs under the chin to the opposite infra-auricular area. Small evacuator bulbs provide the appropriate amount of suction. The drain is removed when the drainage is 25 ml or less in 24 hours. This is usually on the second postoperative day. A dressing is applied for 24 hours after drain removal.

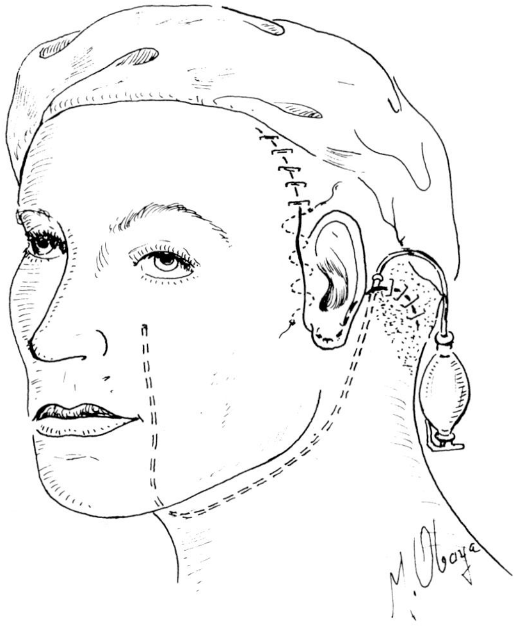

Figure 1-87

The antibiotic ointment is applied to all suture lines (Figure 1-88). Rolled cotton soaked in mineral oil is applied next over the flaps and suture lines. The ointment retards bacterial contamination and, combined with the mineral oil, prevents crusts from forming along the suture tracts and in the incision. The oil facilitates molding of the dressing and prevents adherence of the skin to the dressing. A 4-inch Kling gauze bandage is placed over fluffs that augment the rolled cotton. The next morning the dressing is changed and antibiotic ointment reapplied.

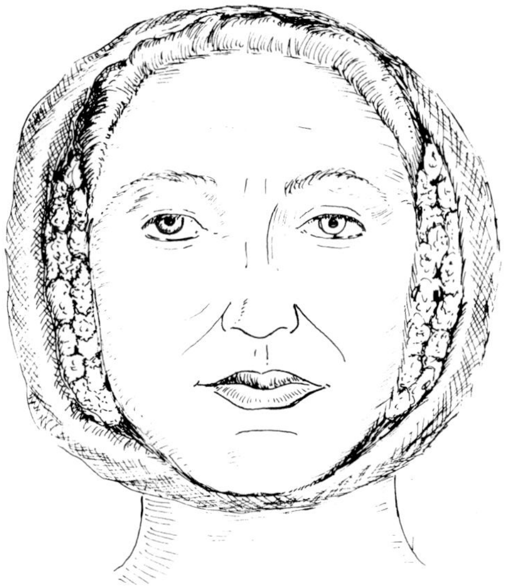

Figure 1-88

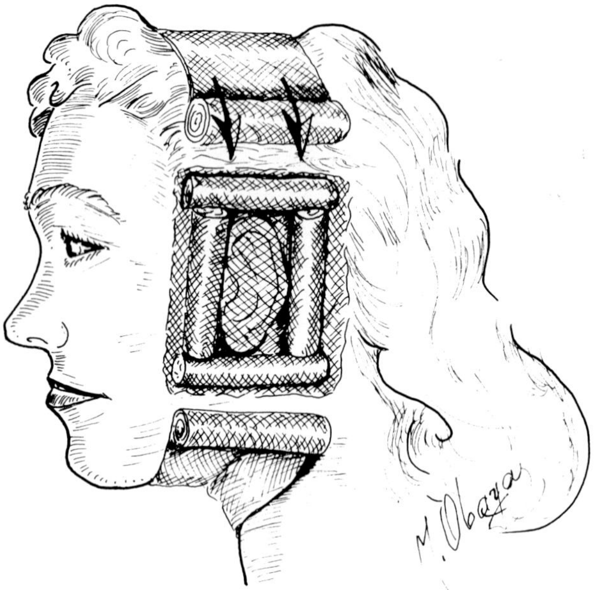

Figure 1-89

A smaller, lighter dressing of folded 4 × 4's is placed in front of and behind the ear and wrapped lightly with a 4-inch Kling (Figure 1-89). This is removed in 24–48 hours.

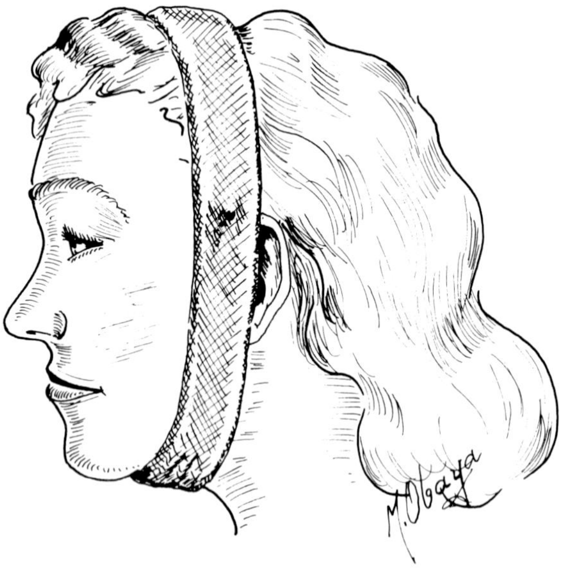

Figure 1-90

For the next week or two, a 6-inch stockinette chin strap is worn at night and around the house to give support to the submental area (Figure 1-90).

COMPLICATIONS

HEMATOMA

Treatment of major hematomas is best accomplished by immediately removing sutures on that portion of the flap under tension (Figure 1-91) and then returning the patient to the operating room for a general anesthetic to explore the suspected area.

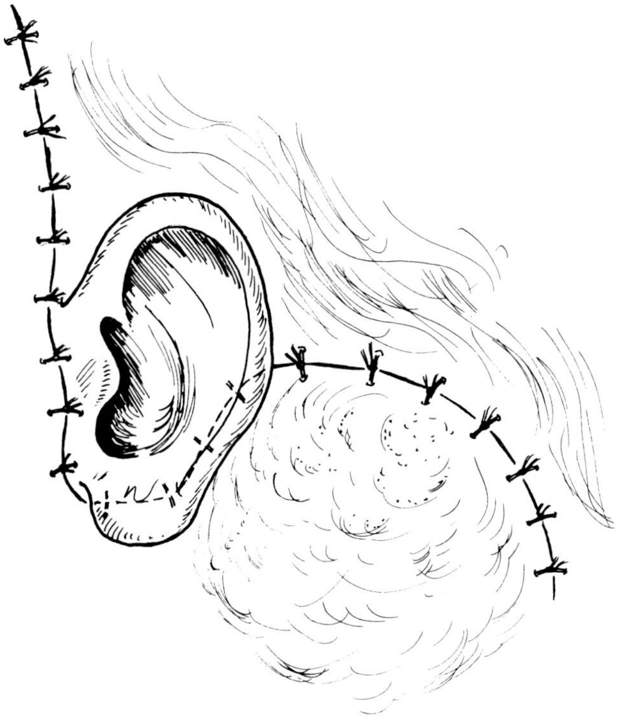

Figure 1-91

Once the flap is elevated, (Figure 1-92) the clot is removed.

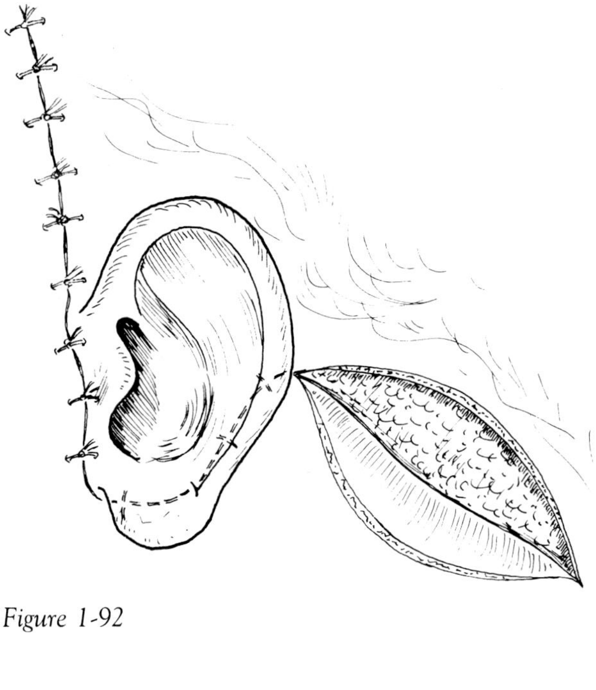

Figure 1-92

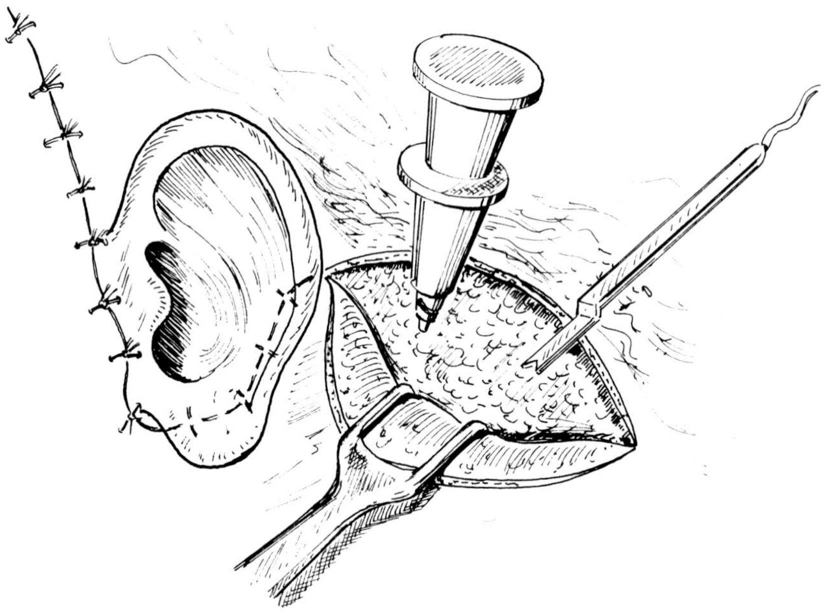

Figure 1-93

The wound is flushed with copious amounts of sterile saline (Figure 1-93). Frequently, specific bleeding points will not be identified but if present may be cauterized or suture-ligated.

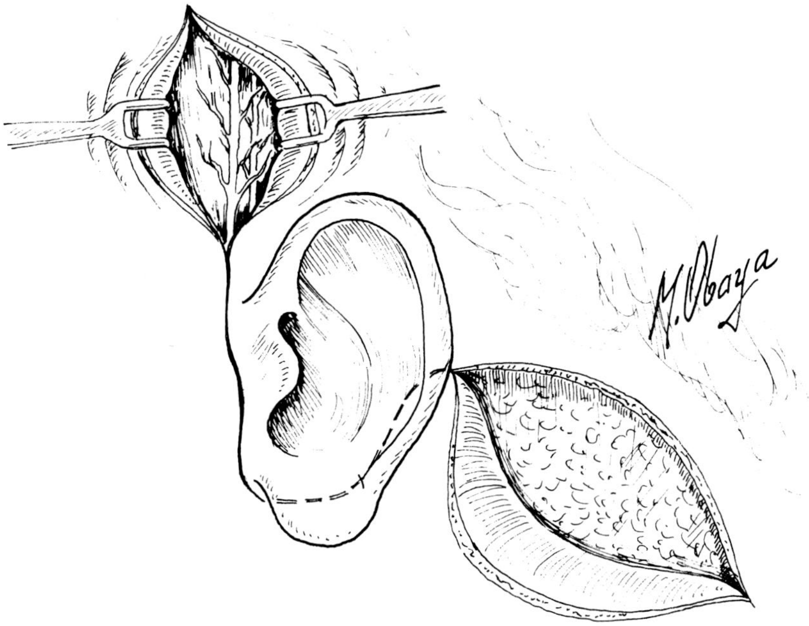

Figure 1-94

If oozing continues, suture removal (Figure 1-94) from the remaining parts of the incision may be necessary to completely explore the entire wound.

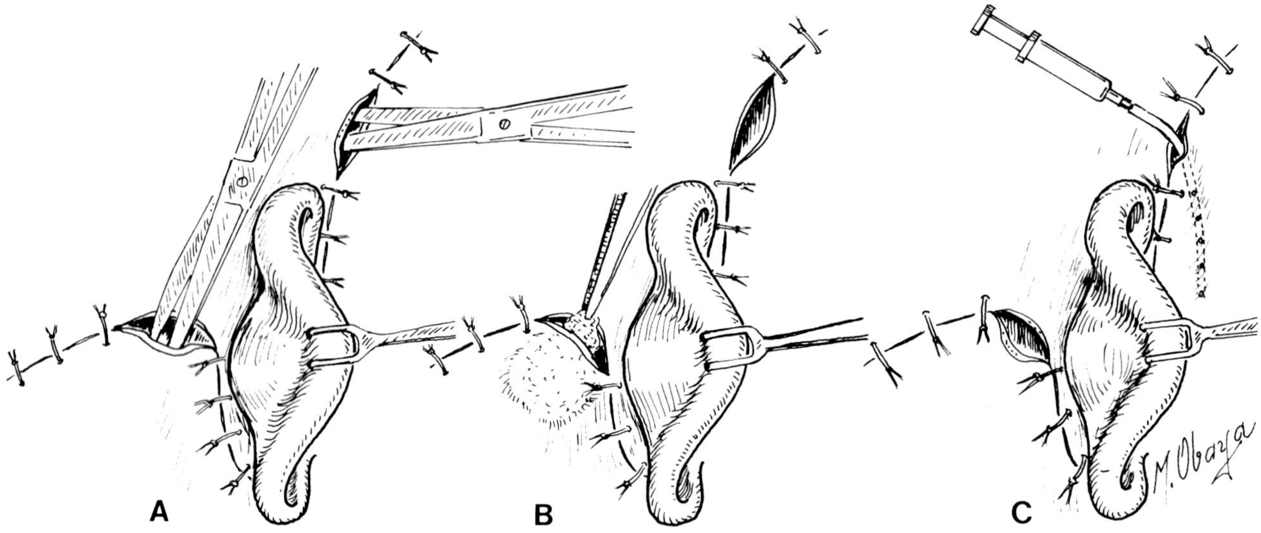

Figure 1-95

An alternative to the above procedure has been described by Pitanguy[7] in which two or three sutures are removed in the temporal and mastoid areas under sterile conditions at the bedside with light analgesia (Figure 1-95A). The clot is extracted with a hemostat (Figure 1-95B) and a 19-gauge nasogastric tube is introduced to irrigate the wound with normal saline (C). The sutures are replaced and the dressing reapplied. If bleeding should persist, the next step is to open the incision under general anesthesia in the operating room. Caution should be exercised in handling the opposite side of the face during evacuation of the clot to prevent a second hematoma from developing on the uninvolved side.

ALOPECIA

Hair loss may occur in the temporal area from excessive tension or damage to the hair follicles during flap elevation. Observation for several months to allow hair regrowth is the initial treatment if the loss is due to follicular shock. For larger areas, punch grafting or local flap transfer may be necessary (Figure 1-96). Wide scars with subsequent hair loss are modified by simple excision and closure.

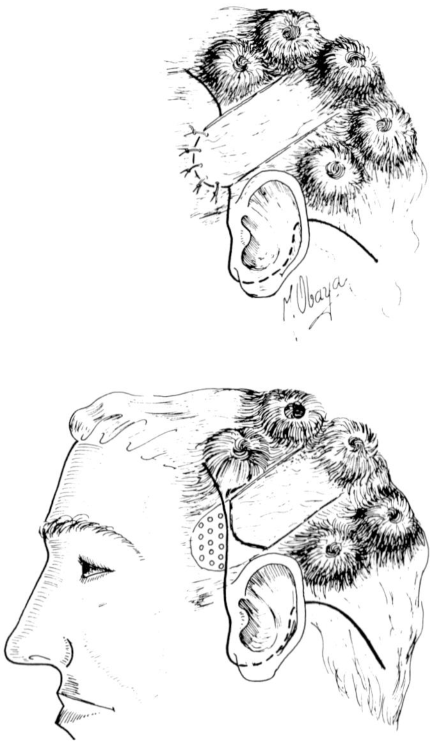

Figure 1-96

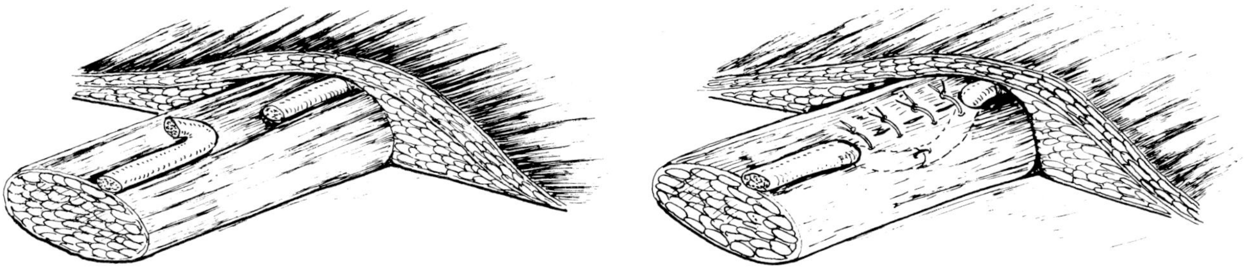

Figure 1-97

NERVE INJURY

If the greater auricular nerve is severed and recognized, it has a strong propensity for regeneration, and the severed ends should be sutured (Figure 1-97). Burying the anastomosis will prevent not only neuroma formation, but also adherence of the nerve to the thin skin flap.

COMPLICATIONS ASSOCIATED WITH SUBMENTAL-SUBMANDIBULAR SCULPTURING AND SMAS-PLATYSMA MANIPULATION

A frequent problem during the immediate postoperative period is recurrent fullness to some degree in the submental area. This will frequently resolve spontaneously as the edema in the subcutaneous tissues is absorbed and the flaps contract (Figure 1-98).

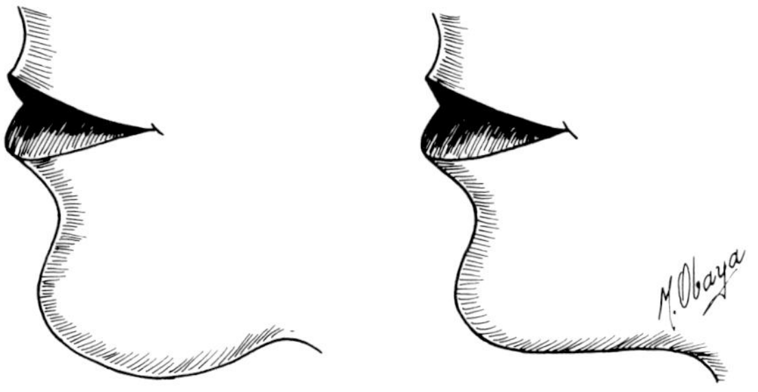

Figure 1-98

Injudicious removal of fat in the submental triangle with overcorrection of the obtuse cervicomental contour will result in an unnatural submental depression or cobra deformity (Figure 1-99).

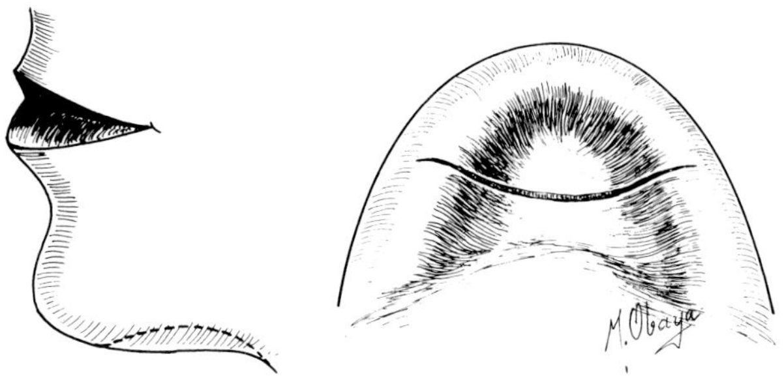

Figure 1-99

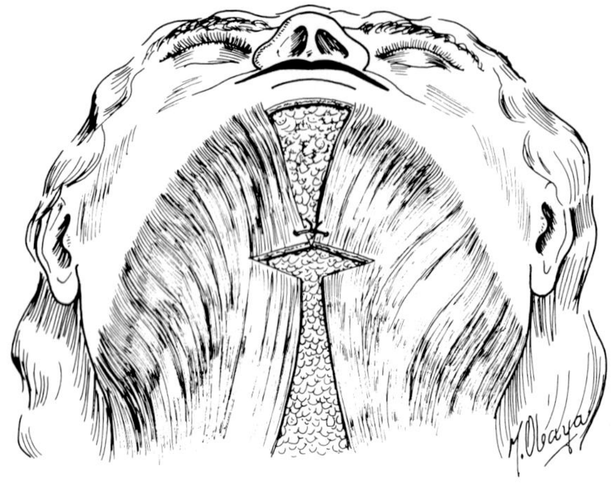

Figure 1-100

Excision of the submental fat pad with exposure of the mylohyoid muscle is to be avoided (Figures 1-23 and 1-24) in most situations. The skin flap becomes adherent to the mylohyoid muscle, thus accentuating the depression and occasionally causing pain on swallowing. Excision of the subcutaneous fat with the concomitant excision of the platysma muscle may also result in an unnatural submental depression. This complication may be prevented by suturing the medial borders of the platysma muscle with permanent buried suture after fat and/or muscle excision. Correction of this depression if unacceptable to the patient postoperatively is done by mobilizing the platysma muscle through the submental incision, creating two muscle flaps and suturing them in the midline (Figure 1-100). A free fat graft to fill in the concavity might be necessary.

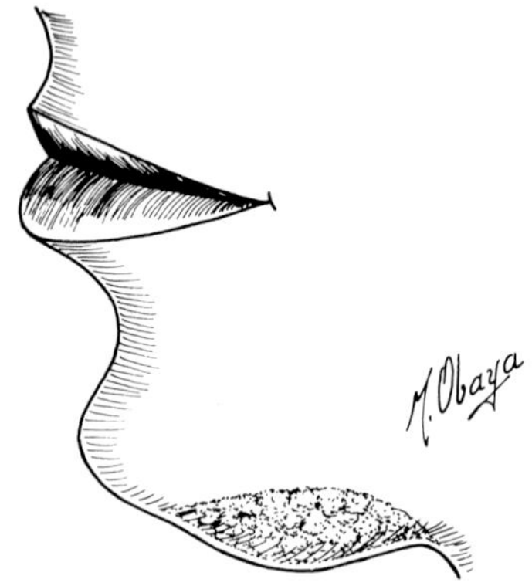

Figure 1-101

Creation of "pseudojowls" in the submaxillary triangles because of excessive submandibular fat excision combined with submental fat and platysma muscle removal is due to ptosis of the submaxillary glands (Figure 1-101). This has been demonstrated on cadaver dissections.

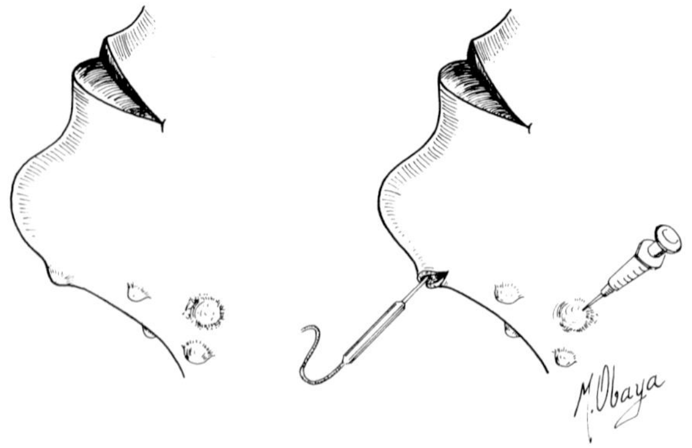

Figure 1-102

Figure 1-102 shows correction of irregular submental or submandibular contour, which is due to uneven removal of fat. These collections of fat may be injected with triamcinolone (10 mg/ml). Excision and/or cauterization through small stab incisions over the lumps can also be done to smooth out the irregularities.

Complete horizontal sectioning of the platysma muscle in thin patients may result in an abnormal step deformity in the neck (Figure 1-103A). In other patients, the superior edge may roll up under the cervical skin (Figure 1-103B).

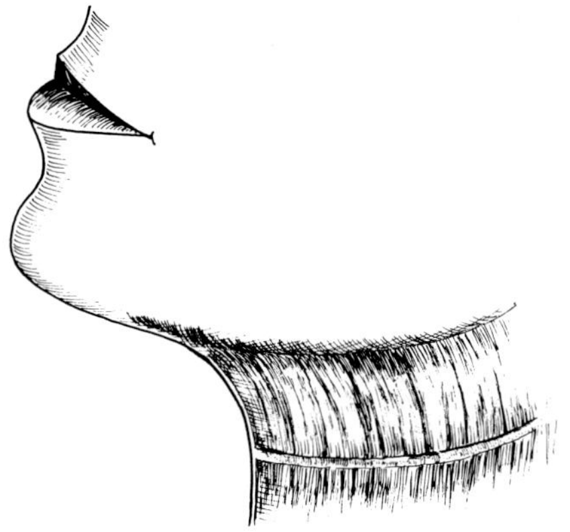

Figure 1-103A

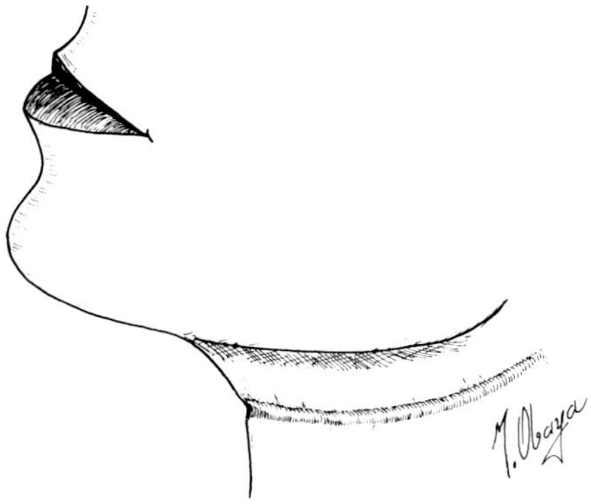

Figure 1-103B

Cadaver dissections and clinical experience have shown a fascial connection between the leaves of the platysma. If left intact, it can transmit the pull of the platysma and form anterior banding in the midline, where no muscle exists (Figure 1-104).

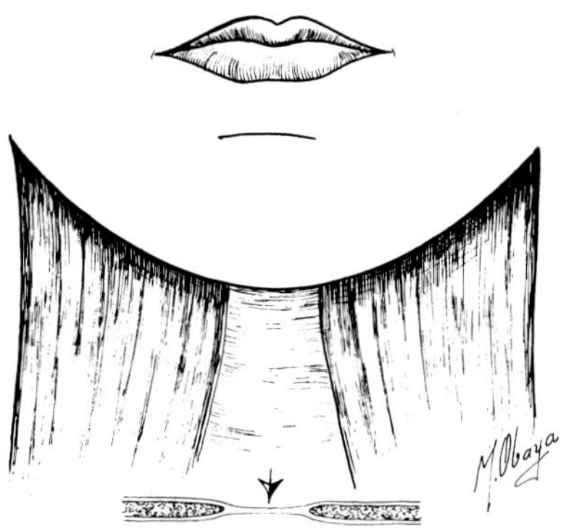

Figure 1-104

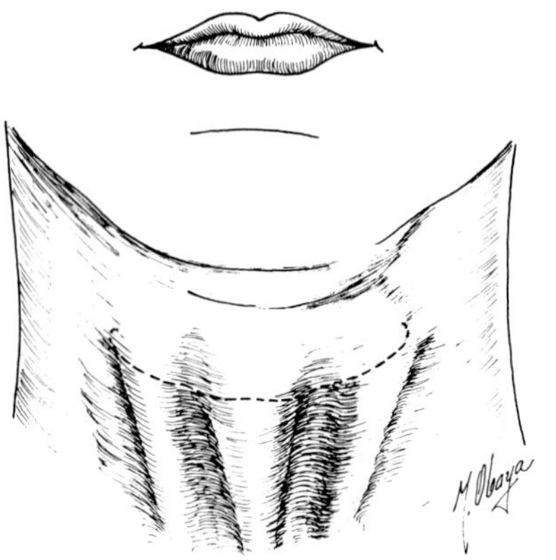

Figure 1-105

Excision of the soft tissues over the thyroid cartilage in an attempt to remove recurrent banding must be avoided (Figure 1-105). The cervical skin will adhere to the thyroid cartilage and create vertical bands and folds as the skin is drawn superiorly with each swallow. The normal anatomy of the larynx with an interposing soft-tissue layer that allows it to slide superiorly with swallowing must be maintained.

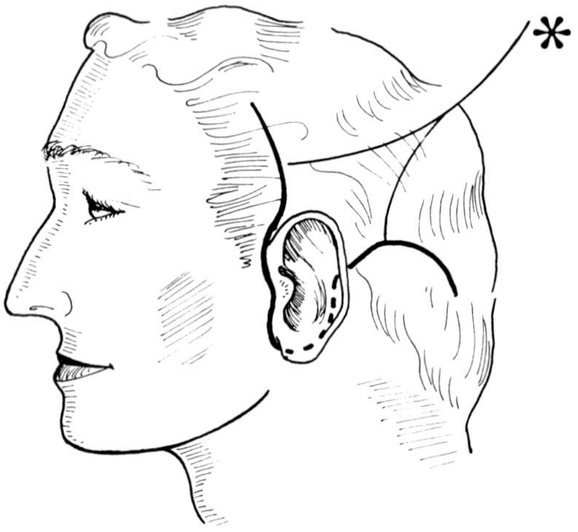

Figure 1-106A

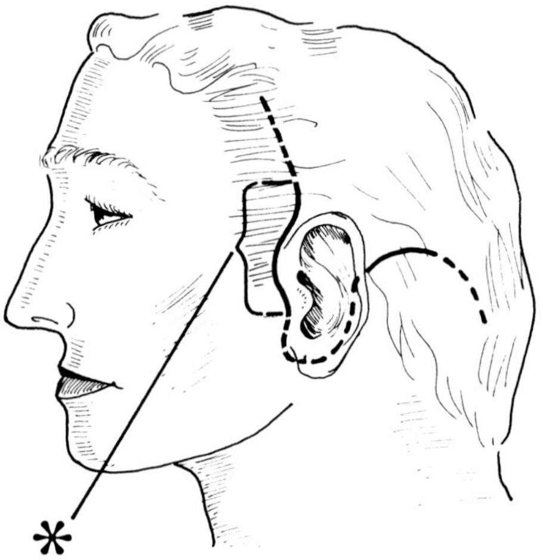

Figure 1-106B

THE TUCK-UP AND SECONDARY FACELIFT

A simple tuck at 6–12 months to correct malar and jowl sagging that develops after the edema subsides is illustrated in Figures 1-106A and B and 1-107A–E. The incision is made around the root of the ear in the previous temporal incision (Figure 1-106B).

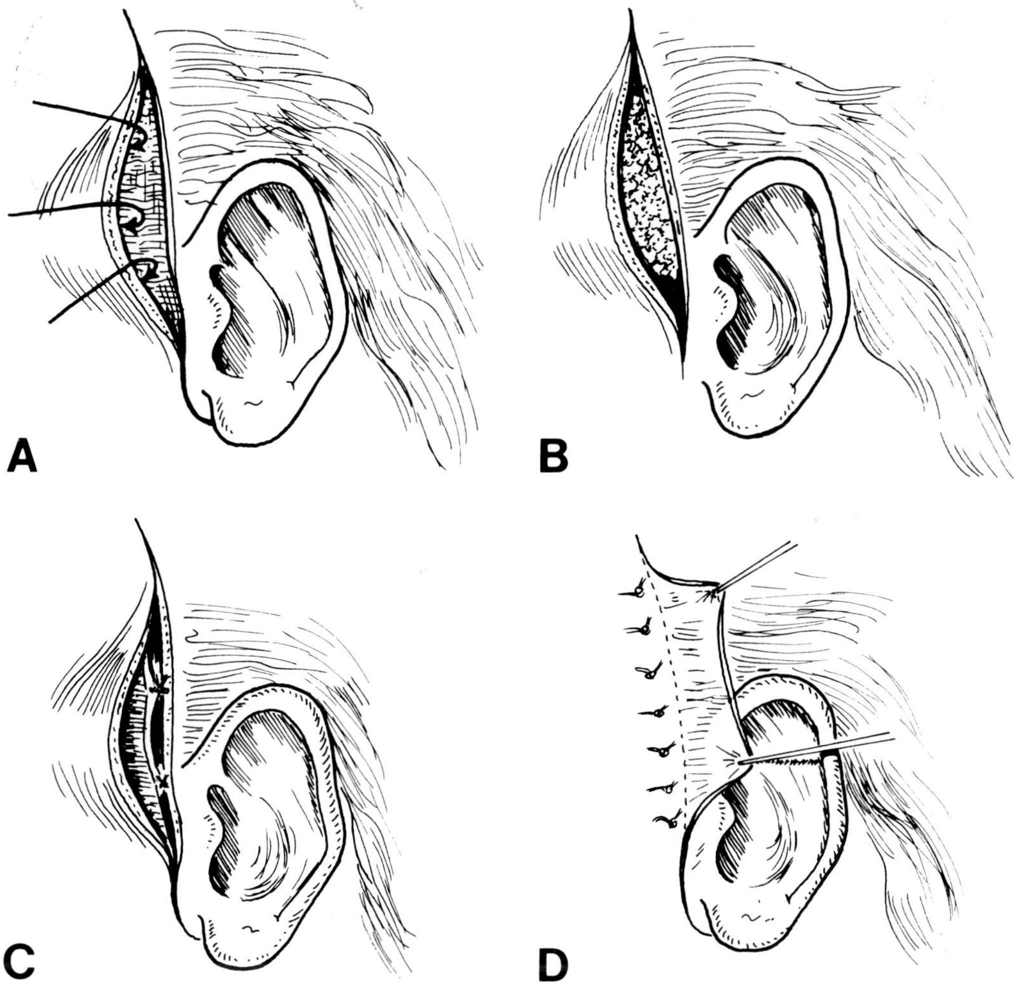

Figure 1-107

The incision is carried down to the fibrotic layer formed from the previous surgery (Figure 1-107A). It is undermined 2–3 cm to correspond to the amount of skin to be excised. The tuckup is thus actually a segmental excision to lift the loose tissue. If any advancement of the fibrotic layer can be achieved, it is incised (Figure 1-107B) and plicated postero-superior (Figure 1-107C). The skin flap is redraped with a moderate amount of tension (Figure 1-107D) and closed in layers using 4-0 Dexon subcutaneously and 4-0 nylon on the skin. Similar tucks may be taken below the lobules (Figure 1-107E).

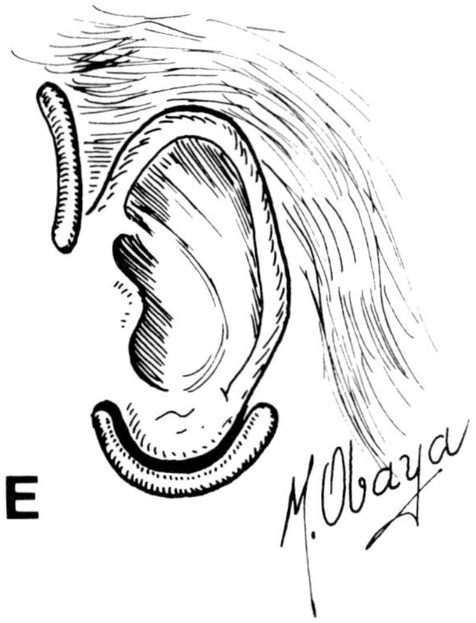

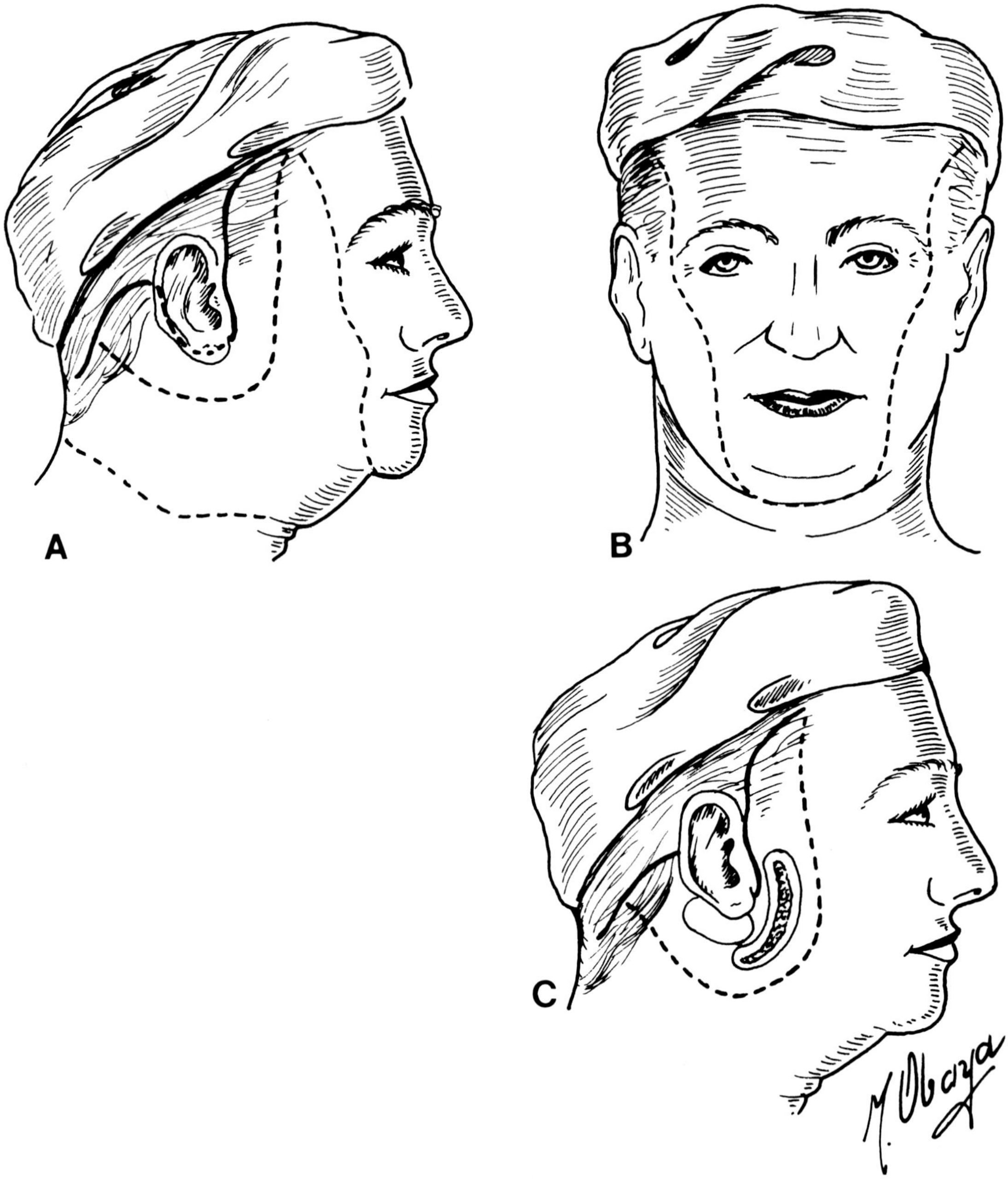

Figure 1-108

Figure 1-108 shows a more extensive secondary rhytidectomy involving wider undermining and a longer incision. The extent of undermining of the first facelift is shown in Figure 1-108A and B. A segment of the fibrotic scar is excised and sutured to support the second lift as shown in Figure 1-108C.

DISCUSSION

ANATOMY

Inferiorly, the SMAS (Figures 1-3–1-11) extends to the platysma muscle. Anterior to the notch of the facial artery, loose fibrous connections between the SMAS and periosteum of the inferior border of the mandible have been identified. The SMAS is believed to be a fibromuscular network located between the dermis and facial musculature to distribute, transmit, and possibly amplify the contractions of the facial musculature. However, the author believes it to be nothing more than a continuation of the superficial cervical fascia.

ANESTHESIA

Local infiltration and/or regional nerve block anesthesia is preferred for all cases (Figures 1-26–1-29). General anesthesia with the hazards of intubation, extubation, draping, and operative contamination usually precludes its use. The recovery phase and bleeding are much less with a local anesthetic, even if the general anesthesia is supplemented with local infiltration. However, certain patients demand a general anesthetic, and if there are no medical contraindications, the procedure may be carried out in this mode.

As the surgical techniques have become more extensive, the operative time has similarly increased. As a result, longer-lasting local anesthetics are required. Marcaine (bupivacaine hydrochloride) has been widely used as a long-acting regional nerve block and infiltrative agent. It is related clinically to lidocaine (Xylocaine) and is metabolized and detoxified in the liver. The onset of action of analgesia requires approximately 10 minutes and may last for up to 6–10 hours. Excessive plasma levels may affect the central nervous system (CNS), resulting in excitation, depression, unconsciousness, and possibly respiratory arrest. Cardiovascular manifestations of toxicity may include depression of the myocardium, hypotension, and cardiac arrest. The maximum dosage of Marcaine is 225 mg with 1 : 200,000 adrenalin in a single dose that is 90 ml of 0.25% solution. A reinjection of another 125 mg (40 ml of 0.25%) may be done 3 hours after the first injection to raise the dose to 400 mg, which should not be exceeded in 24 hours.

For local nerve block anesthesia, 0.5% Marcaine with 1 : 200,000 epinephrine (Adrenalin), may be used to block the infraorbital nerve, superficial cervical plexus, and the third division of the trigeminal nerve. This type of block is effective in patients who cannot have large doses of Adrenalin. It may also be used prior to local infiltration to reduce the discomfort associated with ballooning of the tissues. The incisions are infiltrated with 1% Xylocaine and 1 : 200,000 Adrenalin. A nerve block reduces not only the volume of anesthesia required, but also distortion of tissues. The reduction in the amount of tissue edema may result in less pain postoperatively.

Regarding the procedure illustrated in Figures 1-26–1-29, a total volume of 100 ml of 0.25% Marcaine is sufficient to cover the entire cervical and facial area combined with 20 ml of 1% Xylocaine. The application of one period of infiltration and then waiting for 10 minutes for the local anesthesia and the Adrenalin to take effect allows the patient to calm down prior to starting the procedure. Moreover, the flow of the surgical procedure does not have to be interrupted to infiltrate the opposite side. The prolonged analgesic effect of Marcaine reduces the postoperative requirement for pain medication and prolongs the time before it will be required.

An alternative to using a long-acting local anesthetic would be to use 0.5% Xylocaine with 1 : 200,000 Adrenalin and infiltrate each side just before doing the facelift. Unfortunately, each time Adrenalin is injected and the patient is stimulated, there is a transient rise in pulse and blood pressure that not only increases the risk of bleeding but also requires an offsetting dose of sedation or narcotic.

Some surgeons advocate a hydrodynamic infiltration to facilitate the dissection and elevation of the skin flaps. A total volume of 200–240 ml is used. By using 100 ml of 0.25% Marcaine with 1 : 200,000 Adrenalin and diluting it with 100 ml of normal saline, the tissues are ballooned out. Unfortunately, the distortion and edema of the flaps may be exacerbated by this technique, thereby compromising the amount of tension and excision of the flaps and hence the surgical result. Several weeks later as the edema inevitably subsides, the skin laxity may be more pronounced than those techniques in which a smaller volume of anesthetic is used.

TECHNIQUE: TAILORING THE OPERATION

From an anatomic perspective, the operation depicted in Figures 1-30–1-32 would not resolve nor "lift" all cervicofacial abnormalities. It would be analogous to performing the same rhinoplasty on all patients regardless of the pathologic anatomy. From a surgical view point, the classic "skin flap" myeloplasty contradicts the basic surgical principles. Advancement of skin over a mound of fat creates only a temporary change as the underlying fat will eventually re-create the cosmetic deformity. Similarly, to effect a change in a dermocutaneous junction, the operation and undermining must extend a few millimeters into or beyond the area to produce a permanent change.

In particularly heavy individuals who still have a full or ptotic submental contour after excision of the superficial fat, it may be necessary to remove a portion of the deep submental fat pad. In the young woman who has a congenital collection of submental fat, a simple submental lipectomy may be all that is required to improve the submental contour. The elasticity of the skin in the younger patient allows it to redrape with excellent results.

Figure 1-52 shows chin augmentation to correct congenital microgenia or relative retrognathia from atrophy of the soft tissues and bone absorption. Class V patients (see Table 1-1) have the most spectacular result as the implant acts as a scaffold to maintain stretch of the soft tissues and increase chin projection.

Interestingly, a few patients who were thought to be Class VI were in reality Class III (see Table 1-1) after the submental and submandibular areas were sculptured and tightened. Diagnosis of this class of patient requires an x-ray diagnosis to confirm the level of the hyoid bone. Although no surgical technique is available to elevate the hyoid bone, identification of these patients preoperatively allows surgeons to warn their patients of limited success, regardless of the surgical approach.

An alternative to the widely undermined facelift is the *segmental excision lift.* The advantages of the procedure illustrated in Figures 1-54 and 1-55 are shorter operating time, less chance of hematoma formation, greater tension on skin flaps, and less chance of facial nerve injury. The disadvantages are that movement of skin over a mound of fat is only temporary as the scaffolding of the deeper layers of the face cause the overlying skin that has not been undermined to develop recurrent fullness. The plication sutures (Figure 1-55) will not reduce the fullness in the submandibular or submental areas, and revision and tuck-up facelift procedures will not be as effective since there is no layer of scar tissue to act as a scaffold to tighten. As shown in Figure 1-55, the area of support and pull is 10–12 cm from the pathologic anatomy that needs improvement.

There is controversy regarding manipulation of subcutaneous tissue, particularly the use of plication sutures versus direct undermining with rotation and excision of the SMAS-platysma complex. Plication of the SMAS (Figure 1-36) and posterior border of the platysma is quicker and safer. Subcutaneous bunching in the preauricular area may be a problem postoperatively, but it will usually resolve over a 6-week period.

Direct undermining of SMAS (Figures 1-9 and 1-50) and platysma with or without sectioning of the muscle raises risk of injury to the facial nerve, especially if dissection is anterior to line AB in Figure 1-3, and also introduces the possibility of postoperative salivary fistula when the parotid artery is exposed and/or injured.

There is also controversy concerning subplatysma (Skoog) as opposed to subdermal facelift. The incidence of facial nerve injury and hematoma formation is higher with the subplatysma technique. Careful analysis of the postoperative result with short- and long-term follow-up may reveal that there is no advantage to the increased risks with the subplatysmal lift.

Regarding temporal incisions (illustrated in the Finesse section), an incision similar to that shown in Figure 1-61 has been described for the male patient. If the hair follicles are avulsed with a tweezer and the area in front of the ear lightly cauterized on the undersurface of the flap, hair growth is retarded, if not eliminated.

The incision illustrated in Figures 1-63 and 1-64 does not distort the hairline behind the ear. Unfortunately, the distance between the hairline and the skin of the ear is frequently so small that a very narrow flap of skin is created that will slough if any tension is applied to it. Patients (men included) who have short hair cannot as readily camouflage this scar as it runs along the hairline. An alternative to this problem is an incision that runs posteriorly into the hairline (line c in Figure 1-63). Rotation and anchoring of the flap is a few centimeters further from the area to be corrected. There is frequently a step deformity such as that shown in Figure 1-65, but this usually poses no problems.

COMPLICATIONS

The incidence of hematoma (Figures 1-91–1-95) varies from 1.2 to 15 percent depending on whether small hematomas are included and recognized. For hematomas that necessitate drainage, the percentage varies from 0.9 to 8.0 percent. Prevention is the best therapy, and all patients are instructed to discontinue any aspirin-containing medicine for 2 weeks prior to surgery. Intraoperatively, meticulous hemastasis is both derigueur and the ultimate goal.

Postoperative rise in blood pressure, breakthrough bleeding from loss of the epinephrine (Adrenalin) effect, and blood dyscrasias have been associated with postoperative hematomas. The consequences of hematoma formation are increased patient discomfort, hospitalization and expense, skin necrosis, infection, alopecia, subcutaneous nodules, skin puckering, and pigmentation. The patient will usually complain of deep unilateral facial tightness or pain with a major, slowly expanding hematoma. The smaller hematoma will not be recognized until the flap edema subsides and the subcutaneous collection has been identified. These may be aspirated with an 18-gauge needle at 7 days when the clot liquefies. Ecchymoses of the lips or buccal mucosa or unusual unilateral facial swelling are the physical signs heralding a hematoma. If a hematoma is suspected, prompt dressing removal and examination of the flaps is essential. If a hematoma is present, swelling, discoloration, and tension of the flaps with circulatory compromise will be obvious.

Although there is a risk of skin necrosis, major flap necrosis is quite rare following the facelift operation. However, minor areas of skin slough do occur and usually heal without significant scarring or sequelae. The mastoid skin flap is the most frequent site of minor skin loss. When the flaps are placed under excessive tension due to over zealous skin excision, the vascularity is embarrassed and necrosis results. Postoperatively, hematomas, seromas, and infection can lead to skin necrosis. Fortunately, the majority of cases involve areas that are concealed from view and will not be a problem. When skin necrosis is diagnosed and the wound is demarcating, frequent office visits and reassurance to the patient are of the utmost importance. No attempt should be made to debride, skin-graft, or manipulate the thick eschar that forms other than to have the patient apply an antimicrobial agent 3 times daily. Eventually, the skin will be replaced by a slowly advancing epithelial border. Months later, if scarring is conspicuous, serial advancement and scar excision are appropriate therapy. Split-thickness grafts from the inner arm may be necessary for larger areas of slough.

There is also a risk of infection, but fortunately, postoperative infections are unusual in the well-vascularized facial area. Reaction to the nylon sutures with erythema and swelling is managed with local wound care of moist heat, topical antibiotic ointment, and suture removal. Prevention of infection by having the patient wash the hair and face the night before surgery and the morning of surgery along with strict sterile technique reduces the chance for contamination. Occasionally a localized abscess will develop that requires incision, drainage, and systemic antibiotics.

Scarring may also result. The width of a postoperative scar is directly proportional to the tension placed on the edges of the wound. Reapproximation of the subcutaneous layers with tension-relieving sutures and meticulous closure of the wound edges decrease the likelihood of a gradual spreading incision. Keloid formation or thickening of scars in the postauricular area is treated with intralesional injections of triamcinolone (10 mg/ml) spaced 3–4 weeks apart. Reexcision of the scar with intradermal injection of steroids is rarely necessary.

Regarding the possibility of nerve injury, the most frequently injured nerve during a rhytidectomy is the greater auricular nerve (see Figure 1-97 for corrective procedure). Its superficial location on the sternocleidomastoid muscle with a thin covering of superficial fascia makes it particularly vulnerable to injury. Prevention of a postoperative numb ear is best accomplished by elevating the cervical flap in a superficial plane (see anatomy in Figures 1-3 and 1-4B).

Transient ear pain postoperatively may require strong analgesics for up to 6 weeks. Plication sutures that are placed in or across the nerve may crush it and produce pain. Occasionally, a trigger area is identified below the lobule. An injection of 1% Xylocaine with Adrenalin mixed in equal parts with triamcinolone (10 mg/ml) may help to relieve the pain and hasten resolution of the problem. If pain persists for over 3 months or if the patient complains of a numb ear that does not resolve, exploration of the greater auricular nerve with decompression, reanastomosis of the severed ends (if interrupted), and removal of any constricting sutures may be necessary.

More disconcerting than a numb ear, however, is the presence of a localized seventh nerve injury postoperatively. Fortunately, permanent paralysis is rare, and reports in the literature vary between 0.4 and 2.6 percent.[8] The most frequently injured branches are the zygomaticotemporal and marginal mandibular. In the more extensive facelift with SMAS and platysma muscle manipulation, the likelihood of injury is increased. Frequently, an isolated postoperative paresis will return within 6—12 months because of the interanastomoses between the peripheral branches of the facial nerve. Therefore, patient support, encouragement, and frequent office visits during healing is the best treatment for a paresis recognized postoperatively. For a branch that is severed and recognized intraoperatively, immediate microsurgical anastomosis is the treatment of choice. It has been suggested in the literature that a localized paralysis that does not resolve in 12 months may be treated by sectioning the opposite temporal or mandibular branch to create facial symmetry.[8] Electrical stimulation is helpful to identify the specific branch or branches prior to lysis. Unfortunately, facial symmetry may not result in every case.

Regarding complications associated with SMAS-platysma manipulation, particularly salivary fistula and Frey's syndrome, elevation of the SMAS over the parotid gland with inadvertent penetration of the gland parenchyma could lead to a subcutaneous accumulation of parotid secretions. If recurrent swelling occurs over the parotid, aspiration should be done once to establish the diagnosis. Repeated evacuation of the fluid will only stimulate its recurrence. The problem is usually self limiting if Stensen's duct is patient. The fluid will gradually absorb. Frey's syndrome is avoided by advancing the SMAS posteriorly and using it as an interposing layer between the skin flap and parotid gland. Thus parasympathetic fibers from the parotid will not be able to anastomose with the sweat glands of the skin.

Incomplete horizontal sectioning of the platysma will prevent the two problems illustrated in Figure 1-103A and B (see also Figure 1-45). If complete horizontal transection of the platysma is done, it must be at or below the level of the thyrohyoid membrane in order to create a wide flap that will not roll on itself and be sufficient to give support to the neck when the medial borders are sutured together and the posterior border is advanced and plicated posteriorly. Recurrent anterior banding of the platysma muscle may develop postoperatively regardless of the technique to obliterate them. Incomplete section of the folds must be considered first. However, this does not explain their gradual recurrence 10–16 months after surgery. When the free edges of the platysma are plicated in the midline without concomitant horizontal sectioning, the muscle fibers will continue to contract and form the vertical-bands. Conversely, when the anterior folds are sectioned horizontally and sutured in the midline, the anterior bands are simply moved more laterally. Excision of the anterior folds with or without plication will similarly move the banding more laterally. In patients who develop recurrent banding despite complete horizontal sectioning of the platysma, fibrous connections must form between the cut edges to account for the recurrent anterior folds.

Revision surgery to remove these troublesome folds and that shown in Figure 1-104 must be done with care. Overzealous excision of the bands may create dimpling and a worse cosmetic deformity.

With respect to the tuck-up and secondary facelift procedures (Figures 1-106A and B, 1-107A–E, and 1-108), it is useful to correct the laxity several years after the primary facelift. The lift is achieved by excising and advancing the fibrotic layer from the previous surgery. The more extensive the primary surgery, the more dramatic will be the secondary lift. In patients who have had a minilift or one that involves minimal undermining, the secondary lift will have to be more extensive than previously described if the desired cosmetic result is to be achieved.

Despite extensive undermining, fat sculpturing, and subcutaneous plication, the aging process never stops, and gravity, sun, and genetic predisposition continue to take their toll of even the best postoperative result. The older the patient, the sooner a secondary procedure will be required.

REFERENCES

1. Anderson, J.: The Tuck-Up Operation: A New Technique of Secondary Rhytidectomy. *Arch. Otolaryngol.* 101:739–743, 1975.
2. Dedo, D. D.: Anatomic Basis for Sculpturing the Neck in Myeloplasty. *Arch. Otolaryngol.* 107:439–442, 1981.
3. Dedo D. D.: Management of the Neck in Cervicofacial Rhytidectomy. Transactions of the Third International Symposium of Facial Plastic and Reconstructive Surgery, New York. Grune & Stratton, New York, 1981.
4. Kamer, F. M.: The Two-Stage Concept of Rhytidectomy. *Laryngoscope,* 89:500–503, 1979.
5. Kamer, F. M.: Sequential Rhytidectomy and the Two-Stage Concept. *Otolaryngol. Clin. North Am.* 13: 305–320, 1980.
6. McKinney, P. and Katrana, D. J.: Prevention of Injury to the Great Auricular Nerve During Rhytidectomy. *Plast. Reconstr. Surg.* 66:675–679, 1980.
7. Pitanguy, I., Ceravdo, M. P.: Hematoma Postrhytidectomy: How We Treat It. *Plas. Reconstr. Surg.*, 67:526–529, 1981.
8. Rees, T.: Aesthetic Plastic Surgery, Vol. II, W. B. Saunders Co., Philadelphia, pp. 600–683, 1980.

2
Cosmetic Blepharoplasty

Michael Patipa

UPPER EYELID BLEPHAROPLASTY

Upper eyelid blepharoplasty essentially involves the excision of skin, muscle and/or orbital fat with the goal of restoring a youthful appearance to the eyelids. Each patient, because of personal appearance and desires, requires an operation tailored to goals that the surgeon and patient set.

A basic surgical outline follows, and modifications that will assist in individualizing the operation and result are provided.

EYEBROW PTOSIS

The preoperative evaluation of patients considered for blepharoplasty requires careful examination of the eyebrows. Brow ptosis can masquerade as severe upper eyelid dermatochalasis, and removal of the lax upper eyelid tissues without first recognizing and correcting ptotic eyebrows will result in poor cosmetic results and vertical shortening of the upper lid tissues.

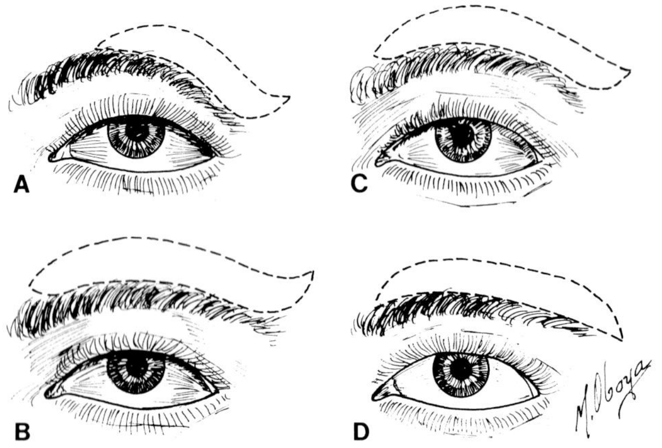

Figure 2-1

A suprabrow elevation is performed as shown in Figure 2-1. The shape and fashion of the excision is determined by the type of brow ptosis. Ptosis of the temporal brow will give an appearance of severe dermatochalasis of the lateral upper eyelid (Figure 2-1A). This is corrected with a temporal brow elevation. If the entire eyebrow is ptotic, but more severely ptotic laterally, a superior curve at the lateral end of the excision will restore a normal appearance (Figure 2-1B). When the eyebrow is most ptotic in its center, a "lazy-S"-shaped excision is performed (Figure 2-1C). Flattening and drooping of the entire brow is corrected by symmetrically elevating the entire length of the eyebrow (Figure 2-1D).

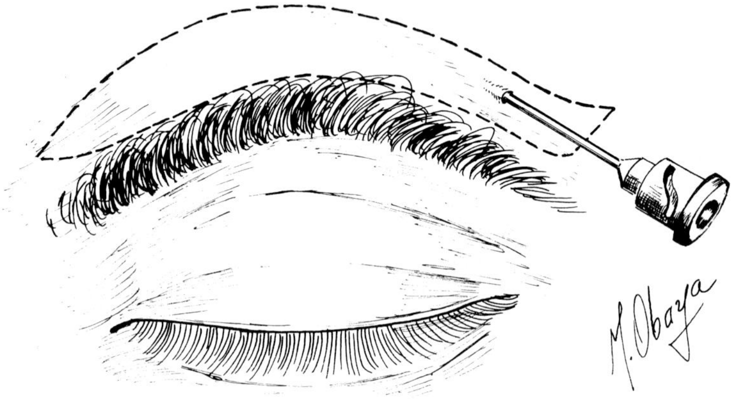

Figure 2-2

Technique

The lower incision line is placed in the uppermost row of the cilia of the eyebrow (Figure 2-2). After marking the proposed incision, infiltrate the subcutaneous tissue with local anesthetic (Xylocaine with 1 : 100,000 epinephrine). The epinephrine reduces the abundant bleeding when operating in this vascular region of the face. The anesthetic should be massaged to allow its diffusion through the tissue.

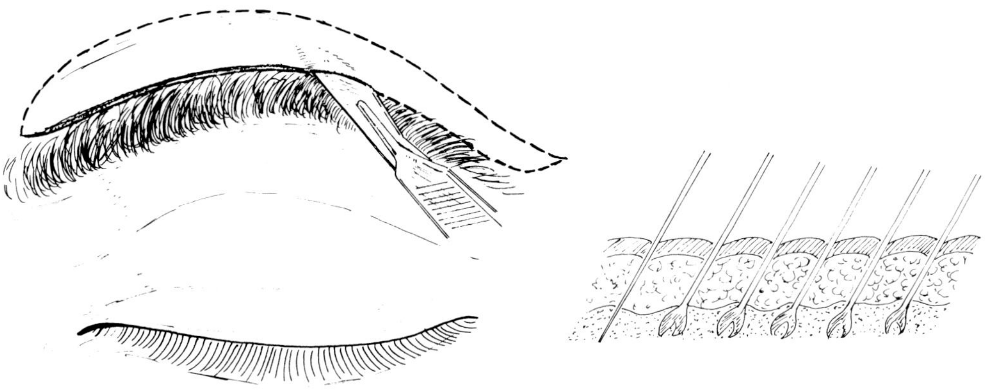

Figure 2-3

The scalpel blade should be angled in the same direction as the eyebrow cilia (Figure 2-3). This is particularly important for the lower incision to help avoid cutting across the hair follicles and damaging the superior eyebrow cilia (see inset to Figure 2–3).

The skin and subcutaneous tissues are excised with scissors (Figure 2-4). Care should be taken to keep the plane of the wound parallel with the skin to avoid migrating deeper into the brow medially. The supraorbital vascular bundle can be avoided by careful dissection, thereby avoiding the severe bleeding encountered when these vessels are cut. If large vessels are cut, they should be cauterized or ligated.

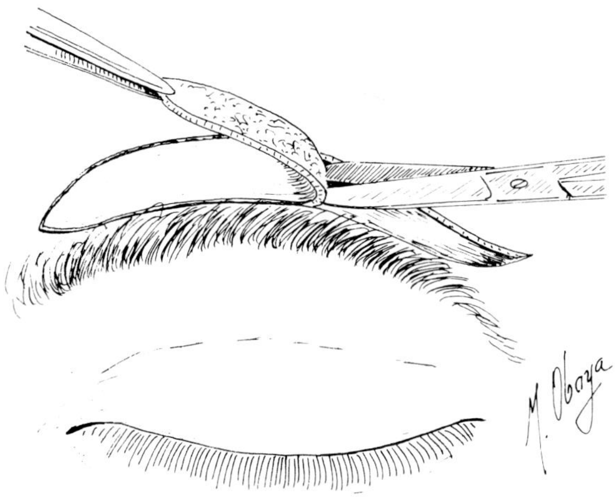

Figure 2-4

Once the brow excision has been completed, the surgeon should reappose the wound edges bimanually (Figure 2-5) and have the assistant mark the sites for wound closure as indicated. There is invariably a temporal shift of the upper wound and careful alignment and marking of your closure will help prevent an unsightly scar.

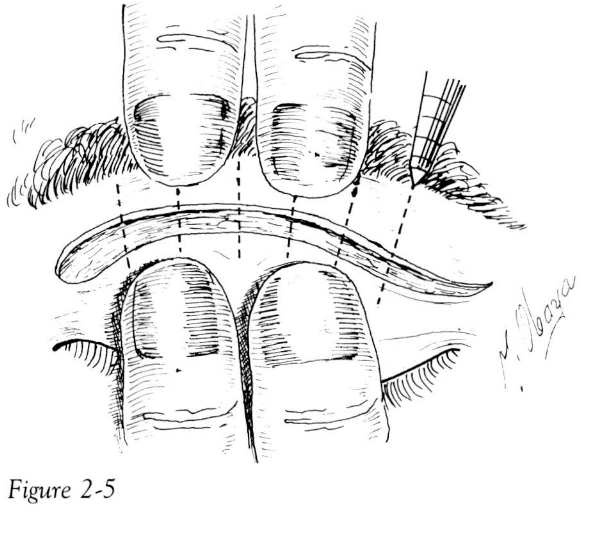

Figure 2-5

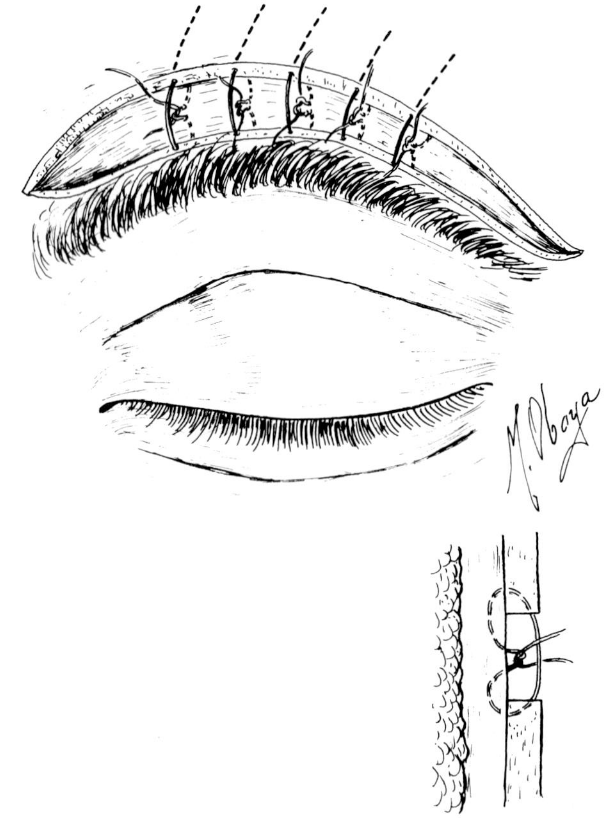

Figure 2-6

The deep eyebrow tissues should be closed with interrupted buried 4-0 nylon sutures (Figure 2-6). The sutures engage the deep subcutaneous tissues and the frontalis muscle with each bite (see inset to Figure 2-6). The periosteum should not be included in the sutures. The marking lines identify the location for each suture bite.

Once all the deep nylon sutures have been tied, there should be no gaping of the wound edges. Otherwise, a scar of corresponding width will remain. The subcutaneous tissue is closed with interrupted 5-0 polyglactin (Vicryl) buried sutures where they are required, and the skin is closed with interrupted 6-0 silk sutures (Figure 2-7). A properly closed wound should appear as if the skin sutures are not required. The skin sutures are removed in 3–4 days.

Modifications

Brow ptosis can be corrected by various other surgical techniques. Temporal brow lifts and midforehead and coronal brow lifts are discussed in Chapter 4.

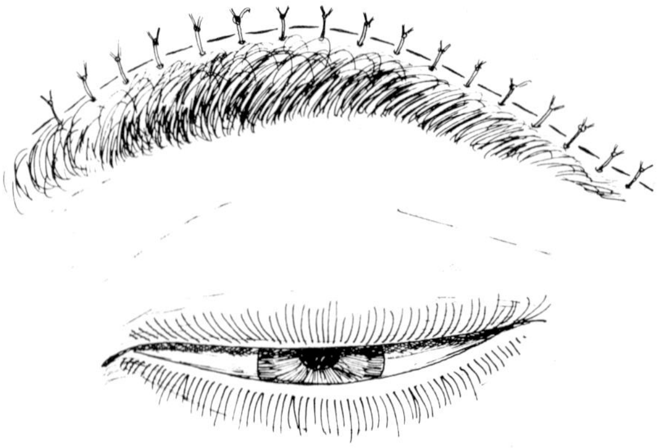

Figure 2-7

Marking the Skin

Marking the area of skin to be excised in the upper eyelid blepharoplasty should be done prior to injection of anesthetic. This will prevent distortion of the anatomy of the eyelids. The patient, under local anesthesia, is asked to move his or her eyes from downgaze to upgaze. The eyelid crease is marked (gentian violet or brilliant green on applicator sticks or fine-tipped marking pen) and individual ink dots are extended laterally and medially and united (Figure 2-8). It is rarely necessary to extend the incision beyond the lateral orbital rim; never beyond the medially located nasocanthal depression.

The center of the lower incision is generally 10 mm from the eyelid margin (Figure 2-9). In women, a higher lid crease (i.e., 11–12 mm) is preferable. In men, the lid crease should be 8–10 mm from the lashes. To avoid canthal webbing, the medial end of the line should be brought no closer than 4–5 mm from the upper punctum. Laterally, the line should be kept 5–6 mm above the lateral canthus to avoid webbing. A caliper is invaluable for careful marking and comparison of the eyelid markings for symmetry.

With the use of fine-toothed forceps, the redundant skin is pinched up and the upper skin incision carefully marked (Figure 2-10). The eyelid should remain just closed or open 1 mm when the upper and lower lines are apposed. It should be remembered that an additional millimeter of skin will be included in both the upper and lower incision marks, thereby excising an additional 2 mm, when the skin edges are sutured together.

Redundant skin in the medial canthus does not *all* have to be removed (Figure 2-11). The concave shape of the skin overlying the protruding fat pockets will become concave following fat removal. Removal of too much skin will cause the skin to tent over the debulked fat pockets in the medial canthus and lead to webbing. In addition, if the surgeon anticipates medial canthal webbing, the lines can be shifted upward, as shown by the dotted line, to prevent webbing.

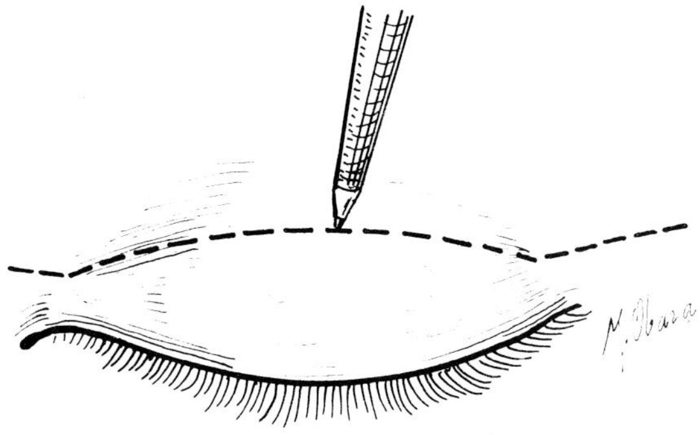

Figure 2-8

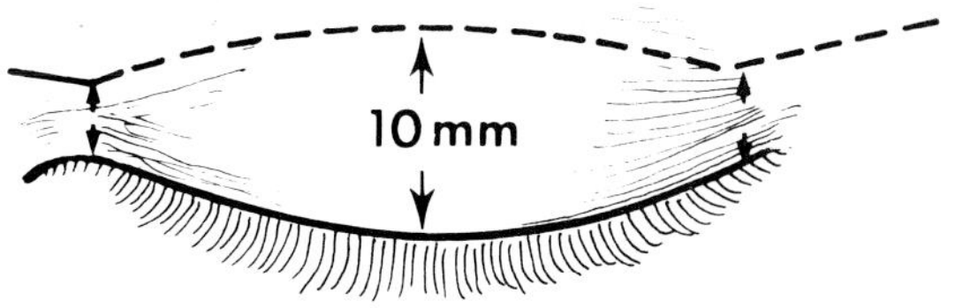

Figure 2-9

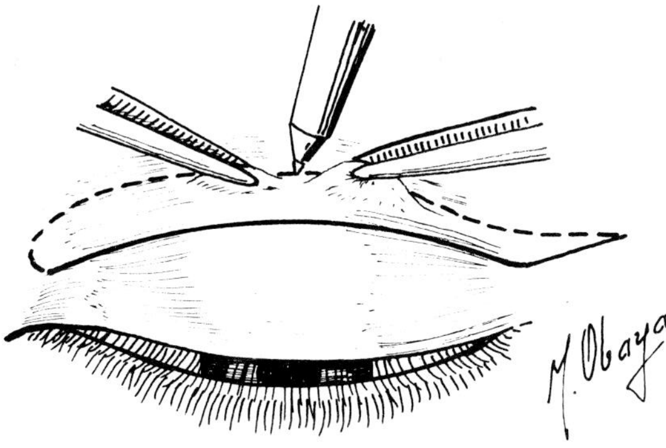

Figure 2-10

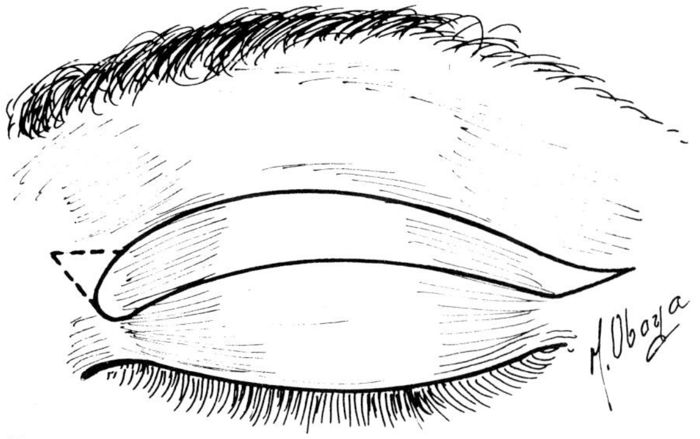

Figure 2-11

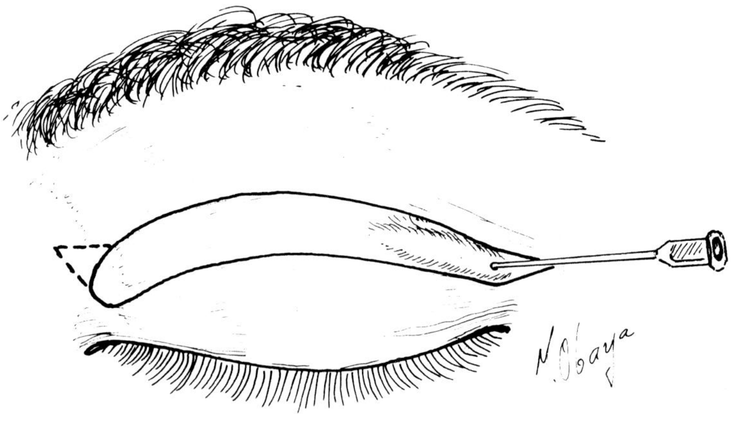

Figure 2-12

Anesthesia

Blepharoplasty surgery is most commonly performed under local anesthesia (injection point shown in Figure 2-12). The patient's awake state allows the surgeon the benefit of taking into consideration the patient's facial animation and dynamic facial appearance. A 27- or 30-gauge needle is used to inject Xylocaine with 1 : 100,000 epinephrine just beneath the skin. Deep injections will cause orbicularis muscle hematomas. The skin is ballooned up and away from the underlying orbicularis muscle using approximately 1.0–1.5 ml per lid. In longer cases (e.g., four-lid blepharoplasty), a longer-acting anesthetic such as bupivacaine 0.75% plain is mixed half and half with the Xylocaine. The anesthetic is massaged for several minutes to allow its spread through the eyelid.

Skin Excision

With the lid tissue on tension, the skin incisions are carefully made along the markings (Figure 2-13). The lower line is incised first to keep the field of view free of blood.

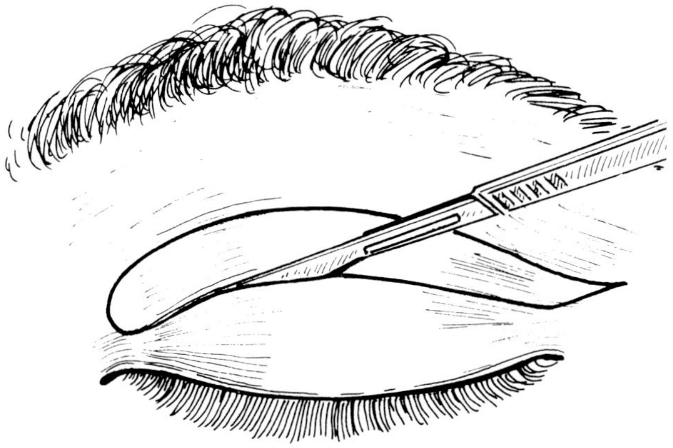

Figure 2-13

The skin is dissected away from the underlying orbicularis muscle (Figure 2-14). Starting laterally, the surgeon uses fine-toothed forceps and a sharp scissor to begin the excision. This prevents traumatizing the lateral edge of the wound. After developing a plane between the skin and orbicularis muscle, the instruments are replaced with larger-toothed forceps and curved blunt scissors. The surgeon first undermines and then cuts along the previously outlined wound edge.

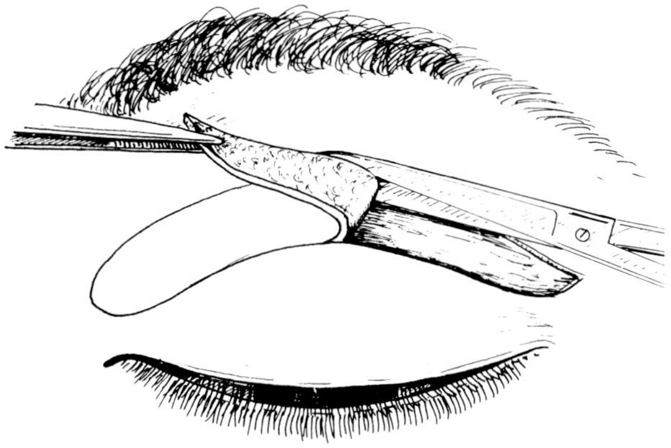

Figure 2-14

To assist with hemostasis, a neurosurgical pattie soaked in local anesthetic with epinephrine is placed on the exposed orbicularis muscle bed (Figure 2-15). The opposite eyelid skin is excised at this time.

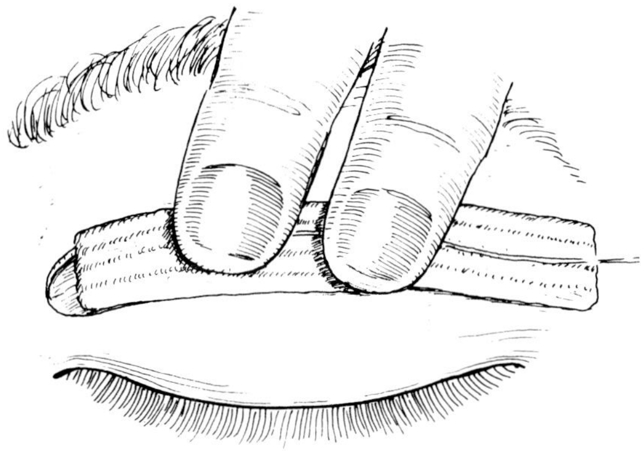

Figure 2-15

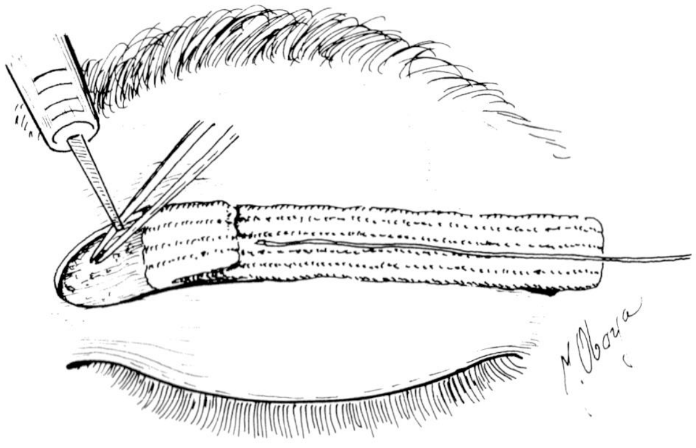

Figure 2-16

With the bovie cautery set *very low,* small bleeding vessels are picked up with a fine-toothed forceps and coagulated (Figure 2-16). A cutting bovie is never used for this fine-tissue dissection. Careful and minimal cauterization will reduce postoperative inflammation.

Fat Excision

Before starting the operation, the surgeon should have a clear mental picture of where excessive fat pockets lie when the patient is seated or standing. Color photoprints taken in the office are of immense assistance in gauging fat excision at the time of surgery. Some surgeons have their patients lie down in the office to compare the appearance of the herniated orbital fat pockets in both erect and supine positions. Digital pressure should be applied to the globe to cause the medial fat pocket to bulge forward (Figure 2-17). The points of a sharp scissor are directed superonasally, and when opened, they spread the orbicularis fibers and tear open the orbital septum. The underlying fat will protrude through the buttonhole opening. The applied pressure keeps the scissor tips away from the underlying levator muscle and superior oblique tendon. The scissor should *never* be blindly plunged deep into the orbit.

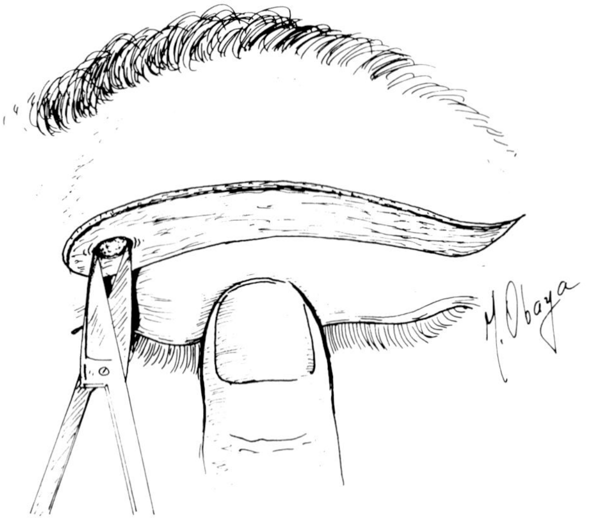

Figure 2-17

Digital pressure is released, and a plane between the orbital septum and orbital fat is cut by lifting both edges of the orbicularis muscle and orbital septum and horizontally opening the entire septum (Figure 2-18). This gives the surgeon an open-sky view of the orbital fat and orbital contents. The edges of the orbicularis muscle and orbital septum will bleed vigorously, and a moment should now be taken to coagulate any bleeding vessels.

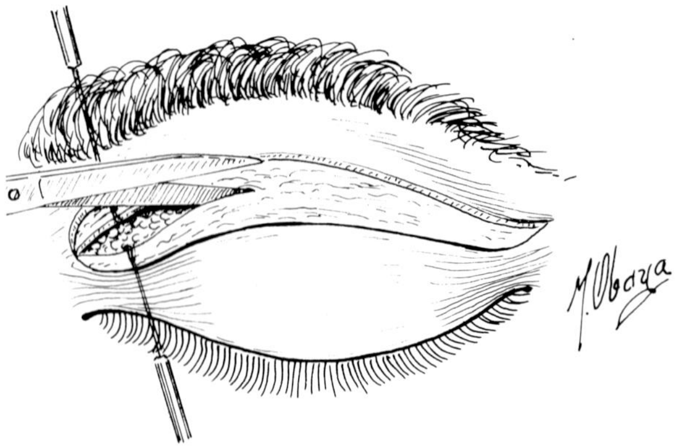

Figure 2-18

Once the orbital fat is exposed, pressure is reapplied to the globe via the lids and the fat lobules are dissected from their membranous capsule (Figure 2-19). The medial fat pocket has a characteristic white appearance, unlike the more yellow central fat pocket.

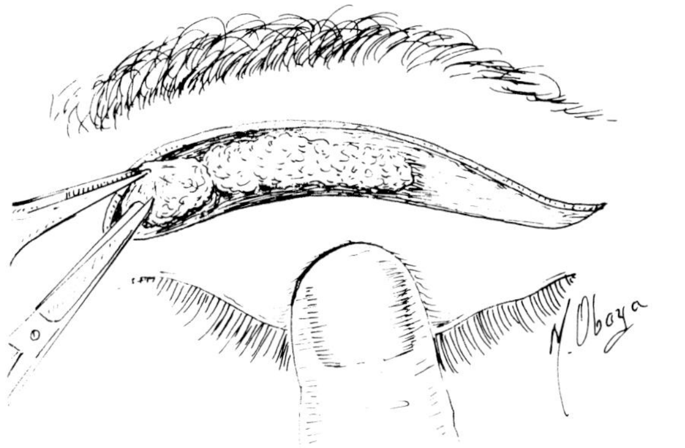

Figure 2-19

The herniated orbital fat is clamped with a hemostat. The surgeon should not tug on the fat, but rather clamp the base of the fat that protrudes from between the edges of the opened orbital septum when there is pressure on the globe (Figure 2-20). The clamped fat is excised with a scalpel (No. 15 blade). The assistant should hold the hemostat in a stable position without pulling on the orbital fat.

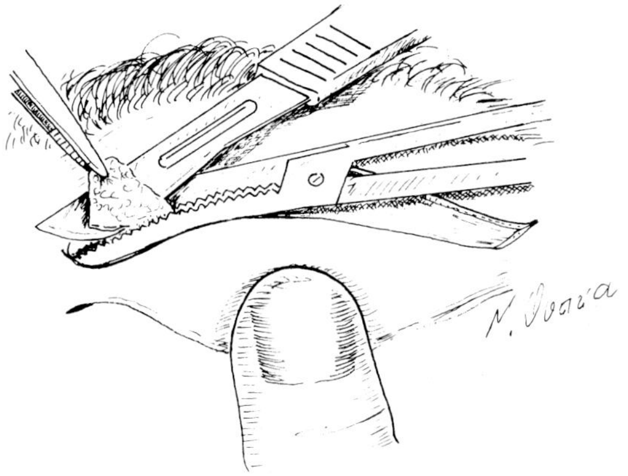

Figure 2-20

The stump of fat that remains in the hemostat is cauterized (Figure 2-21). The patient is warned not to move for a moment and that some pain may be experienced. The bovie should not be set too high to prevent conduction of the electric current to the posterior orbital contents and risk optic nerve damage.

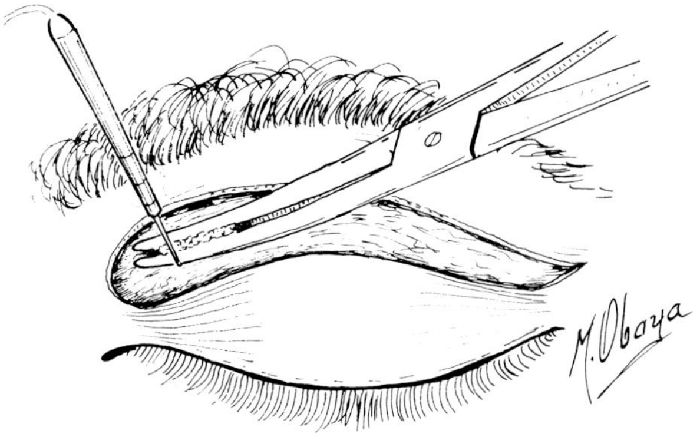

Figure 2-21

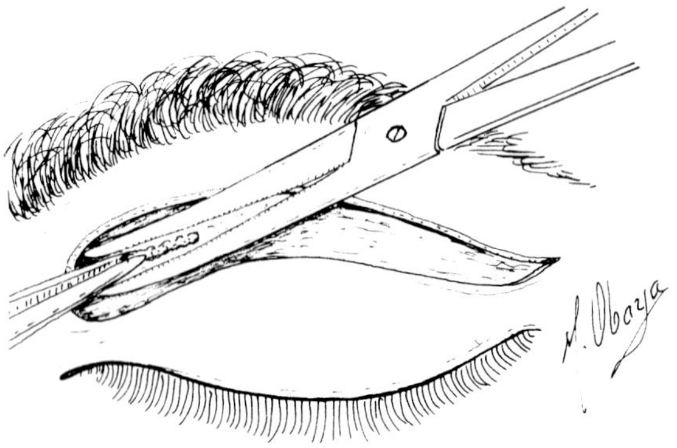

Figure 2-22

Before the hemostat is opened and the orbital fat released, the stump of fat is grasped with a forceps (Figure 2-22). The hemostat is now opened and the fat examined for any residual bleeders. This step will prevent the fat from retracting back into the orbit where it is more difficult to find a bleeding vessel.

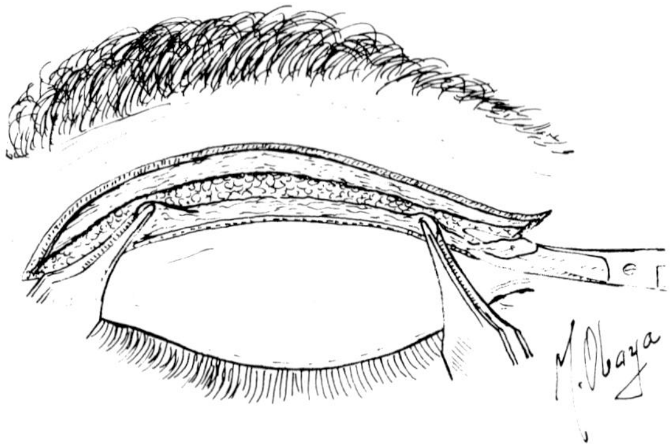

Figure 2-23

Excision of a flap of orbicularis muscle and orbital septum from the distal wound edge may enhance the supratarsal sulcus (Figure 2-23). Again, any bleeding vessels should be carefully cauterized from the edge of the wound.

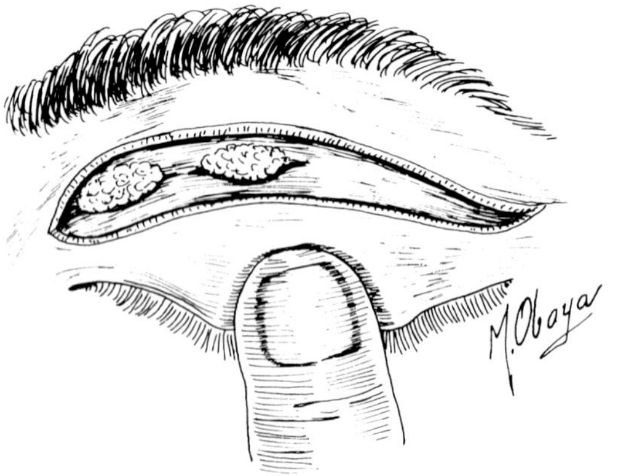

Figure 2-24

An alternative to an open-sky excision of orbital fat is to open two small buttonholes in the orbital septum (Figure 2-24). Pressure on the globe will permit prolapse of fat through the holes, and the fat can be excised. The major disadvantage to this simpler method is the poor visibility the surgeon is provided for observing retroseptal bleeding. Nonetheless, the patient with only a small amount of excessive fat may benefit from this approach.

Closure

Supratarsal fixation is commonly used when a feminine, high supratarsal sulcus is desired (Figure 2-25). This provides a large surface area of exposed eyelid for application of cosmetics.

Three interrupted sutures are placed through the skin and the supratarsal tissues of the levator aponeurosis. One suture is placed in the center of the eyelid, one at the junction of the medial and middle one-third of the lid, and one at the junction of the lateral and middle one-third of the lid. All three sutures should be placed prior to tying to improve visibility.

Another method for obtaining a deep lid crease and supratarsal fixation, illustrated here (Figure 2-26) and in Figure 2-23, is excision of a strip of orbicularis muscle. This leaves a raw surface for adhesion of the skin to the edge of the orbicularis muscle and underlying levator aponeurosis. Supratarsal fixation and orbicularis muscle resection can be used separately or combined. If a deep lid crease is not desired, which is the case particularly in men, then only the skin is closed. There is no reason ever to suture the orbital septum. Suturing the orbital septum, either intentionally or inadvertently by including it in skin sutures, will result in the patient's inability to close their eyelids. To close the skin, an interrupted suture (6-0 silk) is placed at the lateral end of the wound. A hemostat is attached to this lateral suture. This maneuver will straighten and appose the wound edges (see Figure 2-25).

The skin edges must be carefully closed, as shown in Figure 2-27. Some surgeons prefer interrupted 6-0 silk sutures, although a subcuticular running monofilament suture gives fine results. Do not use absorbable sutures on the eyelid skin. Antibiotic ointment and a piece of gauze are placed on the lids. No adhesive dressing should be used. Some surgeons use ice packs for the first 48 hours to reduce postoperative edema.

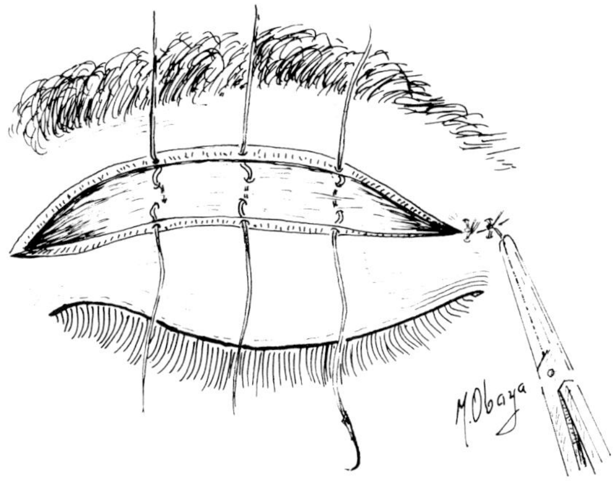

Figure 2-25

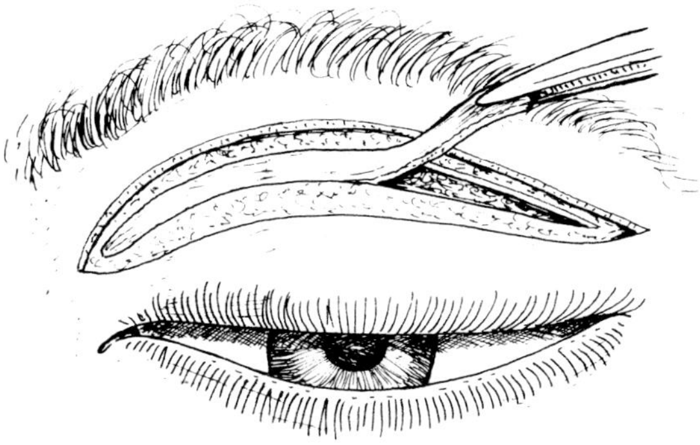

Figure 2-26

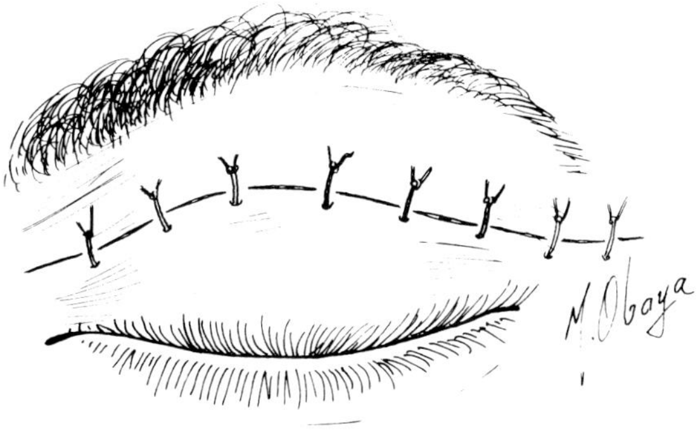

Figure 2-27

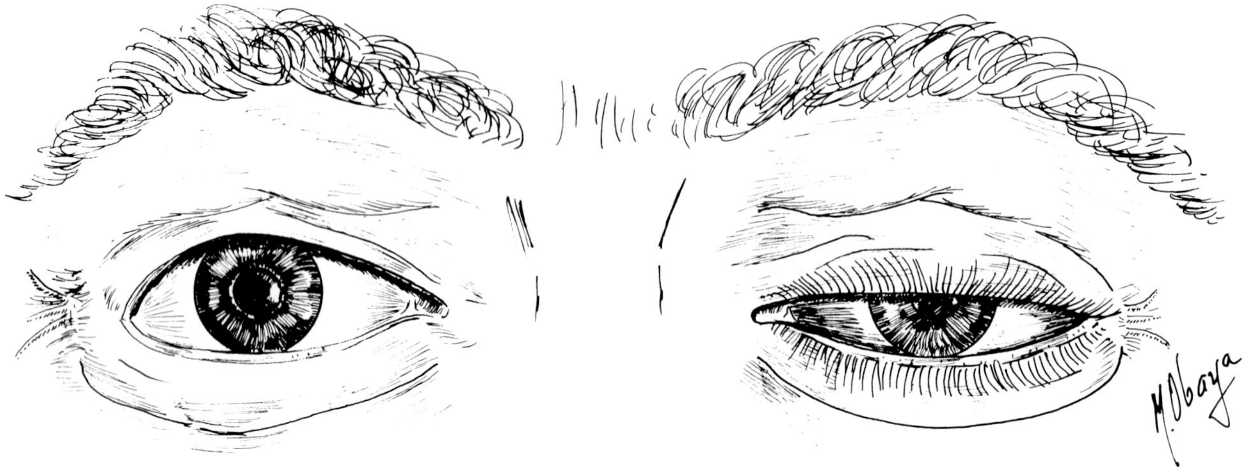

Figure 2-28

EYELID PTOSIS

An appropriate evaluation of a candidate for blepharoplasty surgery requires a careful examination of the eyelids and adjacent adnexa. We have already seen the importance of recognizing and managing brow ptosis. Eyelid ptosis, different problem, needs to be recognized and is illustrated in Figure 2-28.

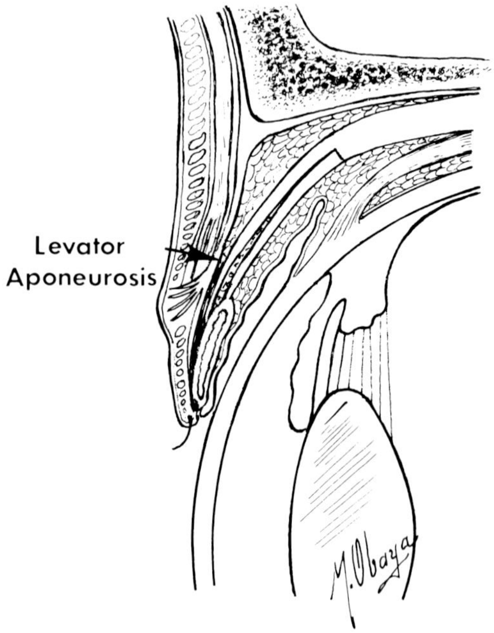

Figure 2-29

As shown in Figure 2-29; the normal levator aponeurosis attaches onto the anterior tarsal plate with fibers transmitted to the eyelid at the lid crease.

A levator dehiscence or disinsertion appears as a thinning or frank separation of the aponeurosis from the tarsus (Figure 2-30). This is the most common cause of upper eyelid ptosis.

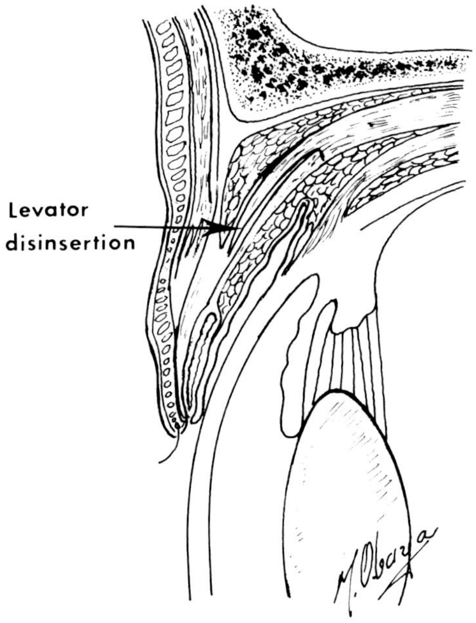

Figure 2-30

The correction of a levator aponeurosis defect can be done at the same time as an upper eyelid blepharoplasty (Figure 2-31). Once the entire orbital septum has been opened, the orbital fat is retracted upward. Normally, the next plane encountered is a white, glistening levator aponeurosis (Figure 2-31).

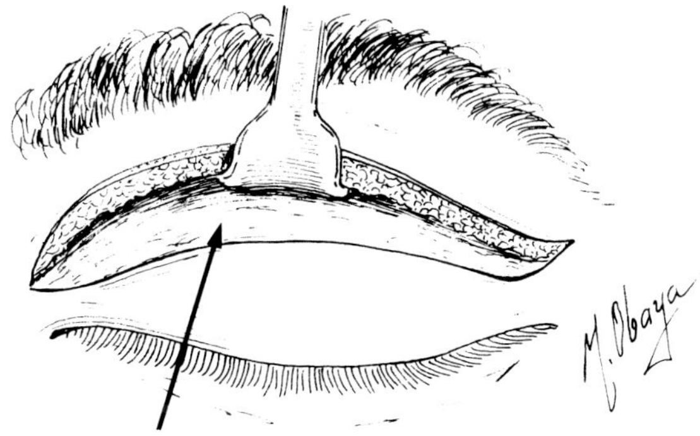

Figure 2-31

The edge of a disinserted levator aponeurosis will appear as a white horizontal margin of tissue superior to and separated from the tarsus (Figure 2-32).

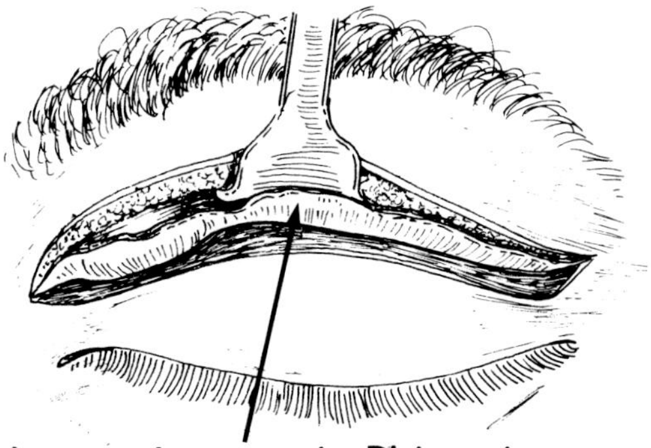

Figure 2-32

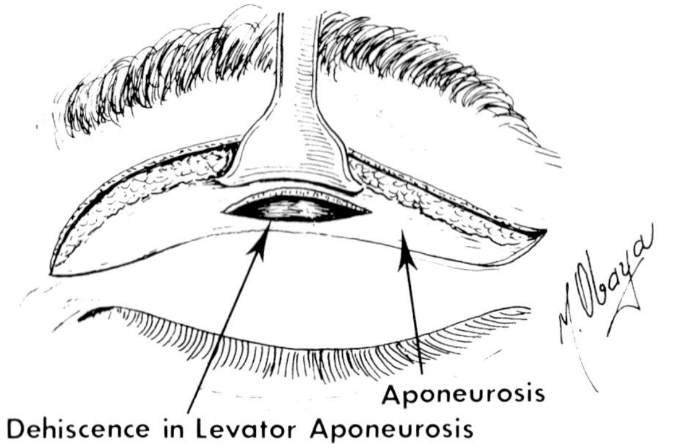

Figure 2-33

A dehiscence in the levator aponeurosis will appear as ragged openings in the white tissue as seen in Figure 2-33.

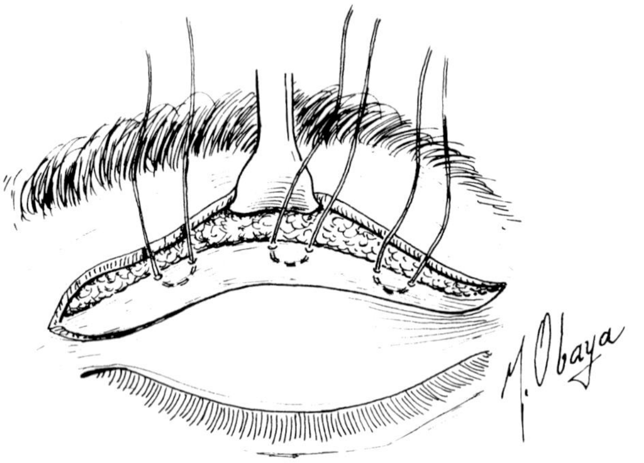

Figure 2-34

Once the levator aponeurosis has been properly identified (i.e., the aponeurosis should move up and down in unison with the patient's eyelid moving up and down), three interrupted nonabsorbable, double-armed sutures are placed 2 mm below the superior edge of the tarsus on the anterior tarsal surface and through the edge of the levator aponeurosis (Figure 2-34). This surgery is preferably done under local anesthesia to permit accurate adjustment of the lid height and curvature.

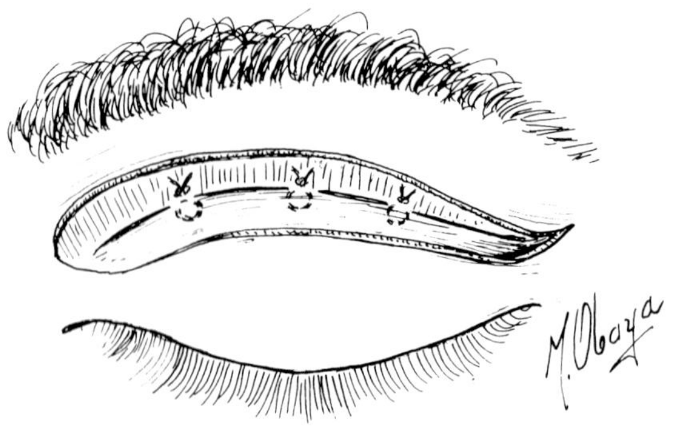

Figure 2-35

When the proper height and lid curvature have been obtained, the sutures reattaching the levator aponeurosis to the tarsus are tied (Figure 2-35). Excessive orbital fat can be excised from the same wound.

The closure should be with three 6-0 silk sutures for supratarsal fixation to reform a lid crease (Figure 2-36). The skin closure is of the surgeon's preference.

Ptosis as a Complication of Blepharoplasty

When ptosis is first recognized *following* surgery, it can be corrected as previously described (Figures 2-20–2-25). Another excellent method of correcting mild, acquired ptosis is a block resection of tarsoconjunctiva-Mueller's muscle (i.e., per Fasanella and Servat).[3] A width of 3.0–3.5 mm is marked at the superior tarsus with a caliper (Figure 2-37A). Two small curved hemostats clamp the block of tissue (Figure 2-37B). To avoid post operative lid notching, the ends of the hemostats must curve toward the superior tarsal edge. Also, the skin must not be included in the clamped tissues. A 5-0 plain suture is knotted at one end. The suture is passed through the skin, run in a serpentine fashion along the convex edge of the hemostats, and brought out onto the skin nasally (Figure 2-37B).

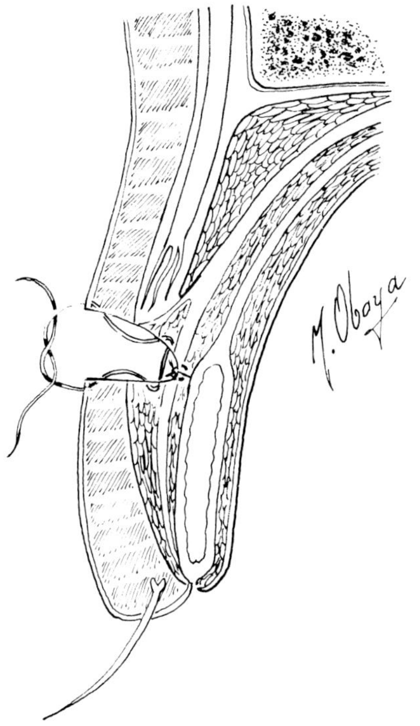

Figure 2-36

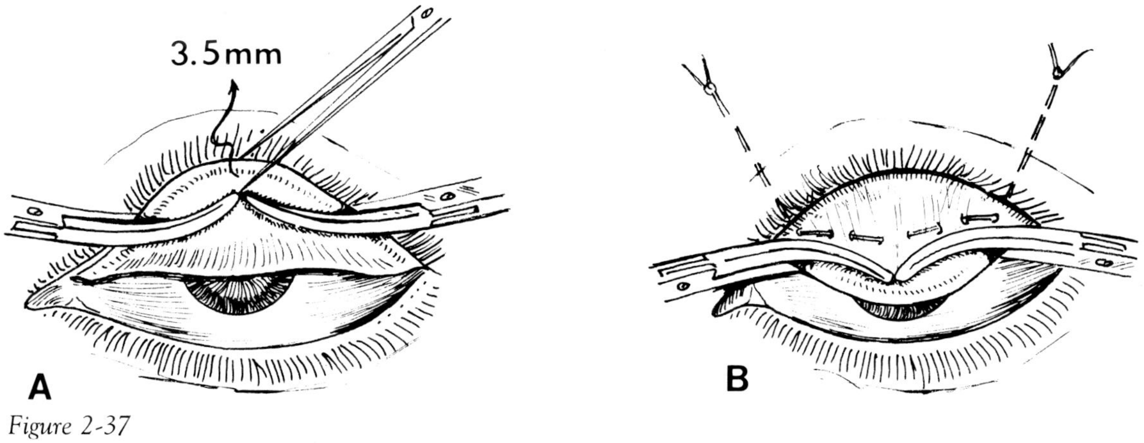

Figure 2-37

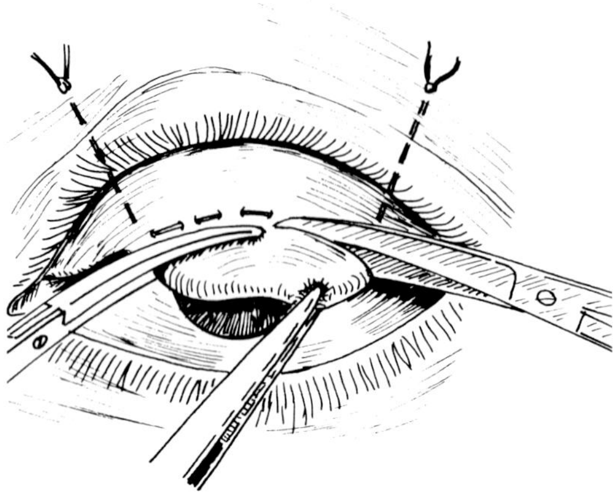

Figure 2-38

The clamps are released and the block of tissue excised (Figure 2-38). Care must be taken not to cut the suture.

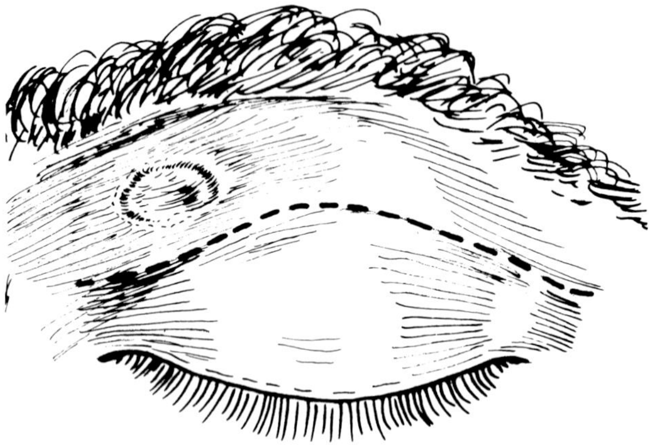

Figure 2-39

CORRECTION OF OVEREXCISION OF ORBITAL FAT

Excessive excision of orbital fat will result in a depression of the overlying skin and a poor cosmetic result (Figure 2-39). The best way to avoid this complication is to carefully gauge the amount of orbital fat removed during a blepharoplasty. In a case of overexcision of fat, a surgical correction can be attempted by filling in the defect with adjacent orbicularis muscle.

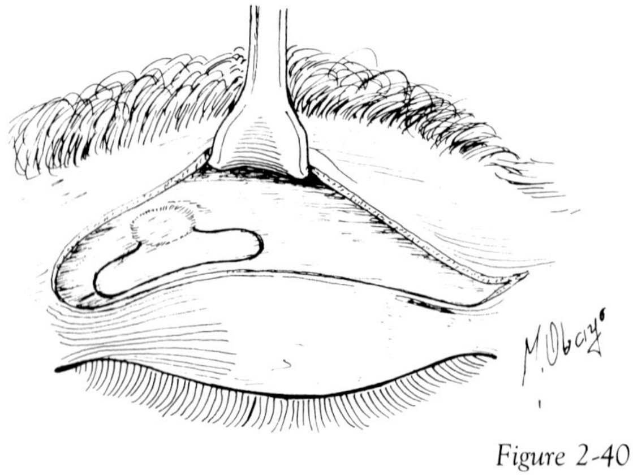

Figure 2-40

The two flaps of orbicularis muscle are fashioned and placed into the defect as shown in Figure 2-40.

The two flaps of orbicularis muscle are then crossed and fixated with absorbable sutures (Figure 2-41).

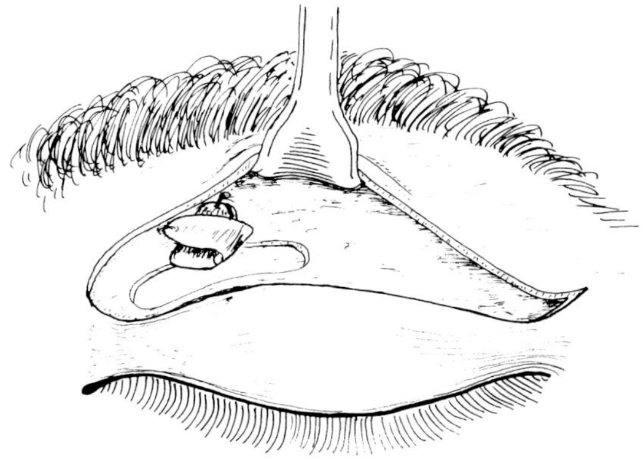

Figure 2-41

CORRECTION OF EXCESS UPPER LID SKIN EXCISION

Lagophthalmos (inability to close one's eye) following an upper-lid blepharoplasty may cause corneal irritation and even ulceration due to chronic drying of the inferior cornea. This may be due to excision of too much upper lid skin during the blepharoplasty or to incarceration of the orbital septum in the wound closure.

Correction of lagophthalmos secondary to excision of too much skin during a blepharoplasty requires replacement of the skin. A standard skin incision is marked at the lid crease (Figure 2-42).

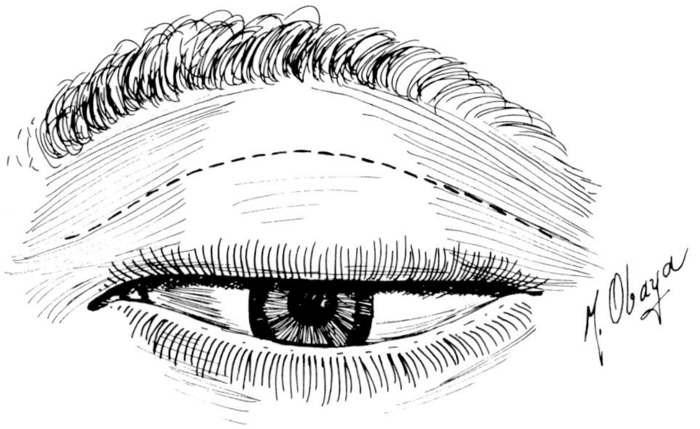

Figure 2-42

The skin is undermined from the underlying orbicularis muscle until the upper lid is easily pulled shut (Figure 2-43). Gentle cautery is used for hemostasis of the orbicularis muscle bed.

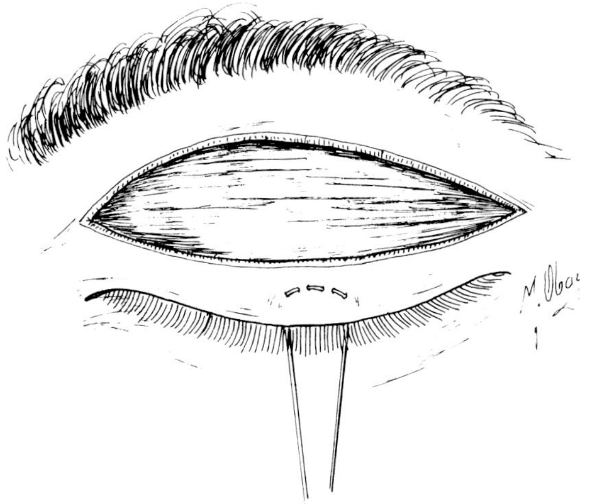

Figure 2-43

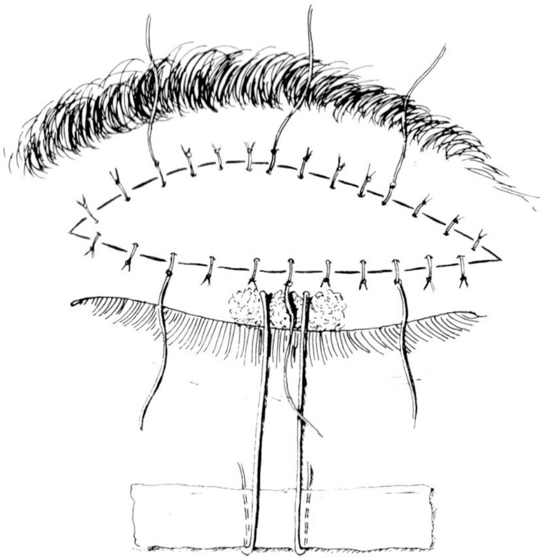

Figure 2-44

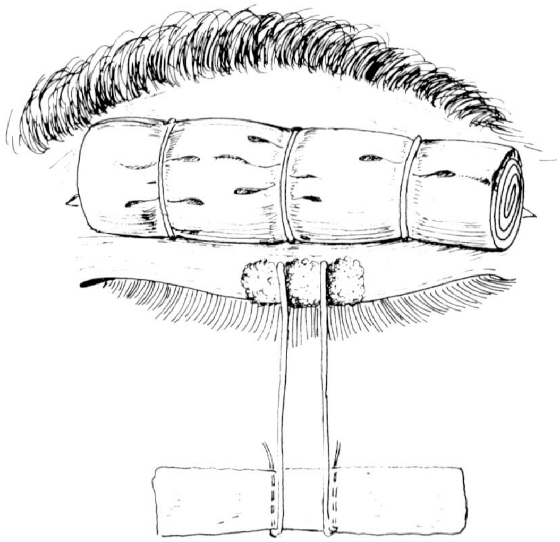

Figure 2-45

A full-thickness skin graft from the opposite upper eyelid is used when available. Otherwise, a retroauricular skin graft is removed. The graft is sutured into place with multiple interrupted 6-0 silk sutures, leaving several ends long to tie over a bolster (Figure 2-44).

A 4-0 silk suture is placed through the lid margin and taped to the cheek for 3–4 days to keep the lid on stretch (Figure 2-45).

LOWER EYELID BLEPHAROPLASTY

A properly performed lower eyelid blepharoplasty can produce a dramatic effect of youth and vigor rather than the sad-eyed, sleepy appearance from droopy lids, large fat pockets, and sagging lax lower eyelids. Lower lid surgery frightens many surgeons because they must contend with intangible variables, including gravity and involutional lid laxity when dealing with lower eyelid surgery. These factors may result in such complications as postoperative ectropion, even though the surgeon considered that the operation had been properly performed.

In order to obtain satisfactory results with minimal complications, the blepharoplasty surgeon's armamentarium must include procedures for fat excision, eyelid laxity repair, and an understanding of skin flaps versus skin-muscle flap procedures. In addition, the surgeon must be capable of managing the possible complications following blepharoplasty.

TECHNIQUE

Marking the Skin

A series of carefully placed ink dots are drawn 1–2 mm below the lower eyelid lash line (Figure 2-46). The dots are connected and the line extends from the punctum medially to the canthal angle laterally. The line should lie close enough to the lashes to allow the surgical scar to be concealed by the shadow of the lashes. The line should not be made too close to the eyelashes, or the lashes may be incised. In addition, carrying the incision too close to the lid margin risks laceration of the lacrimal canaliculus or laceration and scarring of the lid margin. One can also conceal the lid incision in a natural eyelid fold.

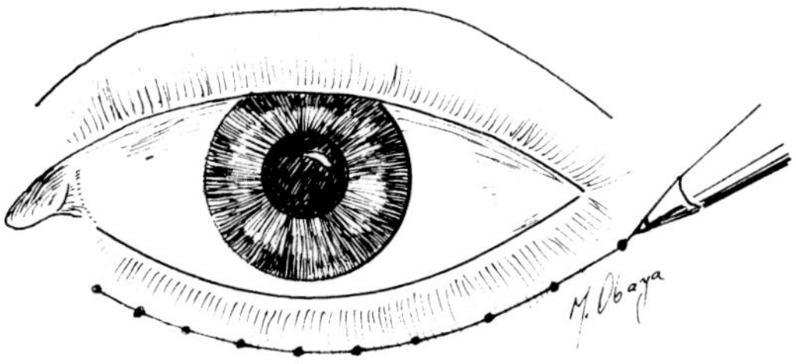
Figure 2-46

If there exists excessive lower eyelid skin which the surgeon intends to remove, a lateral canthal flap is drawn (Figure 2-47). This line can be placed in a crow's-foot in older people. It should form approximately a 30° angle with the lower eyelid and should be a continuation of an imaginary line extending inferiorly from the curve of the upper eyelid. The flap should be approximately 1 cm long and can always be extended later in the operation. The local anesthetic is injected after the lower eyelid is marked.

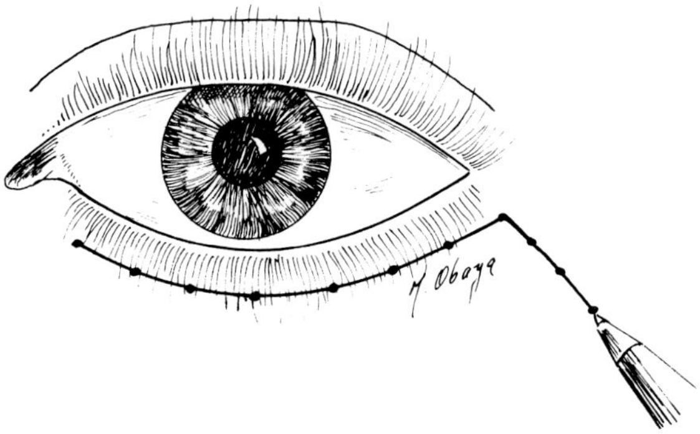
Figure 2-47

Skin Incision

The initial incision in the skin is made along the line drawn for the lateral angle flap (Figure 2-48). A scalpel incision goes just through the skin.

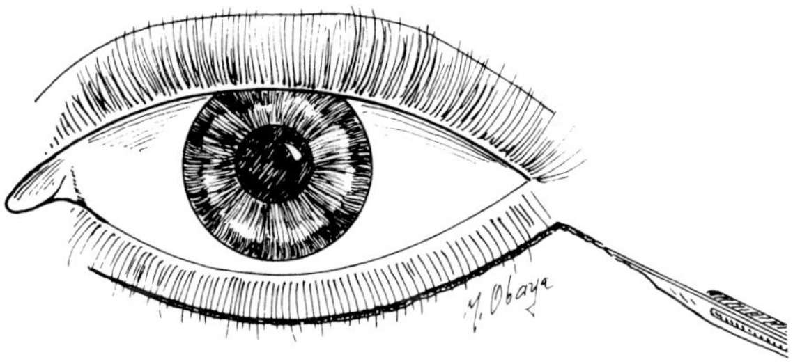
Figure 2-48

Carefully pick up the tissues with a fine-toothed forceps and use scissors to undermine the skin from the underlying orbicularis muscle (Figure 2-49). Then cut along the horizontal line with blunt-tipped scissors, undermining the skin as you progress medially. Try to avoid cutting the eyelashes by having your assistant precede your incision with a moist cotton-tipped applicator and move the lashes out of the way. Eyelashes that are incised and fall in the wound should be removed by copious irrigation with saline or another solution, and attempts should be made to remove the fragments of cut lashes.

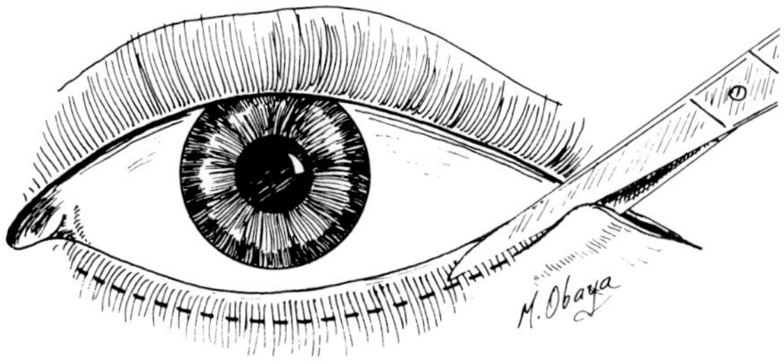
Figure 2-49

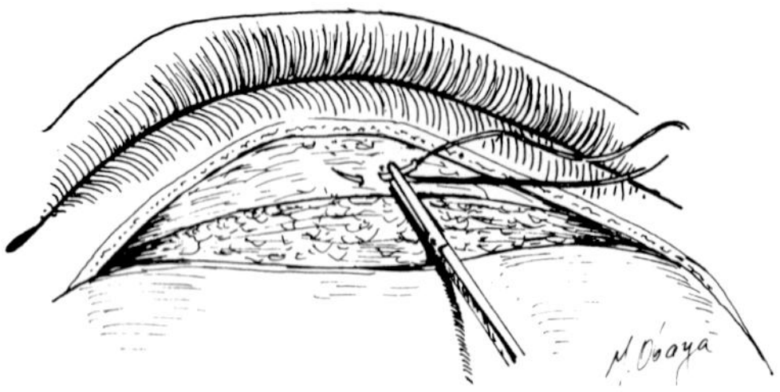

Figure 2-50

A 6-0 silk suture is placed through the orbicularis muscle and tarsus (Figure 2-50).

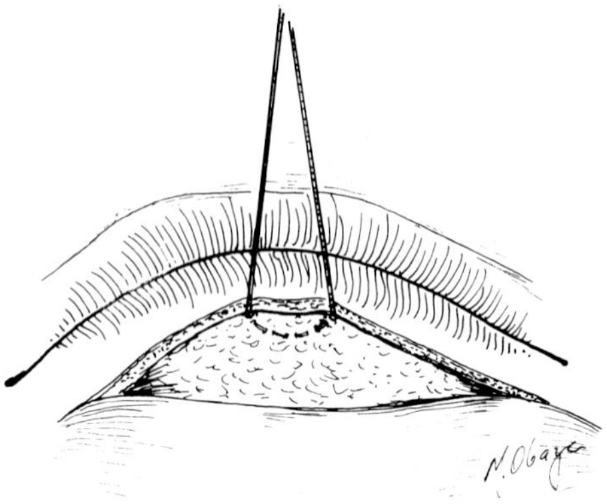

Figure 2-51

The lower eyelid tissues are placed on stretch by clamping the suture to a forehead drape (Figure 2-51).

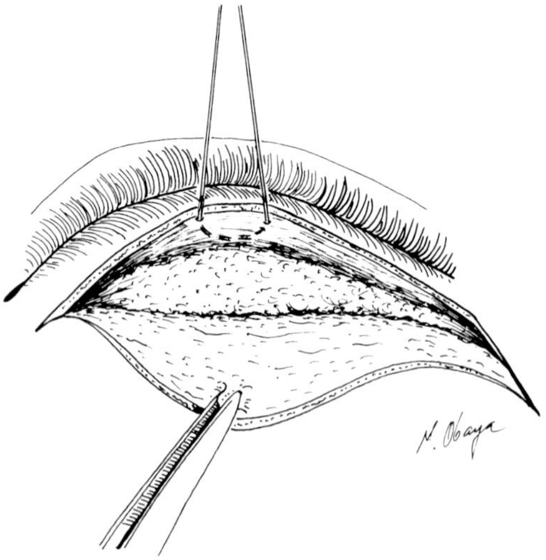

Figure 2-52

This will place the posterior eyelid tissues on stretch and provide a plane for dissection between the skin and underlying structures with good visibility (Figure 2-52).

Carefully dissect the skin away from the orbicularis muscle (Figure 2-53). Hold the eyelid by the deeper tissues (i.e., orbicularis muscle) to avoid tearing the skin with the forceps.

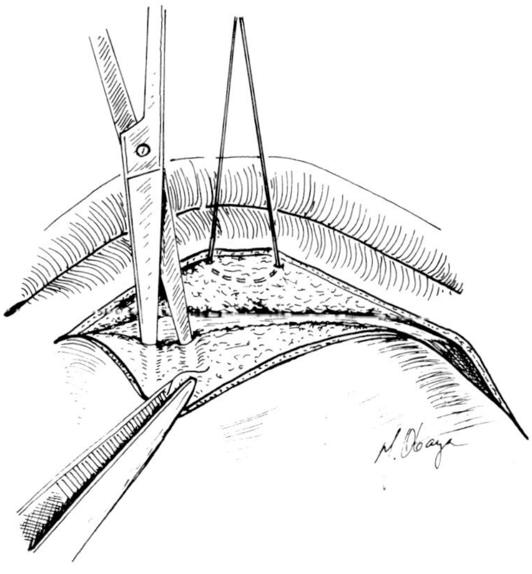

Figure 2-53

An effective method of bluntly dissecting the skin from the orbicularis muscle and deeper orbital septum is to roll a moistened cotton-tipped applicator between the tissues (Figure 2-54). Continue dissecting inferiorly until the edge of the inferior orbital rim is reached. For large festoons of lower eyelid tissue, the dissection can be extended below this point.

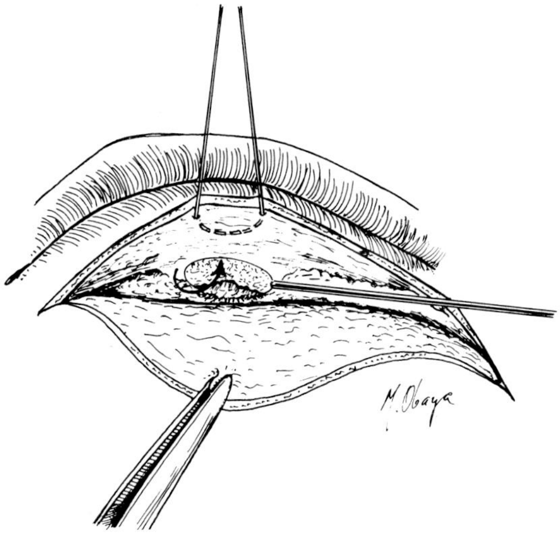

Figure 2-54

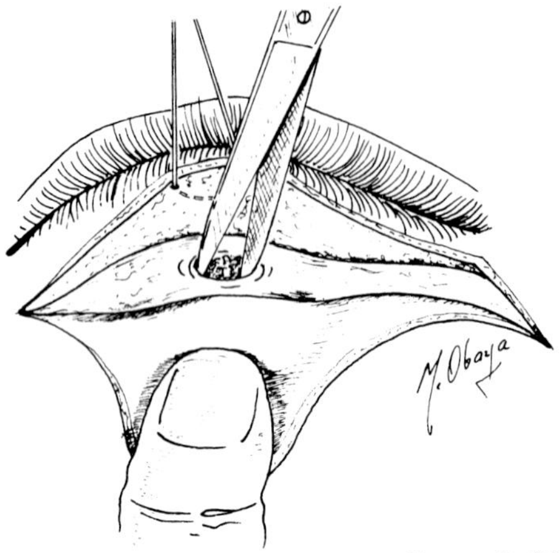

Figure 2-55

Fat Excision

The surgical assistant should place pressure on the globe through the closed eyelids. This will force the orbital contents forward and expose the fat pockets. Place the tips of sharp scissors into the fibers of the orbicularis muscle and open (Figure 2-55). This will spread these horizontally coursing muscle fibers and also tear a buttonhole in the orbital septum, exposing the orbital fat.

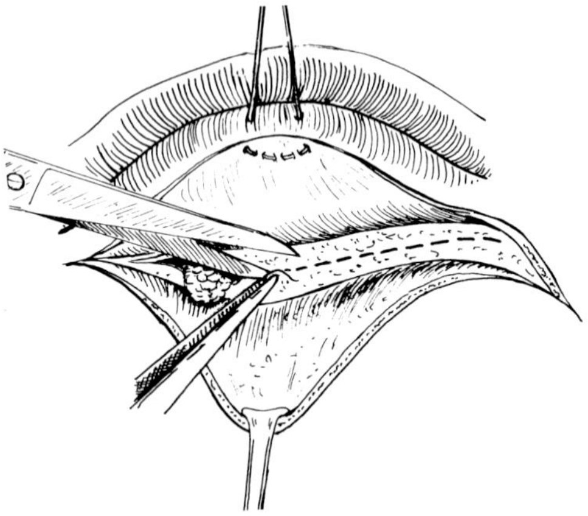

Figure 2-56

Pick up the edge of the buttonholed orbicularis muscle and orbital septum and place one blade of the scissor under the septum (Figure 2-56). No pressure is applied to the globe at this time. Pick the scissors and tissues up and away from the orbit and horizontally open the orbital septum.

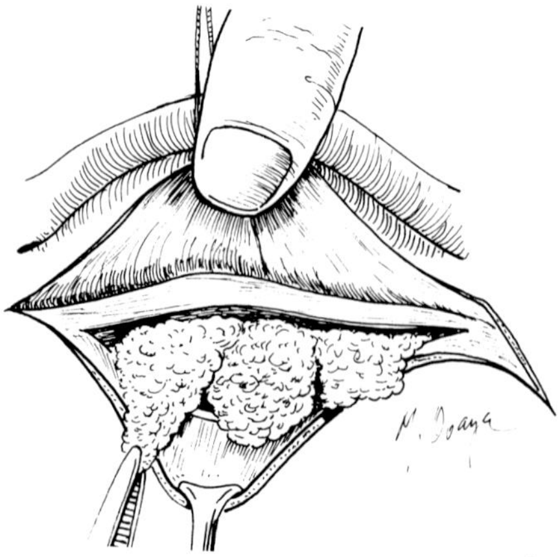

Figure 2-57

Three fat pockets are present in the lower eyelid. The medial fat pocket is separated from the central and lateral fat pockets by the inferior oblique muscle. Carefully dissect the orbital fat from its membranous capsule (Figure 2-57). Avoid tugging on the orbital fat. In order to obtain satisfactory cosmetic results, be certain to note preoperatively whether the patient has extra fat herniation laterally, as this fat pocket is often missed by surgeons. Particular attention should be directed to this lateral fat pocket when indicated.

The assistant applies pressure to the globe. The excess fat that has been dissected free from its membranous capsule is clamped with a hemostat and excised with a scalpel (Figure 2-58). After the fat has been clamped, the assistant should release pressure from the eye to avoid extended periods of elevated intraocular pressure that can reduce blood flow to the eye. Releasing pressure also allows the remaining fat to return to its normal position.

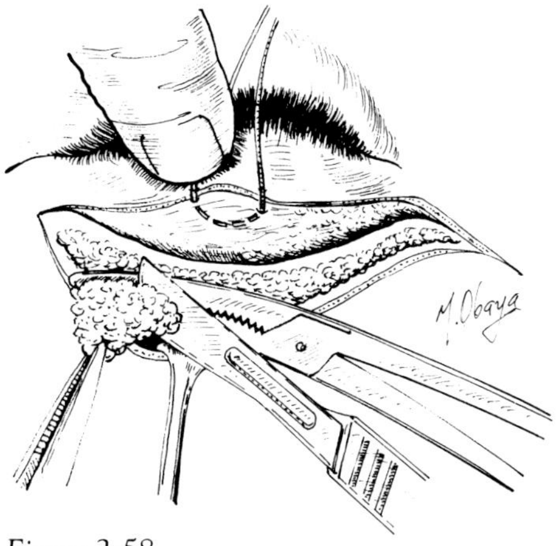

Figure 2-58

The bovie cautery coagulates the stump of fat within the hemostat (Figure 2-59). Be sure that all skin edges are away from the hemostat to avoid accidentally burning the skin.

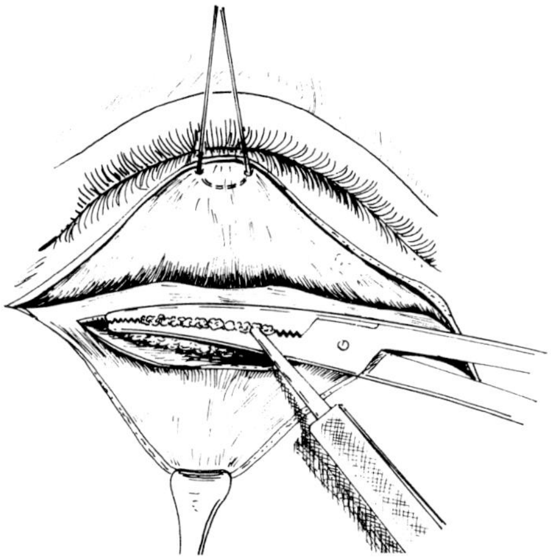

Figure 2-59

The fat is held with forceps as the hemostat releases the cauterized stump (Figure 2-60). If any bleeding persists from the fat pedicle, it should be cauterized. This prevents a bleeding fat stump from retracting into the orbit. When an adequate quantity of fat has been removed, place a neurosurgical cotton pattie soaked in local anesthetic with epinephrine on the field. This will considerably reduce bleeding while operating on the second eye.

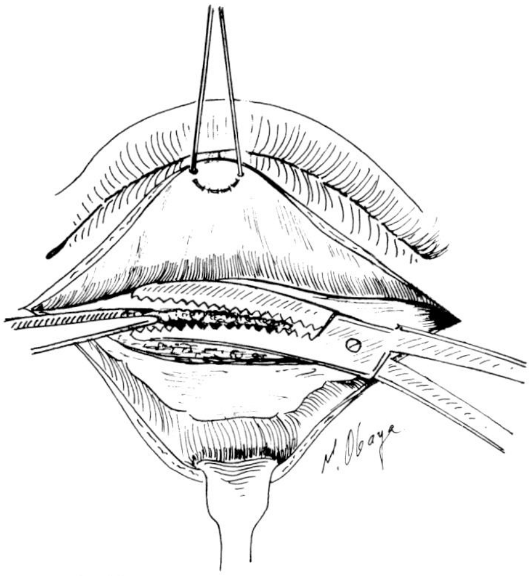

Figure 2-60

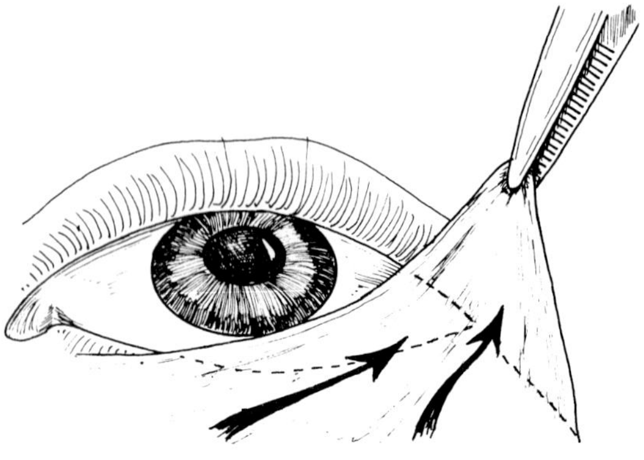

Figure 2-61

Skin Excision

The excess lower eyelid skin is now resected.

The skin flap is draped over the eyelid margin by gentle traction in a superolateral direction (Figure 2-61). The skin can be draped with a wet Q-tip or with forceps. With the patient's mouth open and gaze directed upward toward the 12 o'clock position, maximum stretch is placed on the malar skin; this maneuver helps to prevent excess skin excision and ectropion.

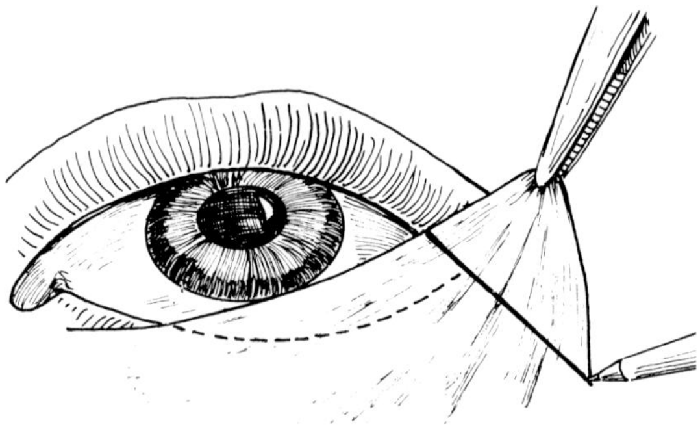

Figure 2-62

A lateral triangle is drawn with its base *up* by marking a line continuous with the upper eyelid margin and connecting it with the end of the lower eyelid skin flap incision (Figure 2-62).

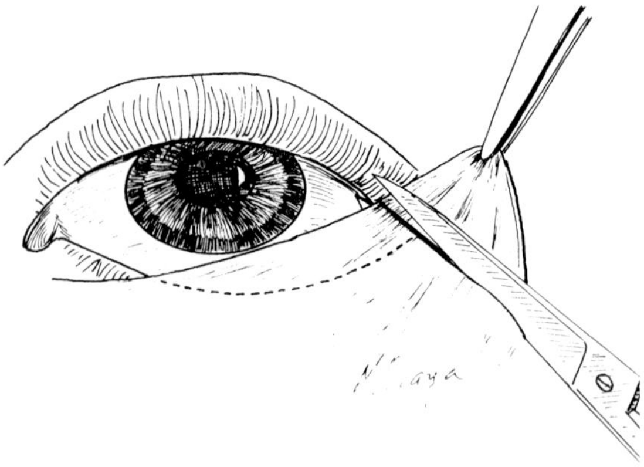

Figure 2-63

The lateral triangle of skin is now cut away with scissors (Figure 2-63).

A second triangle of skin is marked with its base formed by the lateral canthus, with the patient's mouth open and gaze directed upward toward the 12 o'clock position (Figure 2-64).

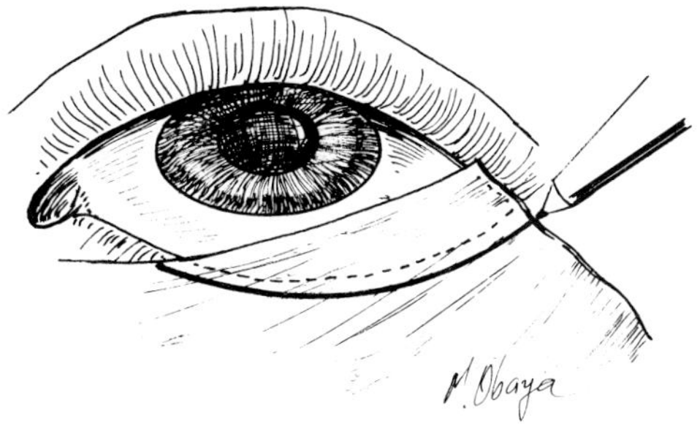

Figure 2-64

A conservative amount of skin is resected along the lid margin (Figure 2-65). Additional skin excision is far easier than correcting for excessive skin resection.

After the skin has been resected, there is often some bleeding from the wound edge, and careful cautery is applied.

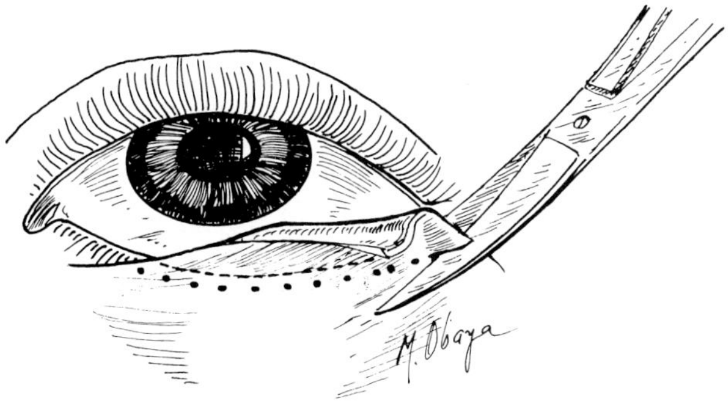

Figure 2-65

The thin skin of the eyelid that has been resected is now replaced by thicker cheek skin. If the skin edges are sutured closed in this state, the wound will heal with lumping and irregular scarring. Therefore, a 1-mm strip of subcutaneous tissue should be excised from the edge of the skin flap to thin the wound edge (Figure 2-66).

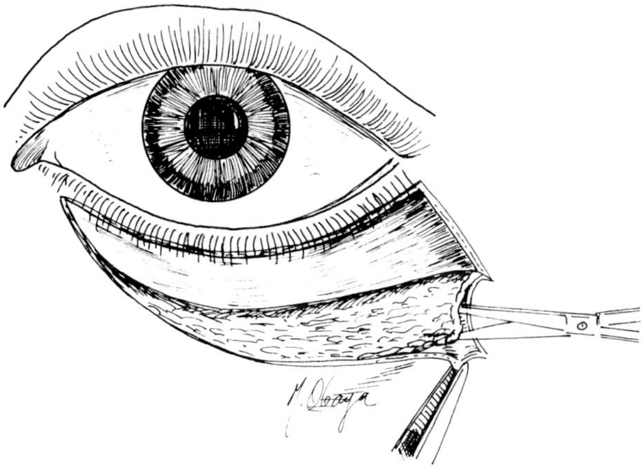

Figure 2-66

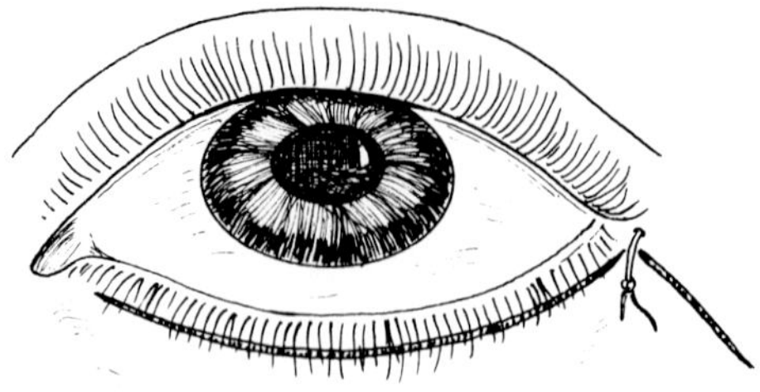

Figure 2-67

If an appropriate amount of skin excision has been done, the edges of the wound should fit together.

The first suture is placed at the lateral canthus (Figure 2-67). This suture aligns the remainder of the wound and should be carefully placed in the proper position. The patient's mouth should again be open and gaze directed upward.

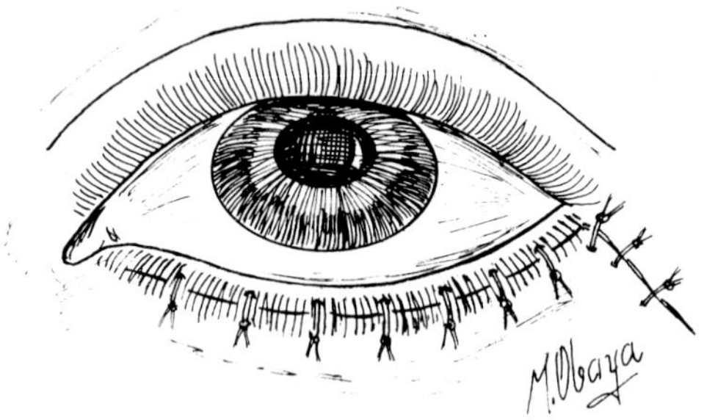

Figure 2-68

When the suture has been placed, the patient can relax and the remainder of the incision is closed with several interrupted sutures (Figure 2-68).

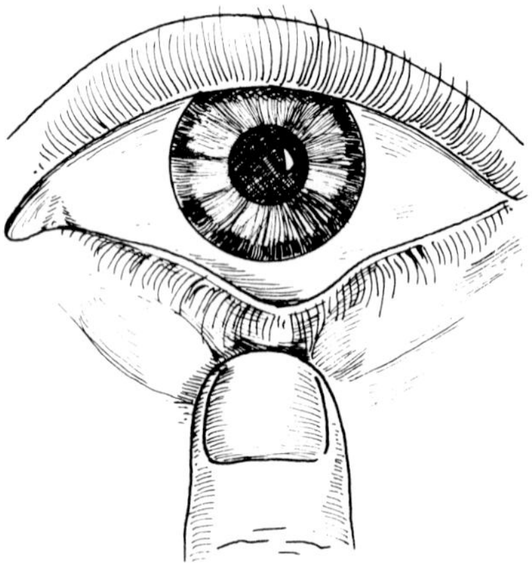

Figure 2-69

EVALUATION OF LOWER EYELID TONE

The lower eyelid should normally rest against the globe (Figure 2-69). The "snapback test" is a simple method of evaluating eyelid tone. If one draws the eyelid away from the globe with an index finger, on releasing the eyelid, it should briskly snap back against the eye.

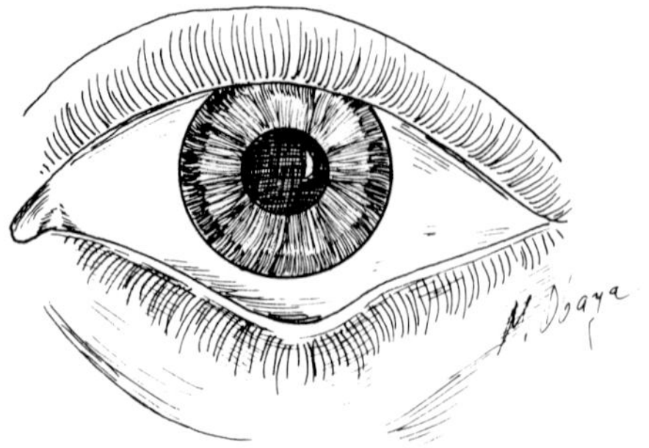

Figure 2-70

If the eyelid is lax, it will remain in a position away from the eye or will very slowly return to the globe (Figure 2-70). The patient should not be permitted to blink when the examiner releases the eyelid or the orbicularis muscle will pull the lid back against the globe. Performing this test on several young patients will give the examiner a good basis of what can be considered normal eyelid tone.

Another simple method of testing lower eyelid tone is performed by pulling the lower lid away from the globe (Figure 2-71). If more than 6 mm is present between the globe and the eyelid, there is lid laxity present, which should be corrected as part of the lower lid blepharoplasty.

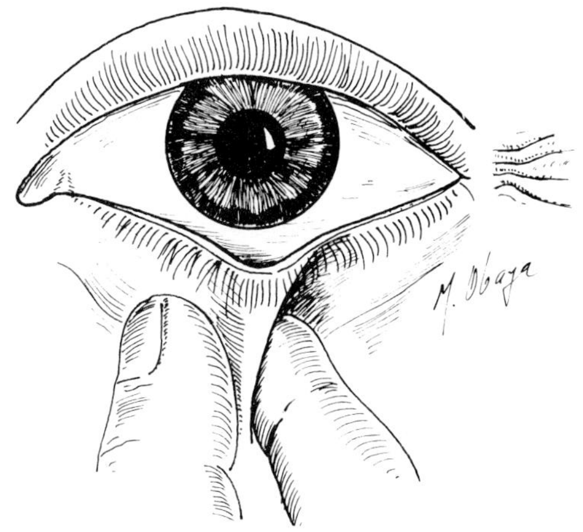

Figure 2-71

LOWER EYELID HORIZONTAL SHORTENING COMBINED WITH BLEPHAROPLASTY

The incision for a lower eyelid blepharoplasty is made in the conventional fashion (Figure 2-72).

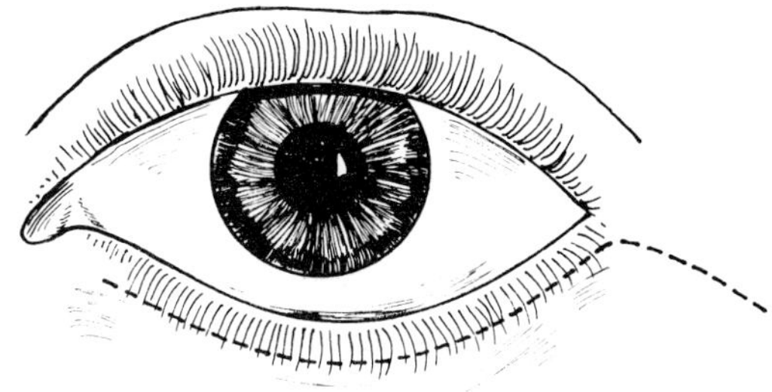

Figure 2-72

As shown in Figure 2-73, prior to horizontally shortening the lower eyelid to correct any eyelid laxity, the skin flap has been completed (see Figures 2-49–2-60) and excess orbital fat removed. The tightening of a horizontally lax eyelid consists of resecting a pentagonal wedge of full-thickness lid margin and reconstructing the eyelid margin. The skin flap is not included in this lid excision. Place one blade of a straight scissors in the inferior fornix, making sure that the blades are perpendicular to the eyelid margin. The eyelid is incised through the entire tarsal plate. The incision is made at the junction of the central one-third and lateral one-third of the eyelid so that the wound is closed at the lateral limbus.

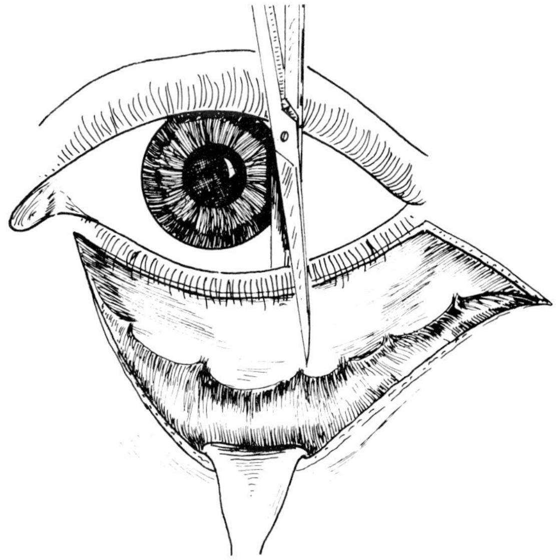

Figure 2-73

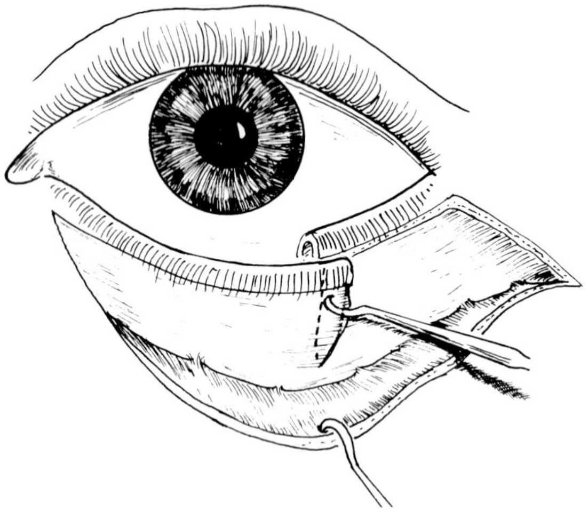

Figure 2-74

A forceps or skin hook is used to overlap the edges of the incised lid margin. This is the amount of excess lid to be resected (Figure 2-74). A second incision is made, again taking care to make the incision perpendicular to the eyelid margin. The two incisions are connected in the lower fornix with two angled incisions. This makes the shape of the defect into an inverted pentagonal wedge. The marginal arteries will bleed and should be carefully coagulated with the bovie cautery. Additional cautery will be necessary to obtain hemostasis of the conjunctiva and orbicularis muscle.

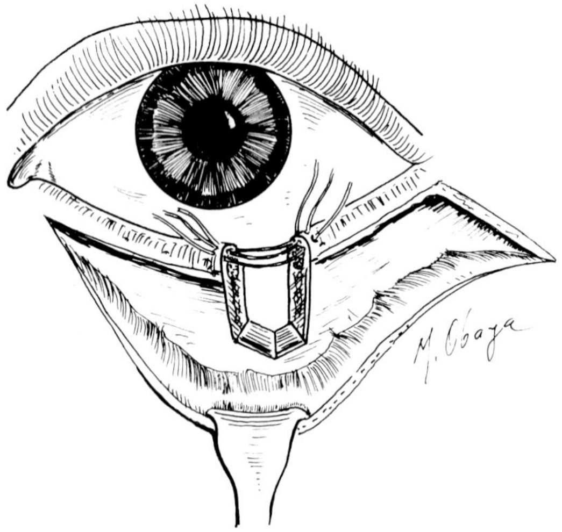

Figure 2-75

The eyelid is reconstructed in a standard fashion.[5] A 6-0 silk suture is placed through the gray-line (i.e., anterior tarsal plate), starting 2 mm from the wound edge, coming out 2 mm below the eyelid margin, and entering in a corresponding position in the opposite eyelid. A second suture is placed at the mucocutaneous junction on the lid margin. A third suture closes the lash line. The ends of the sutures should be left 2 cm long for now so that they can be tied over the anterior eyelid margin (Figure 2-75).

Once the lid margin has been reformed, the tarsal plate is reconstructed. Several interrupted absorbable sutures (5-0 chromic) are used to close the tarsal edges (Figures 2-76).

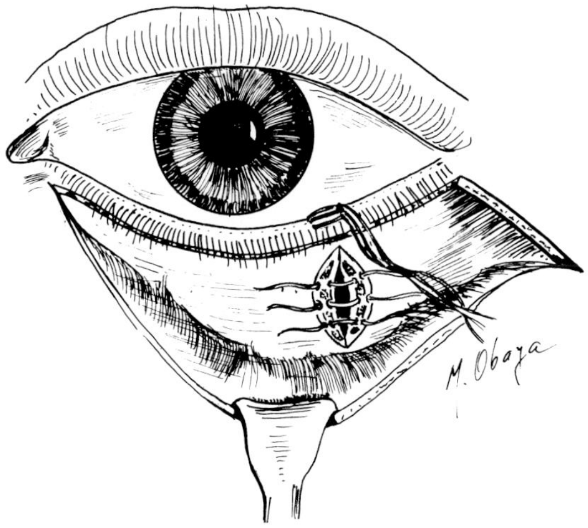

Figure 2-76

A properly reconstructed eyelid margin should have the appearance shown in Figure 2-77. A slight pouting of the edges of the lid margin is acceptable; the edges will flatten as healing progresses.

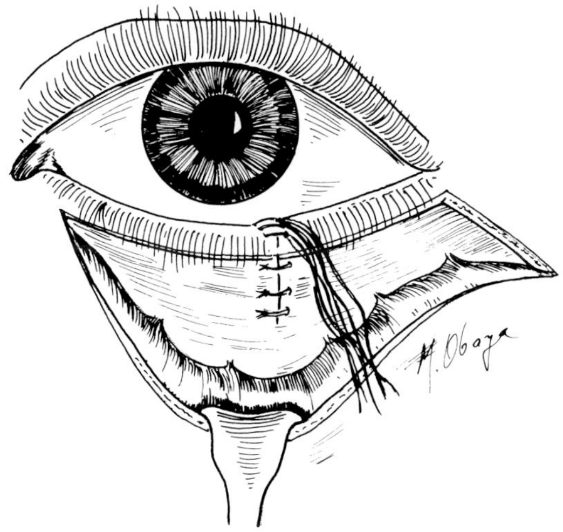

Figure 2-77

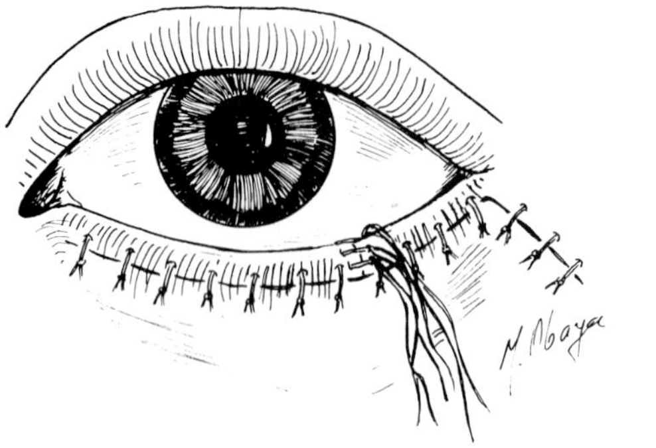

Figure 2-78

The three lid margin sutures are left long (2 cm) and tied under a skin suture (Figure 2-78). The skin excision of the blepharoplasty is completed as described earlier (Figures 2-61–2-68). The lid margin sutures remain for 10–14 days. Incorrect closure of the eyelid margin may result in eyelid notching and chronic corneal irritation.

The Bick procedure for lateral eyelid resection has been used for the correction of involutional entropions and ectropions (Figure 2-79).[2] In order to correct an ectropion due to lower eyelid laxity, a triangle of full-thickness lateral eyelid is resected. This operation can also be performed by resecting a triangle of eyelid tissue behind a blepharoplasty skin flap. A line is drawn at the lateral canthus as a continuation of the curve of the upper lid margin. A hemostat may be applied in this line to clamp the tissues prior to cutting through the lid with scissors. The reduced bleeding from using the hemostat is beneficial, but the crushing effect may damage the lateral lid structures and increase the scarring. The full-thickness eyelid is now cut through with scissors, thereby transecting the lower limb of the lateral canthal tendon. Careful cautery is used to stop the bleeding from the eyelid marginal vessel.

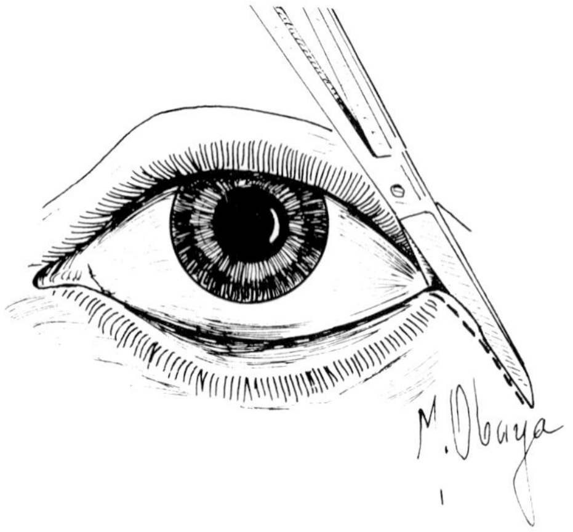

Figure 2-79

The end of the eyelid is drawn laterally to allow the lower lid to rest against the globe (Figure 2-80). The lid tissue extending beyond the lateral canthus is the amount of laxity to be tightened. The excess eyelid is resected as illustrated.

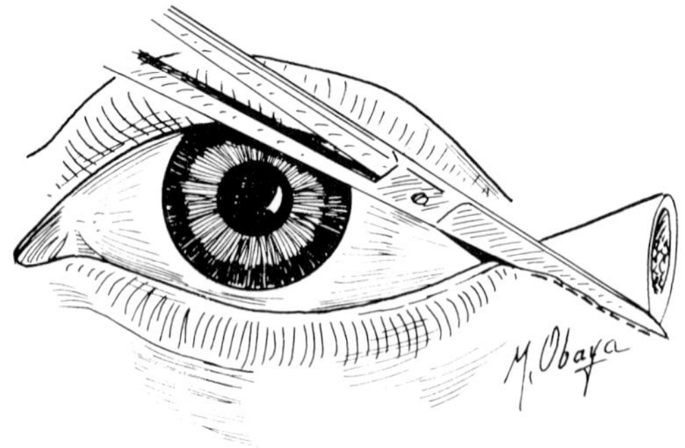

Figure 2-80

A permanent suture (4-0 silk or mersilene) is placed in the lateral tarsal plate and into the periosteum at the lateral canthus (Figure 2-81). The suture should enter the posterior side of the orbital rim 3–4 mm behind the lateral orbital rim, to ensure that the lower eyelid is positioned against the globe. The suture functions as a new lateral canthal tendon for the lower lid and thus should attach the tarsal plate to the orbital tubercle, the anatomic insertion of the lateral canthal tendon. A second nonabsorbable suture is used to reinforce the tarsal-periosteum bond. The subcutaneous tissues are closed with buried absorbable (5-0 chromic) suture, the skin with interrupted 6-0 silk suture. If the lateral lid shortening is done in combination with a lower eyelid blepharoplasty, the blepharoplasty is now continued with the standard skin resection (Figures 2-61–2-68) and wound closure.

The tarsal strip procedure is another effective method of correcting lower lid laxity.[1] In addition, many patients with scleral show and rounded lateral canthi following blepharoplasties can be corrected with this powerful procedure. The principle of the tarsal strip is to form a new lateral canthal tendon (i.e., lower limb) by using a strip of lateral tarsus.

If the operation is used together with a blepharoplasty, the skin flap and fat resection are completed (Figure 2-82).

If the tarsal strip operation is used to correct an involutional ectropion or to reform the lateral canthal angle for correction of postblepharoplasty scleral show or canthal deformity, a lateral canthotomy is performed. A hemostat is placed horizontally at the lateral canthus for a few seconds. It is then removed and the lateral canthus is incised with scissors, thereby dividing the lateral canthal tendon into upper and lower halves (Figures 2-83). In combination with a lower lid blepharoplasty, an identical operation is done behind a skin flap.

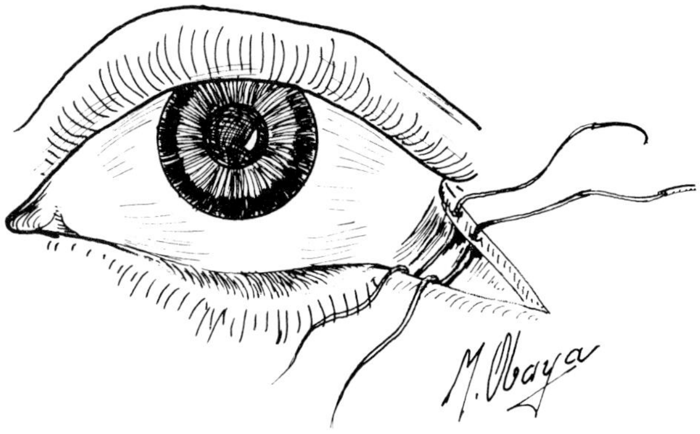

Figure 2-81

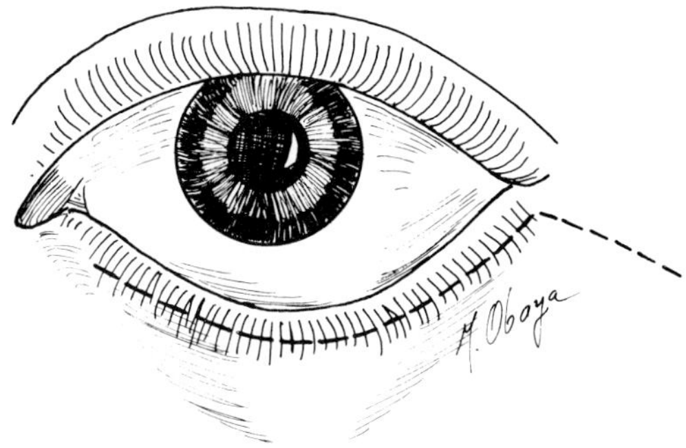

Figure 2-82

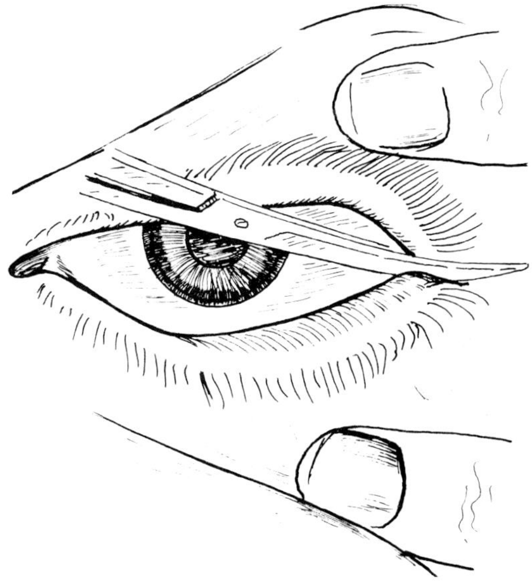

Figure 2-83

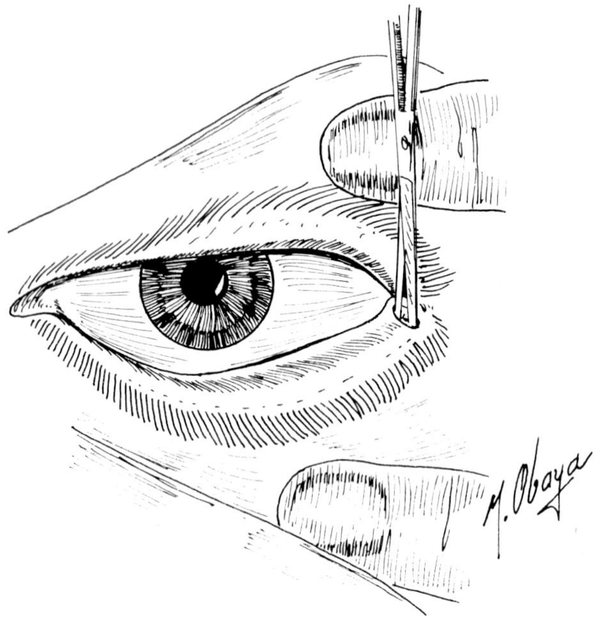

Figure 2-84

The scissor blades are placed between the skin and conjunctiva, and the lower limb of the lateral canthal tendon is cut (Figure 2-84).

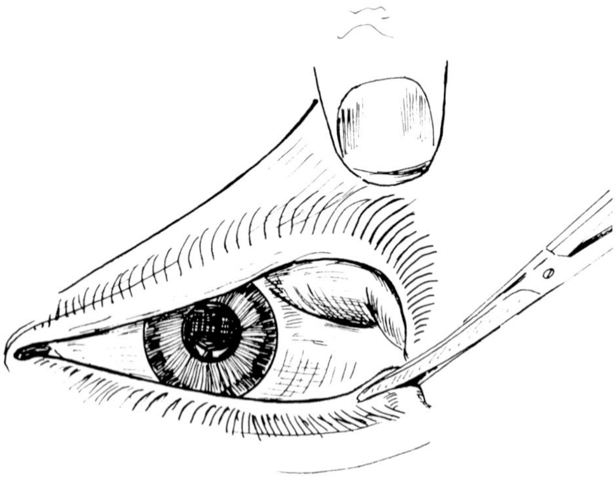

Figure 2-85

The lateral 3–4 mm of eyelid is now divided into anterior lamellae (skin and muscle) and posterior lamellae (tarsus and conjunctiva) (Figure 2-85).

The lateral 3–4 mm of conjunctiva is scraped off the tarsus (Figure 2-86).

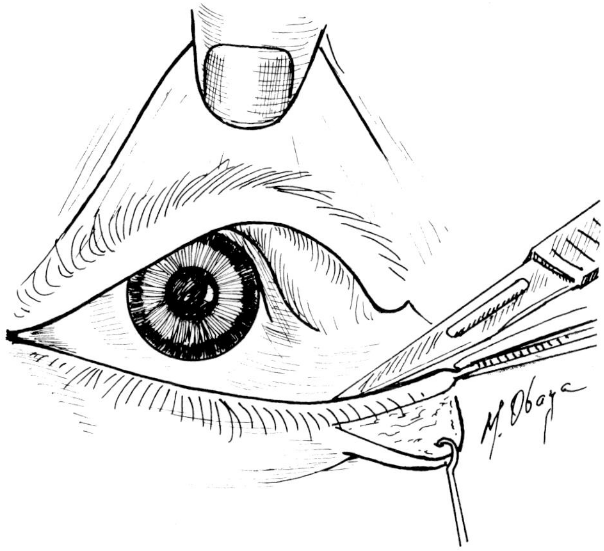

Figure 2-86

Alternatively, the lateral 3–4 mm of conjunctiva can be cut away from the posterior tarsal plate (Figure 2-87).

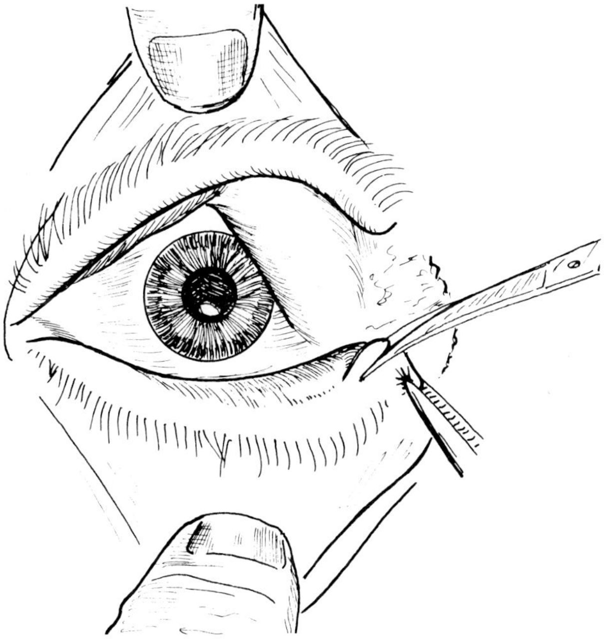

Figure 2-87

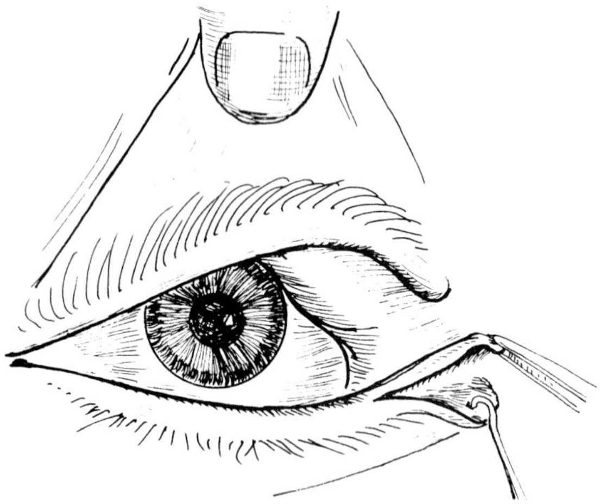

Figure 2-88

A posterior strip of tarsus with lashes remains. The lid margin and eyelashes are excised (Figure 2-88).

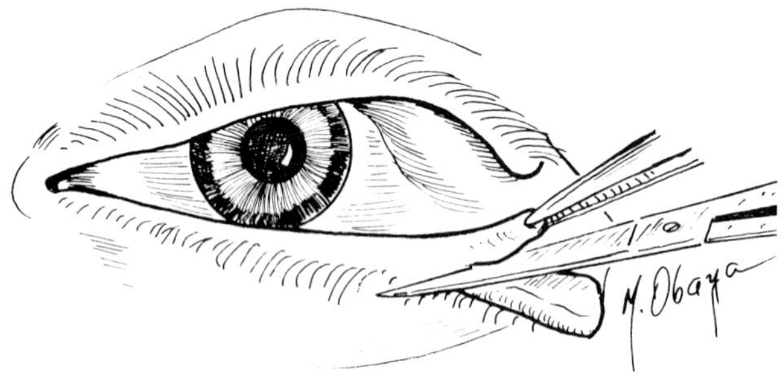

Figure 2-89

The triangle of skin and orbicularis muscle are also excised, leaving a strip of denuded tarsus (Figure 2-89). This strip can be made longer, thereby excising more of the lateral eyelid as determined by the amount of eyelid laxity to be corrected.

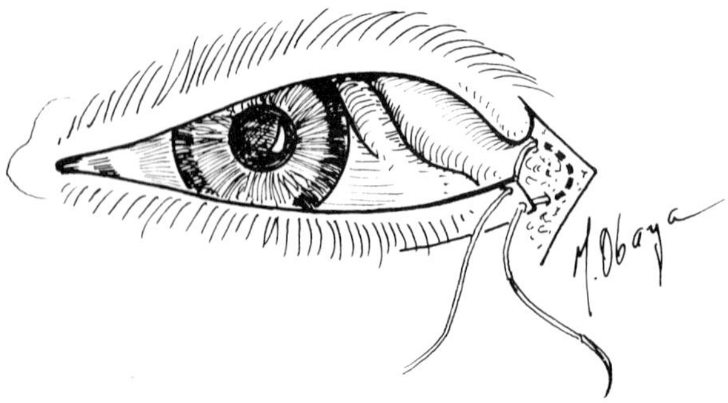

Figure 2-90

A nonabsorbable suture (4-0 suture on a half-circle spatula needle) fixes the tarsal strip to the posterior orbital wall (Figure 2-90). The position of the suture determines the height and angulation of the lateral canthus. Elevation of the insertion of the lower lid also corrects for scleral show by elevating the lid height. A slight overcorrection in tightness and height is desirable to compensate for postoperative stretching and loosening of the fixation.

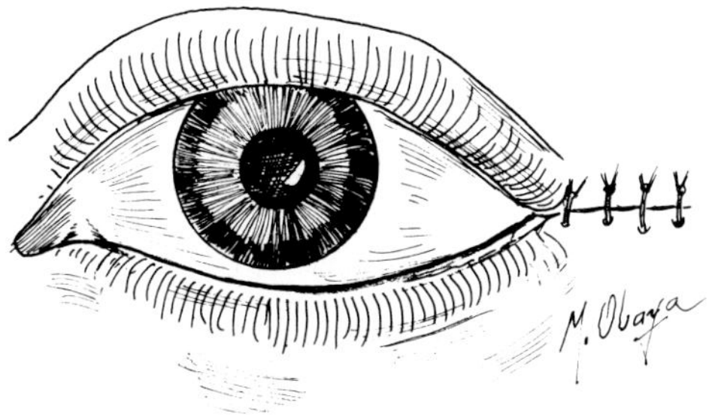

Figure 2-91

The canthotomy is closed with several 6-0 silk sutures (Figure 2-91). If performed with a blepharoplasty, the skin excision is completed and the wound closed.

CORRECTION OF POSTOPERATIVE ECTROPION

A patient who develops an ectropion following a lower eyelid blepharoplasty should be initially managed conservatively with massage and ocular lubricants. After an adequate period of observation, a persistent ectropion should be surgically repaired. The patient should be evaluated to determine whether the ectropion is due to excessive skin excision (i.e., cicatricial ectropion), eyelid laxity not recognized prior to surgery, or a combination of the two.

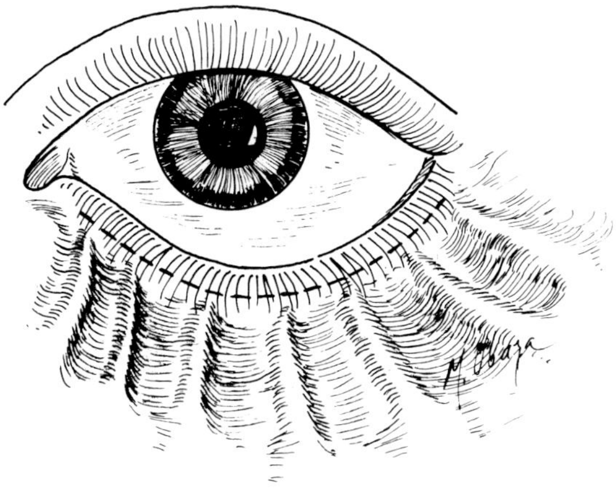

Figure 2-92

If the ectropion is due to excessive skin excision, an incision is made in the blepharoplasty scar. The scar is undermined and scar bands between the skin and orbicularis muscle are released (Figure 2-92).

The lid should be placed on stretch by placing a 6-0 silk suture through the tarsus, as illustrated in Figure 2-93, and clamping it to the head drapes. When the lower lid can be easily pulled up over the cornea, the cicatricial component can be considered released.

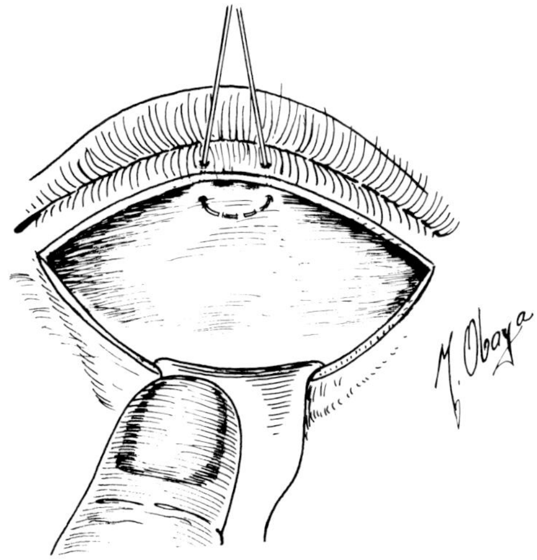

Figure 2-93

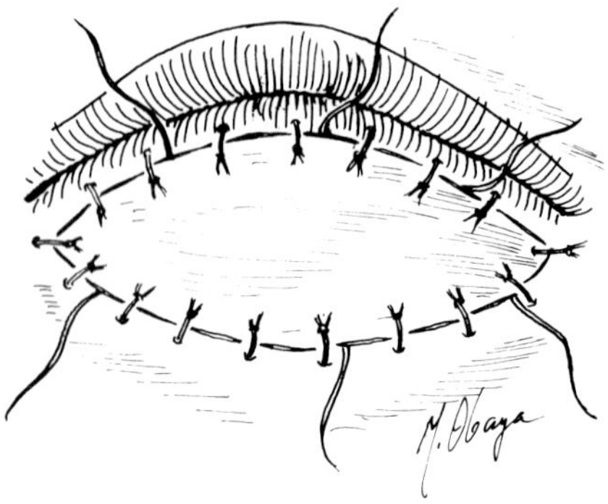

Figure 2-94

A full-thickness skin graft should now be removed from an appropriate donor site and tailored to fit the maximum defect in the lower eyelid (Figure 2-94). The order of preference for skin graft donor sites to be used in the lower eyelid is (1) retroauricular area, (2) upper lid skin if available, (3) supraclavicular area, and (4) inner arm. The graft is sutured into place with multiple interrupted 6-0 silk sutures. Several suture ends are left long and are used to tie over a bolster.

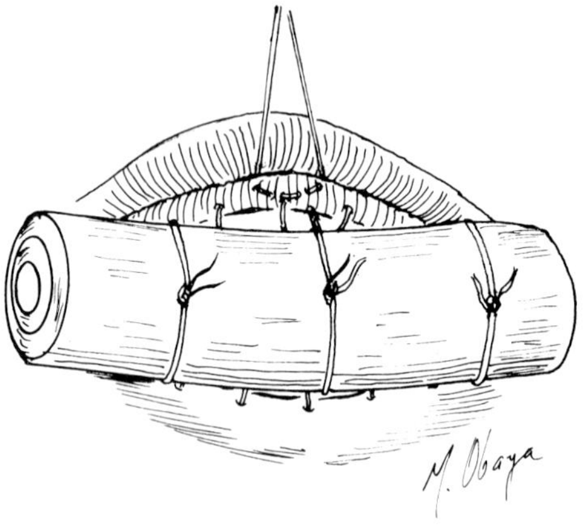

Figure 2-95

A Telfa roll is placed on the graft and secured into place with the long sutures (Figure 2-95). A modified Frost suture is placed through the eyelid margin and taped to the forehead to keep the lid on stretch for 3–4 days.

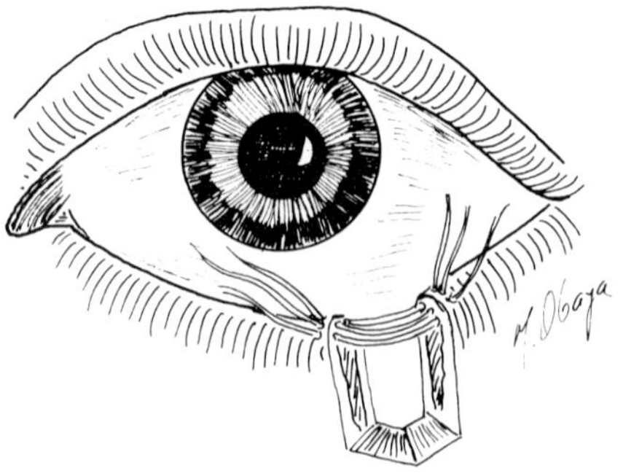

Figure 2-96

A postoperative ectropion due to unrecognized lid laxity is corrected with a standard horizontal shortening (see Figures 2-72–2-78). A full-thickness eyelid excision and reconstruction can be done as illustrated in Figure 2-96, or the wedge resection can be done beneath a skin flap. The latter gives a better cosmetic result, but extreme care should be taken in the handling of the skin edges to prevent any further scarring and vertical contracture.

If there exists a combination of lid laxity and cicatricial ectropion, a horizontal shortening should be done as shown in Figure 2-97 after the scar tissue has been released but before suturing in the skin graft (Figures 2-92–2-95).

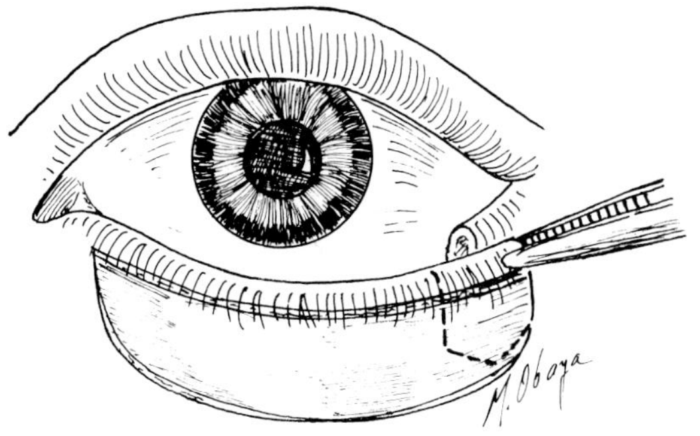

Figure 2-97

TREATMENT OF FESTOONS— "BAGS ON BAGS"

The successful management of lower eyelid dermatochalasis is reasonably straightforward in the patients with moderate amounts of excess skin and orbital fat. However, obtaining a satisfactory result in the patient with large festoons of tissue requires more extensive surgery.

The patient illustrated in Figure 2-98 will have thick rolls of hypertrophic orbicularis muscle, large amounts of herniated orbital fat, and stretched excessive skin covering the tissues. In addition, loss of lid tone will produce scleral show and lid laxity.

A standard blepharoplasty skin incision is marked as shown in Figure 2-99. The lateral vertical line may need to be longer to allow adequate elevation of the skin flap. An extended lower lid blepharoplasty has been described where the lateral incision is continued horizontally.[4] In either case, a skin flap is undermined and extended to or beyond the inferior orbital rim. If additional festoons of tissue lie below the edge of the rim, additional inferiorly directed undermining can be done. Those festoons far below the inferior orbital rim may not be correctible with a blepharoplasty. Festoons or bags remaining following surgery can be excised, but a scar will remain on the cheek.

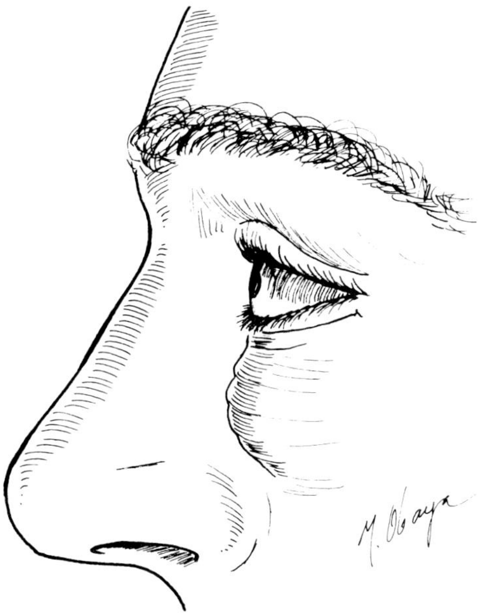

Figure 2-98

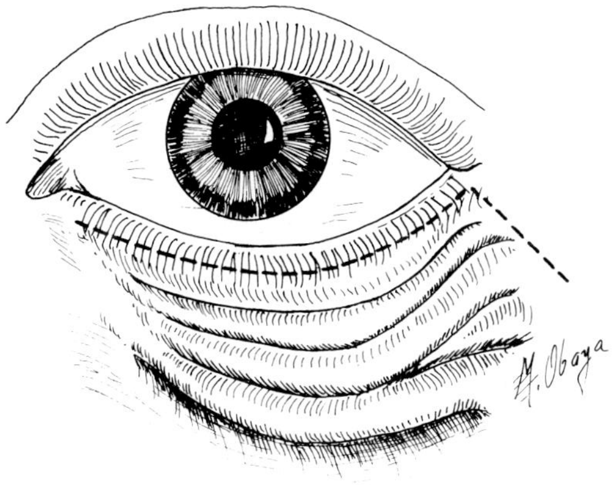

Figure 2-99

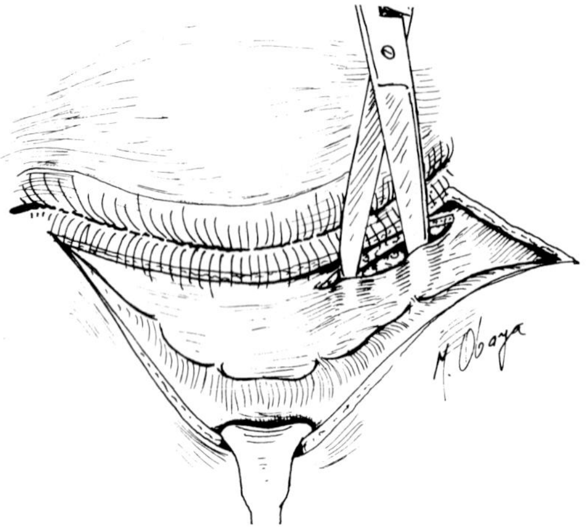

Figure 2-100

Following the skin dissection and fat excision, a second flap of orbicularis muscle is made (Figure 2-100). Scissors are used to undermine the orbicularis muscle from the underlying orbital septum.

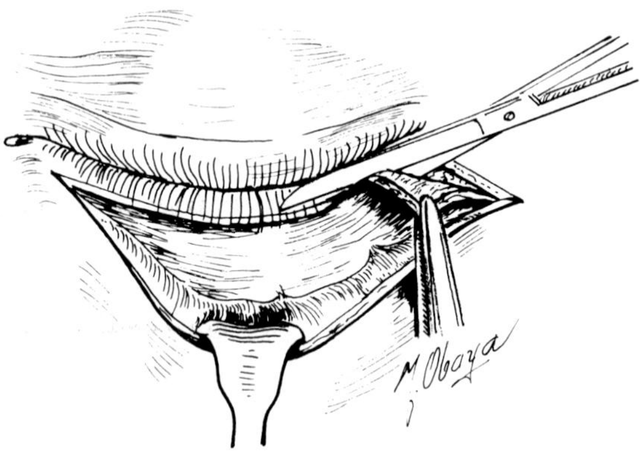

Figure 2-101

The muscle flap is carefully formed by cutting the muscle along the wound margin (Figure 2-101).

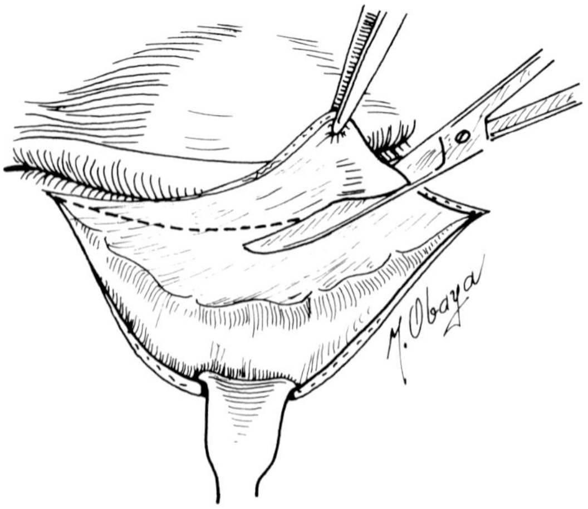

Figure 2-102

The undermined muscle flap is now draped over the edge of the wound and cut away (Figure 2-102).

The edge of the orbicularis muscle may ooze profusely and should be carefully coagulated for hemostasis. The muscle flap should be laid into position along the wound edge (Figure 2-103).

The orbicularis muscle is fixated to the lateral canthal orbicularis muscle with 4-0 absorbable mattress sutures (Figure 2-104). This serves as a support for the lower lid structures. A slight overcorrection is desirable because of postoperative stretching of the orbicularis fibers. The skin is excised as previously described.

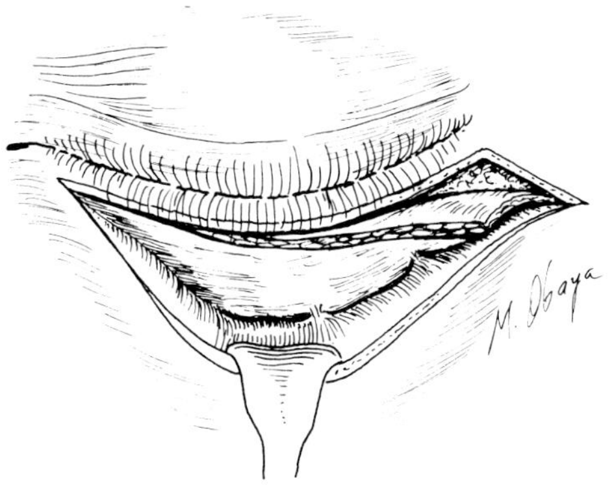

Figure 2-103

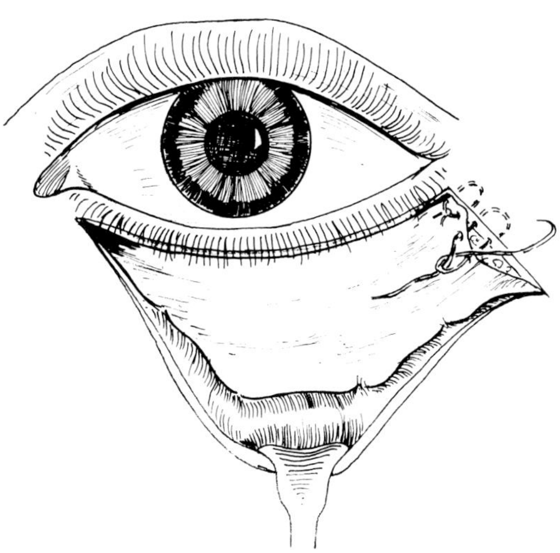

Figure 2-104

WEBBING OF THE LATERAL CANTHUS

The upper eyelid blepharoplasty incision should not be less than 5–6 mm above the lateral canthus. Accordingly, the lower lid incision should also not come closer than 3–4 mm to the lateral canthus. In order to prevent scar bands that contract into webs at the lateral canthus, the surgeon should follow these guidelines and keep the upper and lower incision lines 8–10 mm apart.

If a web develops at the lateral canthus, massage should be attempted initially in hopes of softening or reversing the scar contracture (Figure 2-105). If massage is unsuccessful and at least 3–4 months, but preferably 6 months of observation have elapsed, a Y- to V-plasty will correct the scar. The Y-plasty is placed with the long arm horizontal and the two arms overlying the scar.

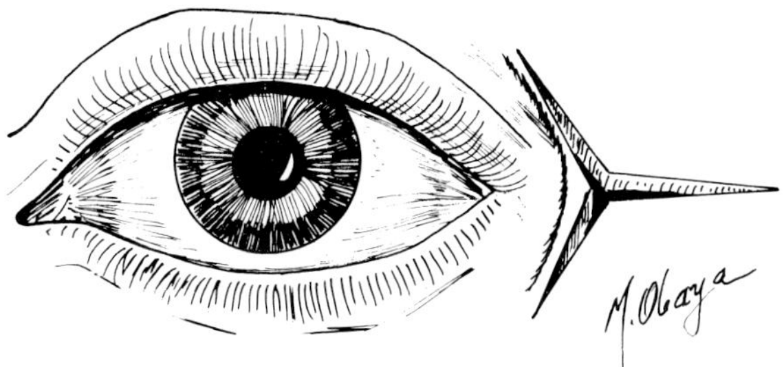

Figure 2-105

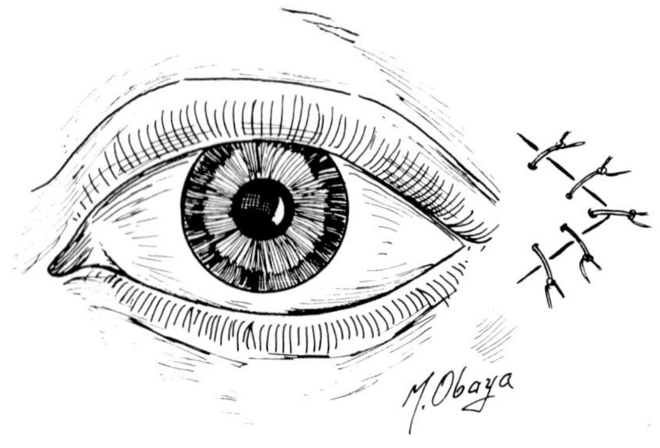

Figure 2-106

The Y-plasty is converted into a V-plasty and closed with 5-0 chromic sutures deep and 6-0 silk skin sutures (Figure 2-106).

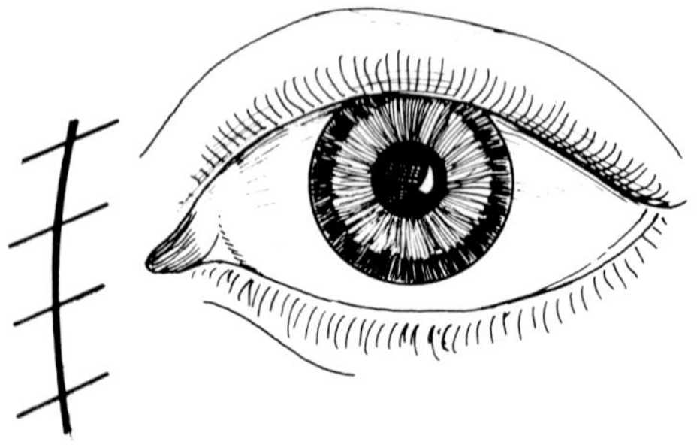

Figure 2-107

A web at the medial canthus most commonly develops from extending the eyelid incision through the nasocanthal depression and onto the nose (Figure 2-107). To prevent this complication, the following guidelines are recommended:

1. Bring the medial upper eyelid line no closer than 4–5 mm from the punctum.
2. Enter but do not traverse and leave the nasocanthal depression. The skin incision should not include the skin of the nose.
3. Do not progress more medially than the lower punctum for the lower lid blepharoplasty.

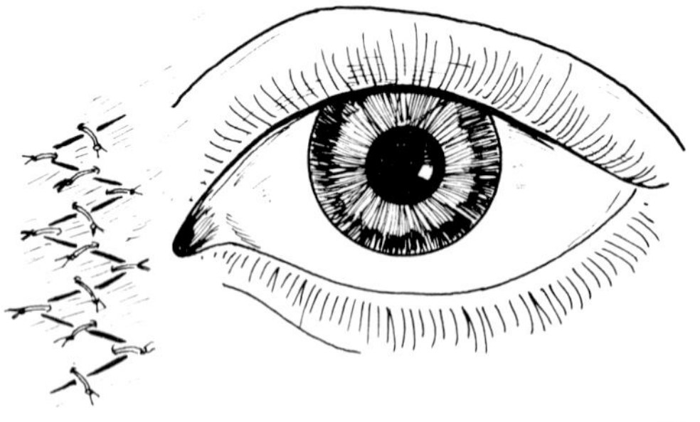

Figure 2-108

If webbing occurs, a Z-plasty or multiple Z-plasties will correct this complication (Figure 2-108).

MANAGEMENT OF ORBITAL HEMORRHAGE

The occurrence of an intraoperative orbital hemorrhage during a blepharoplasty would be an infrequent and unusual complication. This problem might occur from inadvertent injection of local anesthetic posterior to the orbital septum with damage to an orbital vessel. It is also possible to have a lacerated vessel in the orbital fat retract during fat excision and hemorrhage in the posterior orbit. Finally, a person suffering from a bleeding dyscrasia, having severe vascular pathology, or taking anticoagulants might suffer a massive hemorrhage during the injection of anesthetic or during surgery. A careful review of systems and medications being taken prior to surgery is vital.

An intraoperative hemorrhage is managed by intermittent digital pressure applied to the globe. The closed eyelids are alternately compressed with ones' fingers for 10 seconds and pressure then released for 5 seconds in attempt to stop the bleeding. A $\frac{1}{2} \times 3$-inch neurosurgical pattie soaked in 1 : 100,000 epinephrine laid on the orbicularis muscle may also be of assistance in obtaining hemostasis of surface bleeding. Gentle cauterization of the small vessels in the orbicularis muscle and in the orbital septum controls the bleeding. Rarely do these anterior vessels dissect posteriorly and cause a retroorbital hemorrhage with increased intraorbital pressure.

A lacerated vessel in the orbital fat pad is the most likely cause for a massive orbital hemorrhage. The fat pedicle must be well cauterized and examined before allowing the fat to retract back into the orbit. If the fat pedicle begins to bleed after the fat has been released, the bleeding vessel must be visualized and cauterized.

If bleeding is uncontrollable, the operation is terminated and a penrose drain is left in the wound when the latter is closed. Only several interrupted sutures should be used to close the skin incision and by no means should the orbital septum be sutured.

A postoperative hemorrhage that may potentially result in visual loss is the most feared complication of cosmetic eyelid surgery. Similar precautions regarding evaluation of the patient's medical status must be taken. Aspirin consumption should be stopped a minimum of 7–10 days before surgery. Hypertensive patients should have their blood pressures controlled. Patients with thyroid related ocular disease should have adequately stable thyroid functions.

A postoperative orbital hemorrhage characteristically produces deep orbital or ocular pain. This is most likely due to ocular compression from an enlarging orbital hematoma producing increased intraorbital and therefore intraocular pressure. The elevated intraocular pressure may occlude the central retinal artery and cause visual loss.

Any complaint of severe or unusual ocular or periorbital pain following eyelid surgery warrants immediate investigation. Tight dressing should not be used to patch the eyes following surgery. If an orbital hemorrhage occurs, the eye is moved forward by the expanding orbital volume and a firm dressing prevents this natural attempt at decompression, thereby raising the intraocular pressure.

If pain develops, the dressing or patch should be removed. Decreased vision; proptosis; signs of severe conjunctival chemosis or severe periocular ecchymosis; a nonreactive pupillary response to bright light; and findings of optic nerve edema, retinal hemorrhages, and central retinal artery occlusion may all represent an imminent threat of visual loss.

The suture line is immediately opened at the bedside and an attempt is made to evacuate blood clots. It is very difficult to find an isolated bleeding vessel. Acetazolamide (Diamox) 500 mg orally and 500 mg intravenously (IV) is administered. A hyperosmotic agent such as mannitol (20% concentration given IV at 2 g/kg body weight) over 20 minutes is administered if there is no medical contraindication. These maneuvers ae intended to lower the intraocular pressure.

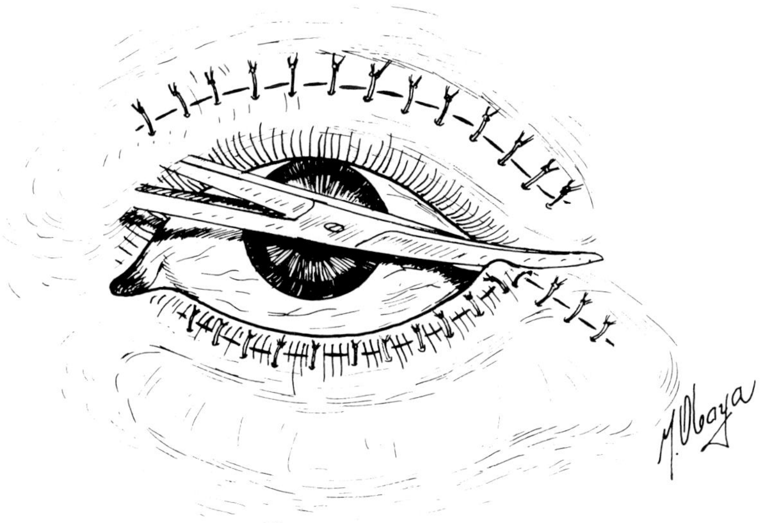

Figure 2-109

If the globe is still proptosed, a lateral canthotomy is performed (Figure 2-109). A hemostat is placed horizontally at the lateral canthus, clamped, and released after a few seconds. Scissors are then used to divide the lateral canthal tendon.

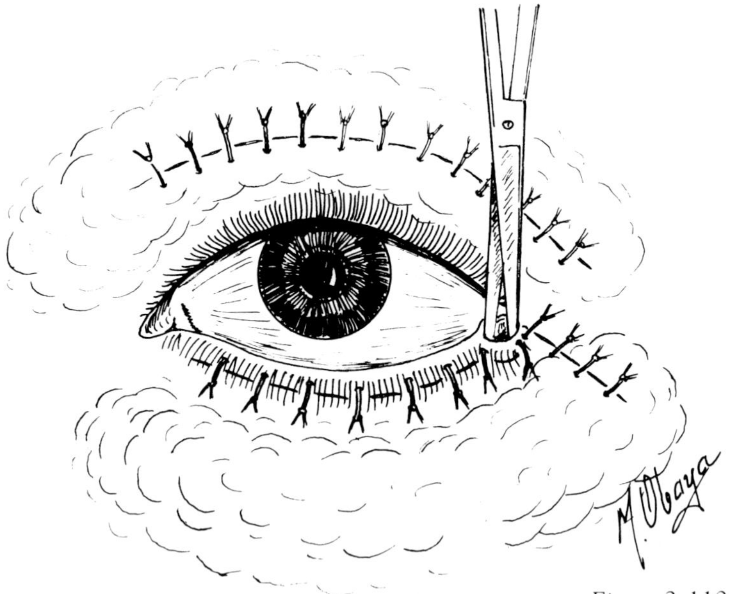

Figure 2-110

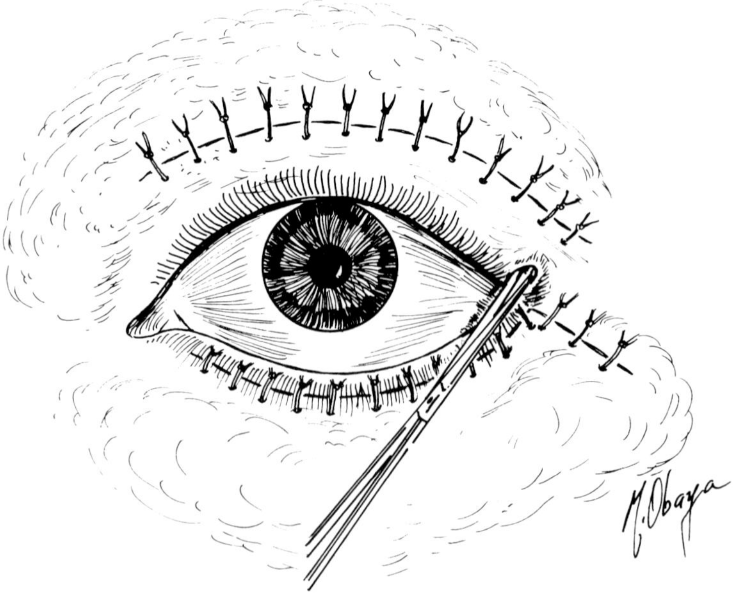

Figure 2-111

The upper and lower limbs of the lateral canthal tendon are now cut, thereby releasing the attachment of the lateral eyelid to the orbital rim (Figures 2-110 and 2-111). This is the most rapid method of orbital decompression and allows the globe to move anteriorly. Assistance should be promptly obtained from an ophthalmologist in the management of a central retinal artery occlusion and orbital hemorrhage.

A postoperative hypertensive crisis may cause severe postoperative hemorrhage. This may occur unilaterally or bilaterally. The patient should be taken back to surgery, the wound opened, and the blood clots evacuated. If individual bleeding vessels are seen, they should be cauterized. As in the case of other hemorrhages, a drain should be placed in the orbit and left for 24–48 hours.

DISCUSSION

Blepharoptosis can be attributed to excessive skin pushing the eyelids down (pseudoptosis); however, other etiologies must first be ruled out. The most common cause of acquired ptosis is due to a defect of the levator aponeurosis, a delicate tissue attachment between the levator muscle (principal eyelid elevator) and the tarsal plate. The clinical signs of acquired ptosis in a clinical setting are a high lid crease, thinning of the eyelid tissues, and good levator function. The normal vertical palpebral fissure measures 10 mm. The normal upper eyelid should cover 1 mm of the superior limbus.[4,6] The patient illustrated in Figure 2-28 has ptosis of the left eyelid.

There are slight variations to the procedures described for fat excision earlier in this chapter (see Figures 2-55–2-60). Some surgeons excise the clamped fat with scissors, as they feel that the crushing of the scissor blades reduces bleeding. In addition, some surgeons will excise excessive lower eyelid fat without paying particular attention to clamping the fat, as they feel that they can monitor hemostasis by careful dissection. This is appropriate for the medial and central fat pockets if the surgeon feels confident in the ability to find a bleeding vessel within the orbital fat. After the fat has been clamped, the assistant should release pressure from the eye to avoid extended periods of elevated intraocular pressure that can reduce blood flow to the eye. Releasing pressure also allows the remaining fat to return to its normal position.

The ability to gauge the proper amount of fat to excise improves with surgical experience in blepharoplasty operations. Removing the fat that protrudes through the edges of the opened orbital septum while pressure is placed on the globe is a general guideline. Other surgeons excise any fat that protrudes anterior to the level of the inferior orbital rim. An important step while removing orbital fat is to compare the amount removed from each lid.

The examination of patients considered for lower lid blepharoplasty surgery should include a careful evaluation of lower eyelid tone. The chronic effects of aging and gravity cause a loss of tone of the lid tissues with increasing lower eyelid laxity. The recognition of lower eyelid laxity is an important indication of a potential postoperative ectropion. The effects of postoperative swelling and tightening of the eyelid skin can tip an incipient ectropion into a frank ectropion condition.

There are numerous methods of tightening the lower eyelid laxity during a blepharoplasty (Figures 2-72–78). In addition to a horizontal shortening of the eyelid, surgery can be directed to the lateral canthus. Many surgeons feel that the lid laxity is due to stretching or dehiscence of the lateral canthal tendon. Repositioning the lateral tarsal plate at the posterior lateral orbital rim combined with shortening of the lid laterally will also correct ectropion.

REFERENCES

1. Anderson, R. A. and Gordy, D. D.: The Tarsal Strip Procedure. *Arch. Ophthalmol.*, 97:2192, 1969.
2. Bick, M. W.: Orbital Tarsal Disparity. *Arch. Ophthalmol.*, 75:386, 1966.
3. Fasanella, R. H. and Servat, J.: Levator Resection for Minimal Ptosis, Another Simplified Operation. *Arch. Ophthalmol.*, 65:493, 1961.
4. Small, R. G.: Extended Lower Eyelid Blepharoplasty. *Arch. Ophthalmol.*, 99:1402, 1981.
5. Wilkins, R. B. and Patipa, M.: Acquired Ptosis and Current Treatment. Symposium on Disease and Surgery of the Lids, Lacrimal Apparatus, and Orbit. Transactions of the New Orleans Academy of Ophthalmology, Mosby, St. Louis, 1982.
6. Wilkins, R. B. and Patipa, M.: Ectropion. Symposium on Disease and Surgery of the Lids, Lacrimal Apparatus, and Orbit. Transactions of the New Orleans Academy of Ophthalmology. Mosby, St. Louis, 1982, p. 205.
7. Wilkins, R. B. and Patipa, M.: The Recognition of Acquired Ptosis in Patients Considered for Upper Eyelid Blepharoplasty. *Plast. Reconstr. Surg.*, 70:431, 1982.

3

Oriental Eyelid Blepharoplasty

John A. McCurdy, Jr.
Douglas D. Dedo

Surgical modification of the Oriental eyelid gained popularity in the Far East following World War II, and at the present time is the most frequently performed aesthetic operation in the Orient. As such surgery is being requested with increasing frequency in North American areas with large Asian populations, the facial plastic surgeon should be familiar with the Oriental eyelid and various methods of surgical modification.

Approximately 50 percent of Orientals demonstrate the "single eyelid," so called because in the absence of a superior palpebral fold, the lid hangs like a curtain from the supraorbital ridge. Creation of a sulcus divides the lid into well-defined pretarsal and palpebral portions, producing the "double eyelid" desired by many Oriental women. The single lid is genetically determined, expressed as an autosomal dominant trait with essentially complete penetrance; thus, if one parent manifests the trait, almost all offspring will exhibit the single eyelid.

Many young Oriental women produce double eyelids by using various tapes and glues to encourage adherence of the pretarsal and orbital skin resulting in a palpebral fold. As such, rituals are time-consuming and temporary; however, surgery is frequently requested after reaching the age of 15–16.

ANATOMY

There are anatomic differences between the Oriental and occidental eyelid.

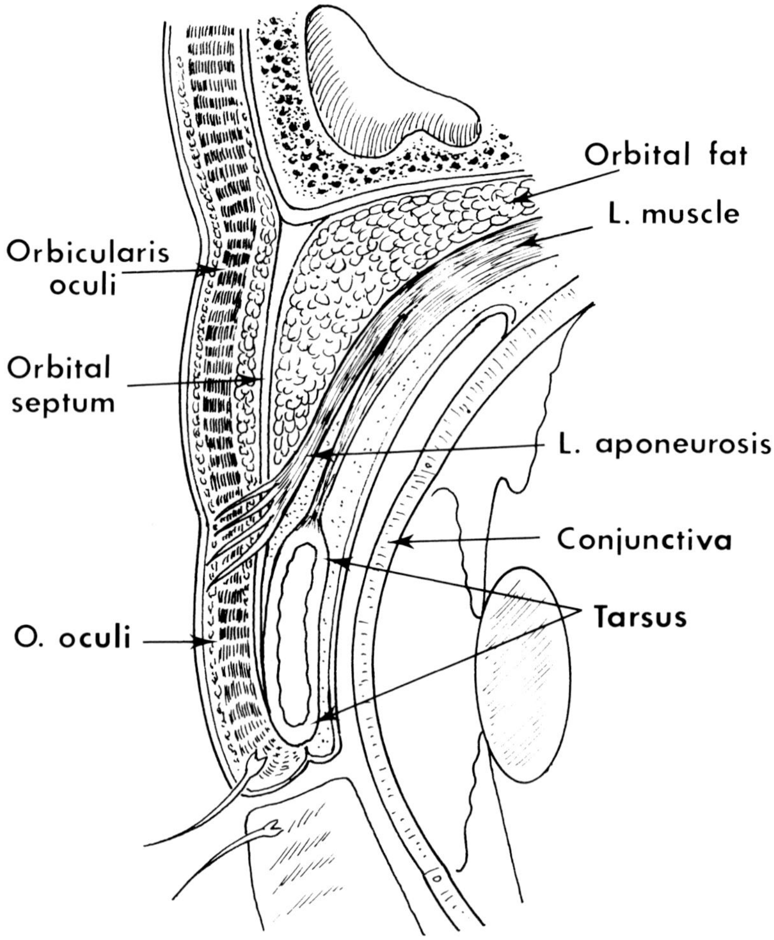

Figure 3-1

In the Caucasian eyelid, filaments of the levator expansion penetrate the orbital septum and orbicularis muscle to attach to the pretarsal dermis (Figure 3-1). This attachment results in formation of a palpebral fold on opening the lid.

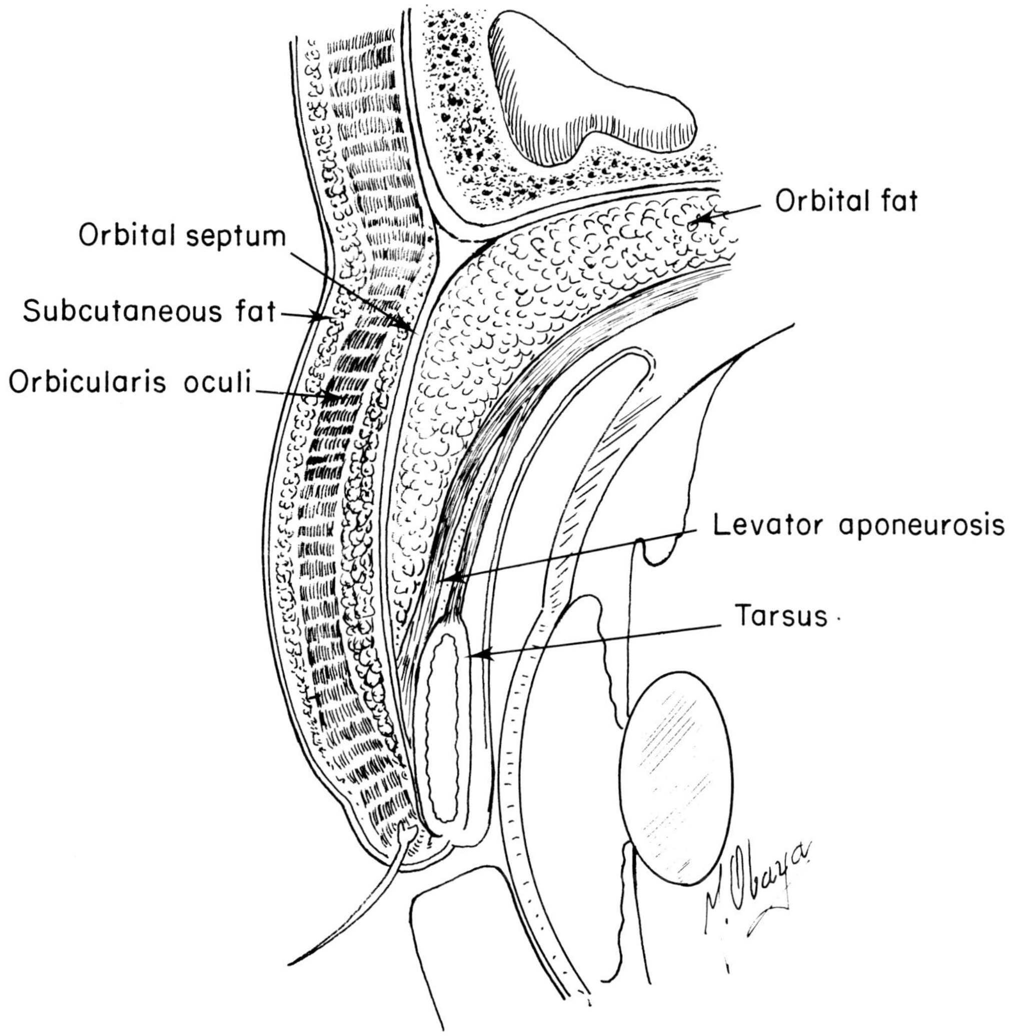

Figure 3-2

In the Oriental eyelid, the levator aponeurosis attaches to the superior margin of the tarsus and does not penetrate the orbital septum nor the orbicularis oculi muscle (Figure 3-2).

The orbital fat compartment bounded by the orbital septum descends inferiorly anterior to the tarsus. Variable amounts of subcutaneous fat and suborbicularis (central) fat as well as pretarsal fat contribute to the puffiness of the Oriental eyelid. The Caucasian eyelid lacks the subcutaneous and central fat accumulations. The anatomic basis for absence of a superior palpebral fold in the Oriental eyelid is therefore that the levator expansion does not penetrate the orbital septum and orbicularis oculi and attach to the pretarsal dermis as occurs in the Caucasian eyelid. In the single lid, the levator expansion terminates as a ridge of fascia on the superior border of the tarsal plate. The Oriental lid is characterized by an abundance of adipose tissue that results in fullness or puffiness characteristic of the single lid. This fat is classified according to its location as noted in Figure 3-2. As a consequence of loose skin and fat protrusion, the width of the palpebral fissure in single eyelids is less than that of double lids. This may give the Oriental eye an air of mystery and stoicism and occasionally gives the suggestion of ptosis (pseudoptosis). A prominent epicanthal (or Mongolian) fold is present in approximately 70 percent of Oriental upper eyelids. As this web may blunt the medial canthus and obscure the lacrimal caruncle, surgical modification is often a goal of Oriental blepharoplasty.

TECHNIQUE

ANESTHESIA

Oriental blepharoplasty is performed under local anesthesia (0.5 % Marcaine or 1 % lidocaine with epinephrine 1 : 100,00) with intravenous (IV) sedation. The vast majority of cases are performed as outpatient procedures in an office surgical facility. As frequent opening and closing of the eyes during surgery are helpful in evaluating symmetry, general anesthesia is not recommended.

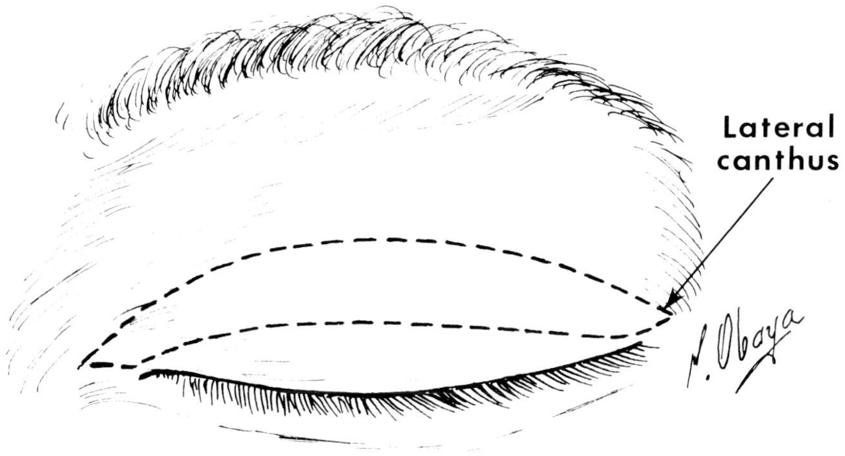

Figure 3-3

WESTERNIZATION OF THE EYELID

The desired level of the superior palpebral fold is marked at midpupillary level (Figure 3-3). The entire fold is then drawn following the natural curve of the lid. In general, this line will be approximately 2 mm more inferior at the medial canthus while remaining at approximately the same level at the lateral canthus as in the center of the lid. If an epicanthal fold is present, the incision must split this fold or course slightly inferior to it. The position of the palpebral fold may be varied by altering the level of the incision with respect to the ciliary margin at the midpupillary level, depending on the desired eyelid size. In the younger patient who does not desire westernization, the incision stops at the lateral canthus as depicted.

The level of the superior incision, which determines the amount of skin to be excised, is determined by pinching the skin with forceps and asking the patient to open and close the eyes as in a standard blepharoplasty procedure. In practice the incision is marked 1–2 mm inferior to this point in order to avoid lagophthalmos.

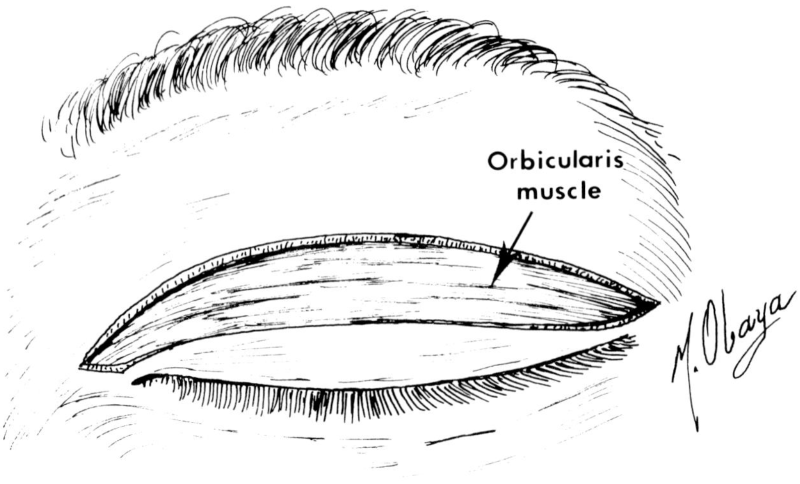

Figure 3-4

Following infiltration of local anesthetic, skin and subcutaneous tissue is excised, exposing the orbicularis muscle (Figure 3-4). Oriental lids generally demonstrate large amounts of subcutaneous areolar tissue.

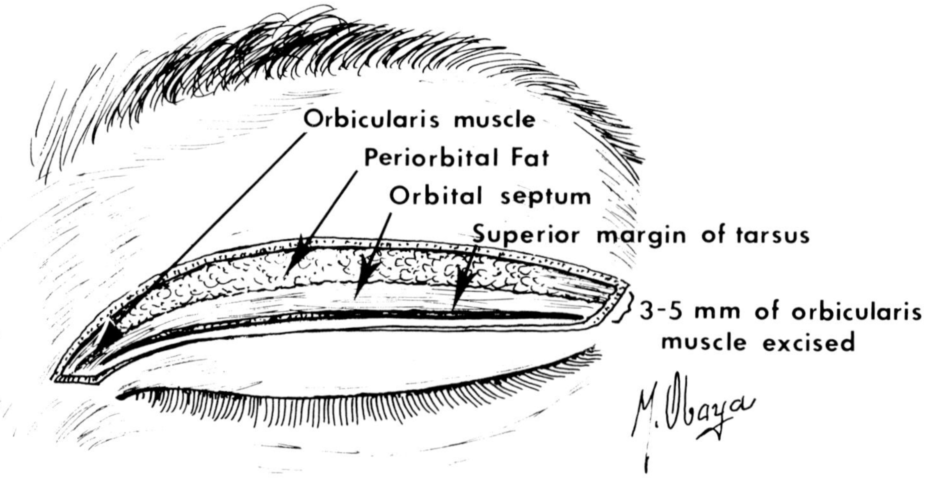

Figure 3-5

Following removal of the subcutaneous fat, a 3–5 mm strip of orbicularis muscle is excised just above the tarsal plate (Figure 3-5). In puffy lids excess muscle is trimmed from the lateral and middle portions of the wound, but muscle tissue must be preserved medially in order to prevent excessive depth of the fold in this area.

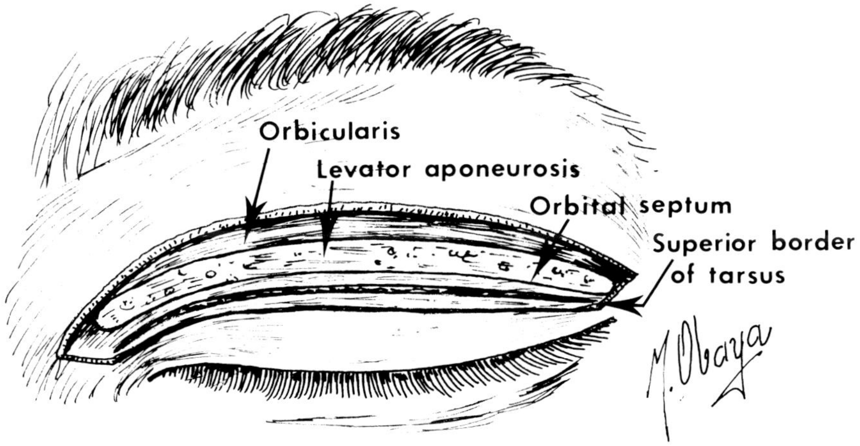

Figure 3-6

The orbital septum is then incised. The structure is generally thick in the Oriental eyelid, as shown in Figure 3-6. In order to create a deep "western" palpebral sulcus, a large fusiform strip of fat is removed, completely exposing the aponeurosis of the levator palpebrae muscle.

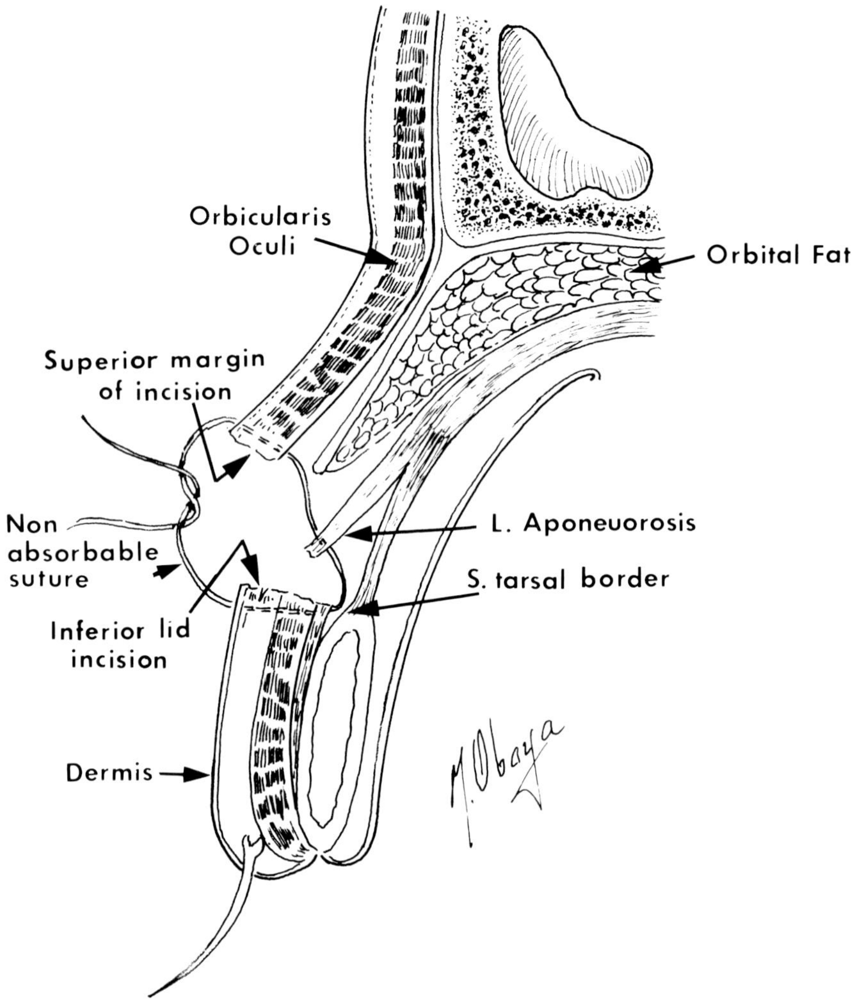

Figure 3-7

The superior border of the tarsal plate is identified and the central portion of the inferior lid incision secured to the adventitia overlying the levator aponeurosis just above its attachment to the tarsal plate (Figure 3-7). As the level of the palpebral fold varies with the level at which this fixation occurs, care must be taken to ensure symmetry. Three fixation sutures of 6-0 nylon are employed to incorporate the skin and underlying orbicularis oculi to the adventitia. (*Note:* The suture does not pass through the tarsal plate.) These sutures also include the skin of the superior aspect of the incision and are tied externally, thus obviating the need for buried sutures. An adhesion is created between the orbicularis oculi and levator aponeurosis rather than between the levator and the dermis per se, producing a softer and more natural fold. Fixation sutures in the more medial and lateral aspect of the incision are unnecessary.

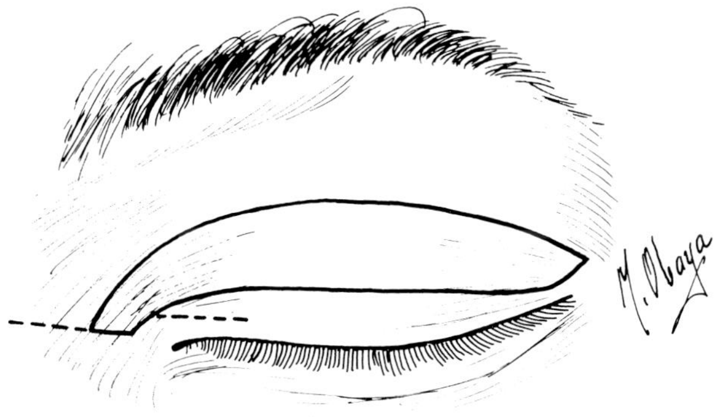

Figure 3-8

If elimination of the epicanthal fold is desired, a Z-plasty is performed (Figure 3-8). Elimination of the fold exposes the lacrimal caruncle, producing a more western appearance.

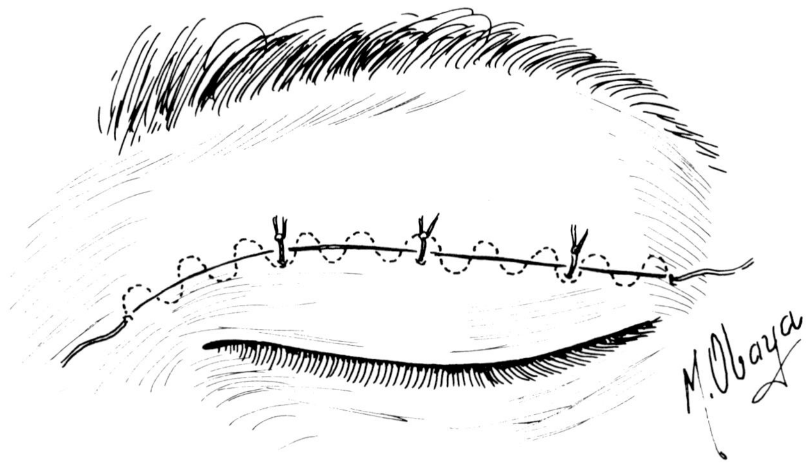

Figure 3-9

The remainder of the incision is closed with a running subcutitular suture of 6-0 nylon as shown in Figure 3-9. All sutures except the deep fixation sutures are removed in 3 days. These sutures are removed on the seventh postoperative day. Makeup can be applied 24 hours after final suture removal and is helpful in camouflaging resolving edema and ecchymosis.

CREATION OF A DOUBLE LID WITHOUT WESTERNIZATION

The palpebral fold is marked at midpupillary level 7–8 mm above the ciliary margin and then drawn on the entire lid as described in the previous technique (Figures 3-3–3-9). Again, the most desirable results are achieved when the arch of the fold is approximately 2 mm more inferior at the medial canthus while approximating the level centrally of the lateral canthus. As in the westernization procedure, the maximum amount of skin that can be excised is determined by pinching with forceps while the patient's eyes are opening and closing alternately. If westernization is not desired, however, less skin is excised. The actual amount of skin that is removed varies from patient to patient according to individual skin laxity but in general approximates 2–4 mm. Following infiltration of the local anesthetic, the skin and subcutaneous tissue are excised, exposing the orbicularis muscle. A 2–3 mm strip of orbicularis is excised above the tarsal plate. Pretarsal fat is removed, but the periorbital fat is preserved in order to maintain the Oriental characteristic of the lid. The superior margin of the tarsal plate is identified, and three central fixation sutures are placed as in the westernization procedure but again go through the adventia of the aponeurosis just above the tarsal plate and not through the plate itself (Figure 3-7). The incision is then approximated with running intradermal suture of 6-0 nylon (Figure 3-9).

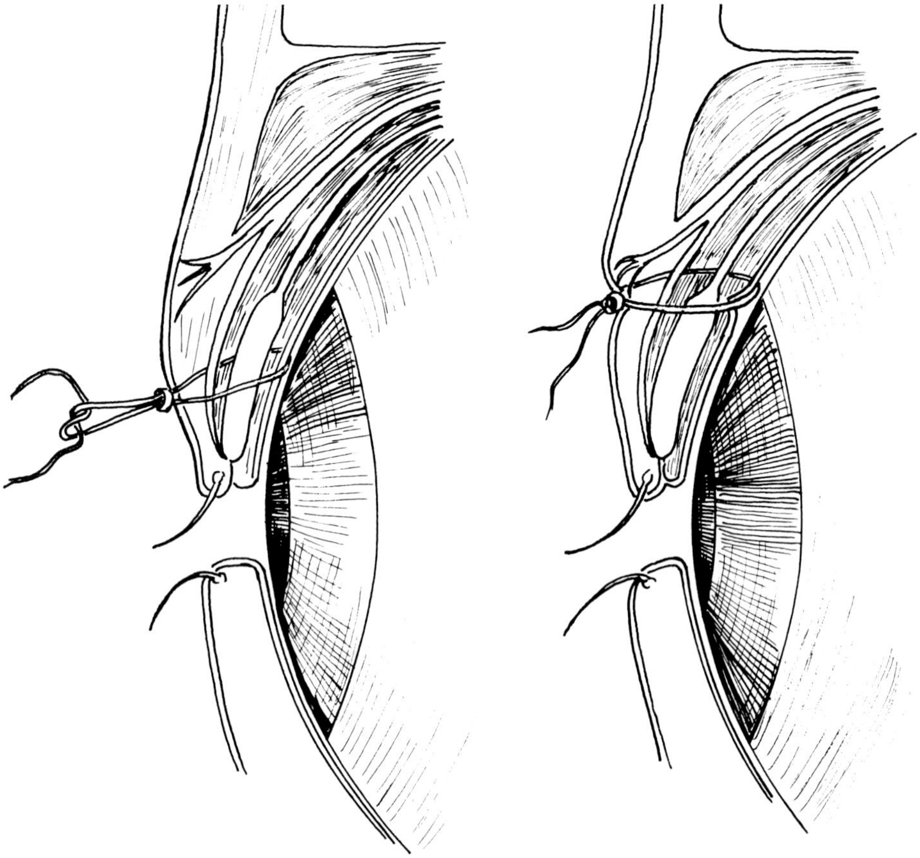

Figure 3-10

Suture removal proceeds as noted in the westernization procedure. Figure 3-10 illustrates suture technique without skin incision. The level of the palpebral fold is marked as described earlier (see Figures 3-3–3-9). A small amount of anesthetic is injected into the area of the fold, with care being taken to avoid distortion of the tissues. The lid is everted and the conjunctiva just above the superior border of the tarsus is injected with anesthetic solution. A suture of 4-0 silk or mersilene is inserted through the skin at the center of the lid, exiting on the conjunctival surface approximately 2 mm above the superior tarsal border. This suture is then reinserted through the conjunctiva, exiting through the skin at a point approximately 3–4 mm lateral to the point of its initial entrance. This suture is then tied over a small rubber band. Three such sutures are placed and remain for 10–12 days. This procedure creates an adhesion between the levator, orbicularis, and skin at the superior tarsal border.

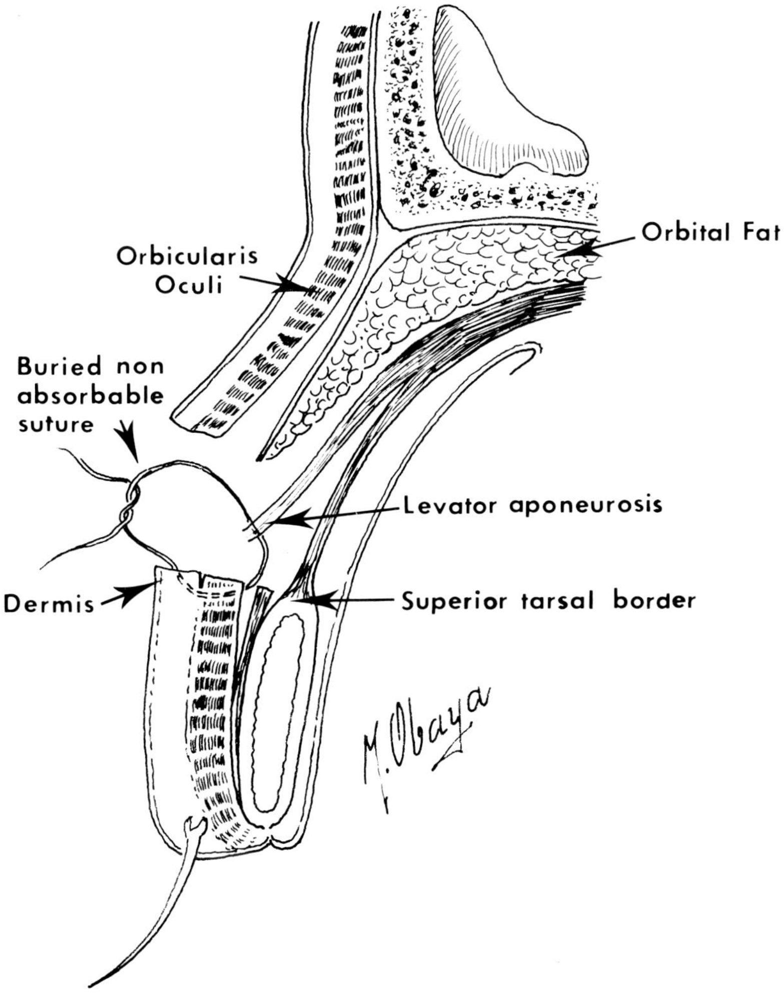

Figure 3-11

Creation of a permanent palpebral fold is accomplished with buried nonabsorbable sutures which fix the dermis to the superior tarsal border (Figure 3-11).

FINESSE

When marking the level of the palpebral fold, the eyelid skin should be stretched upward. If this is not done, the resulting fold will be at a higher level than the surgeon desires, particularly if significant amounts of skin are excised. The fold produced by the use of tape and glue is often an excellent guide in ascertaining the level at which each patient desires the palpebral fold. The arc of the fold is important and has been stressed previously.

Particular care must be exercised in the area of the medial canthus. In order to avoid scar and/or webbing in this area, only a small amount of skin should be resected. Fat removal in this area should also be conservative as the hollow above the medial canthus that is aesthetically pleasing in the Caucasian eye may not be pleasing in the Oriental eye.

Skin, muscle, and fat excision should be performed in both lids prior to placement of the fixation sutures. In order to encourage symmetry, the fixation sutures should be placed sequentially in each lid while the patient's eyes are opening and closing in order to assess symmetry. If there is any doubt about the height and depth of the fold desired by each patient, the surgeon should be conservative. Although the lid can be revised at a later time if the patient desires additional westernization, restoration of Oriental characteristics in a westernized lid is difficult, if not impossible.

COMPLICATIONS

Complications associated with all blepharoplasty procedures (bleeding, hematoma, scar formation, milia, etc.) may follow blepharoplasty in the Oriental eyelid. Complications specific to Oriental blepharoplasty include asymmetry of the eyelids, loss of the lidfold, and scar formation in the medial canthal area.

Because of differential swelling of the eyelids as well as the slight degree of ptosis that may temporarily follow supra tarsal fixation procedures, slight asymmetry in the early postoperative period is very common following Oriental blepharoplasty. Although many patients are concerned about such minor asymmetry, the surgeon should be firm in refusing to consider revision before 3 months as most minor asymmetries will spontaneously resolve within this period. Occasionally more marked lid asymmetry deserves earlier correction. In general, asymmetry is more common in patients with preoperative asymmetry of the eyebrows.

Loss of the lid fold may occur following inaccurate fixation, suture placement, or premature removal of fixation sutures. It may also occur if the fixation sutures are displaced secondary to excessive swelling or hematoma. Revision surgery is necessary in such cases. Extreme caution is advised in such cases in order to avoid damage to the levator complex.

Hypertrophic scarring in the medial canthal region is common, particularly in patients who have skin excision in this area to produce westernization of the lid. Scarring commonly follows attempts to modify the epicanthal fold by Z-plasty or other maneuvers. Most such scars resolve spontaneously in 6–9 months. In some cases scar maturation may be accelerated by judicious use of intralesional steroids.

DISCUSSION

There are preoperative considerations in blepharoplasty for Orientals. Variations in the level of the superior palpebral fold and the depth of the palpebral sulcus result in significant differences in the appearance of the upper eyelid. As both of these variables can be controlled by modifications in surgical technique, careful preoperative evaluation of each prospective candidate is mandatory in planning the double eyelid operation. Many patients desire only creation of a palpebral fold and wish to retain the other characteristics of the Oriental eyelid, whereas others prefer "westernization." The patient should be allowed to study pre- and postoperative photographs of various double-lid procedures in order to select the type of eyelid transformation desired.

As in all blepharoplasty evaluations, asymmetry in brow position, palpebral fissure widths, and other considerations should be pointed out to the patient preoperatively. Ophthalmologic evaluation pertinent to standard blepharoplasty is likewise important in evaluating the patient requesting the double eyelid operation.

There is some controversy regarding the suture technique versus standard surgical procedure. Although the suture technique offers the advantage of speed, convenience, and the avoidance of a healing wound, the fold created by this technique is often temporary. Proponents of this procedure, however, point out that it is easily repeated should the fold disappear. This procedure does not allow removal of the excess skin and fat that is present in many Oriental eyelids and does not allow modification of the epicanthal fold. Moreover, suture marks are often present for prolonged periods of time, and the amount of tension on the suture necessary to crush tissue and produce an adhesion is often difficult to determine.

There is also controversy concerning the application of permanent fixation sutures versus skin sutures. Many surgeons feel that in order to ensure permanence of the fold, the dermis should be fixed to the superior tarsal border with buried sutures of nonabsorbable material (see Figure 3-11). Experience, however, has shown that if skin sutures incorporating this fixation are left in place for 7 days, the fold remains permanent. Buried fixation sutures are often palpable beneath the thin eyelid skin and occasionally produce localized inflammation and extrusion.

Regarding fixation of the pretarsal dermis versus orbicularis oculi, although many surgeons advocate fixation of the dermis per se to the superior tarsal margin or levator aponeurosis, fixation of the orbicularis oculi line immediately beneath the pretarsal dermis produces a softer, more natural fold and encourages more satisfactory approximation of skin edges.

REFERENCES

1. Boo-chai K.: Plastic Construction of the Superior Palpebral Fold. *Plast. Reconstr. Surg.*, 31:74–78, 1963.
2. Fernandez L. R.: Double Eyelid Operation in the Oriental in Hawaii. *Plast. Reconstr. Surg.*, 25:257–264, 1960.
3. McCurdy J. A., Jr.: Westernization of the Oriental Eyelid. *Otolaryngol. Head. Neck. Surg.* 90:142–145, 1982.
4. Millard D. R.: The Oriental Eyelid and its Surgical Revision. *Am. J. Ophthalmol.* 66:646–649, 1964.
5. Pang H. G.: Surgical Formation of the Upper Lid. *Arch. Ophthalmol.* 63:783–784, 1961.

4
Rejuvenation of the Forehead and Brow

Rejuvenation of the forehead and brow areas has involved many different techniques, such as direct excision, nerve lysis, prehairline excision, posthairline excision, chemical peel, silicone or collagen augmentation, muscle excision, and any combination thereof.

The coronal lift provides the most versatile and satisfactory method for eliminating the vagaries of aging seen in the upper third of the face, while at the same time providing effective camouflaging of the incision.

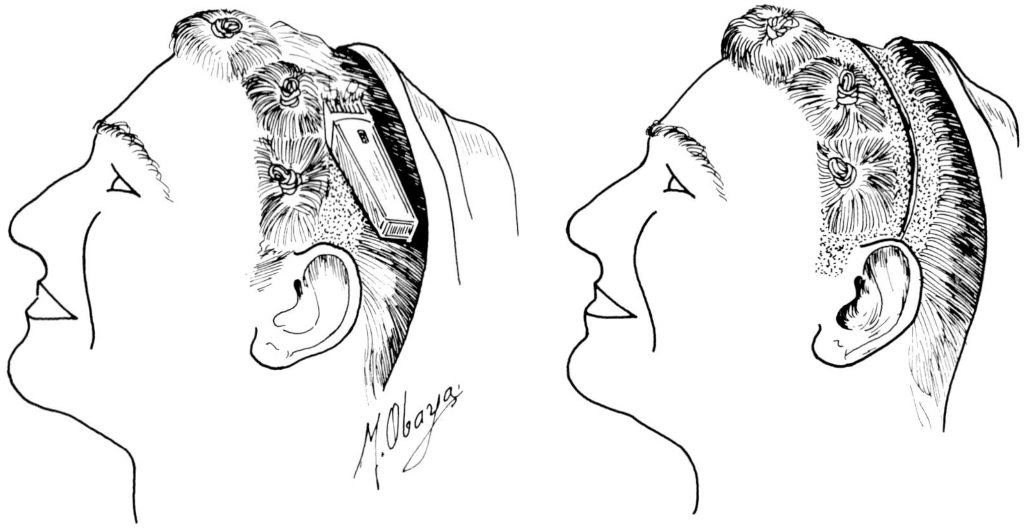

Figure 4-1

TECHNIQUE

CORONAL LIFT

The incision begins at the top of the auricle and runs across the top of the head to the opposite auricle as shown in Figure 4-1. A $\frac{3}{4}$-inch portable electric hair trimmer not only removes the hair from the incision, but provides a premeasured guide to subsequent scalp excision at the time of closure. The hair anterior to the incision is divided into locks and secured with rubber bands.

The rhytids of the frontalis, corrugator, and procerus muscles are marked in methylene blue (Figure 4-2). Do not extend the markings of the frontalis lines lateral to the pupil of each eye to avoid injury to the frontal branch of the facial nerve. The extent of undermining is marked to identify the boundaries for anesthetic infiltration.

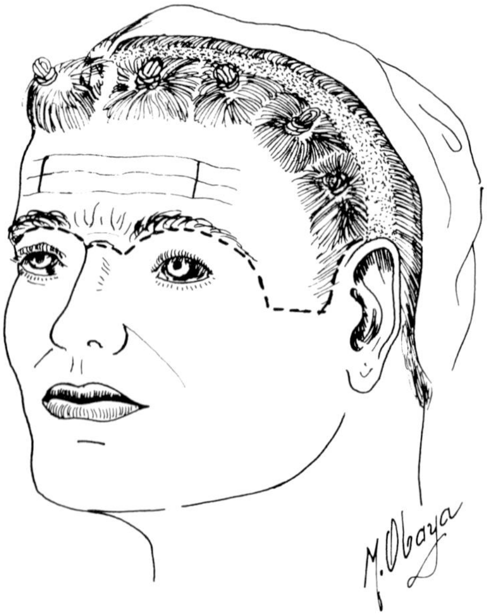

Figure 4-2

Nerve block anesthesia of the forehead is obtained by infiltrating the incision and periphery of undermining with 1% lidocaine (Xylocaine) with 1 : 100,000 epinephrine (Adrenalin), using a 27-gauge needle and a 10-ml Luer lock syringe (Figure 4-3). The area to be undermined is anesthetized with 0.5% bupivacaine (Marcaine) with 1 : 200,000 Adrenalin by means of a 22-gauge spinal needle. Even though the Xylocaine provides a peripheral nerve block to the flap, there are perforating sensory fibers from the periosteum that need to be anesthetized with the Marcaine.

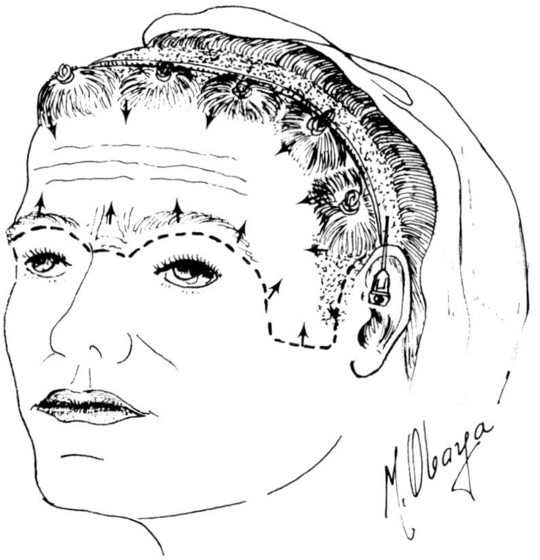

Figure 4-3

The face and scalp are prepped with povidone iodine and the head drape is secured to the scalp with wide staples. By placing the towel in the trimmed area and pulling it posteriorly (Figure 4-4), the hair roots are exposed and the staples placed. The operative field is now isolated in a quick, efficient manner.

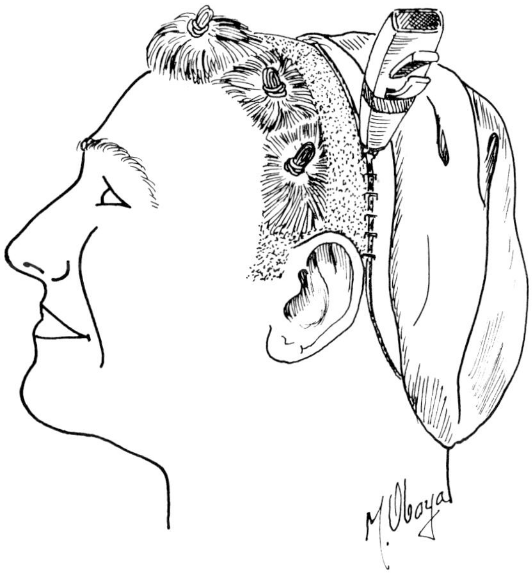

Figure 4-4

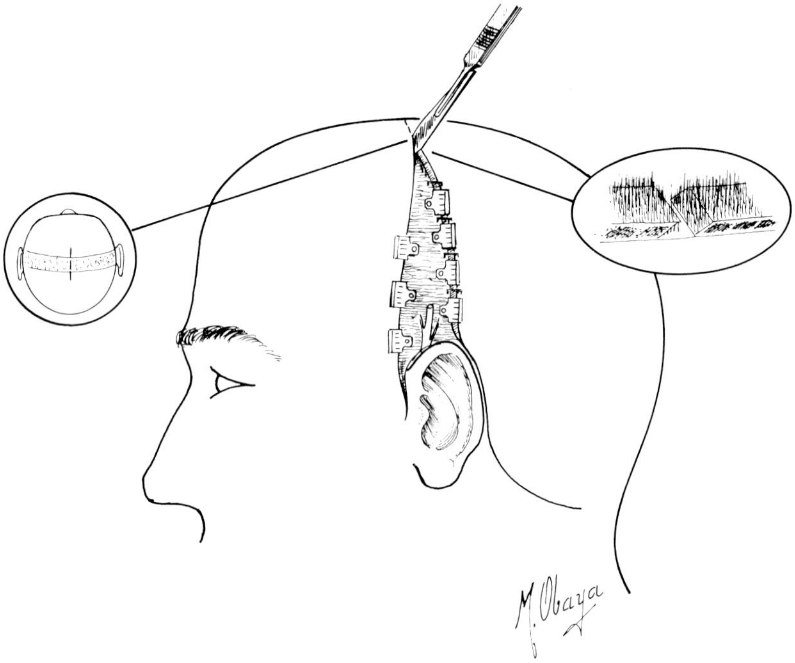

Figure 4-5

The midline of the flap is scored with the scalpel to facilitate closure before beginning the coronal incision. The scalp incision is beveled parallel to the hair follicles (Figure 4-5). Once the complete incision is made and carried down to the subaponeurotic plane, wide paper holders are quickly placed on both sides of the incision to minimize bleeding. The superifical temporal artery, vein, and associated branches are usually transected above the auricle and are cauterized.

A filmy, fibrous layer separates the periosteum from the aponeurosis (a tendon stretching between the frontalis and occipitalis muscles), which identifies the correct layer of undermining (Figure 4-6). Broad sweeping motions with a scalpel or scissor dissection will quickly elevate the initial two-thirds of the flap, thus exposing each temporalis fascia laterally. As the supraorbital rims are approached, the forehead becomes more adherent to the periosteum and the flap is turned on itself over the eyes.

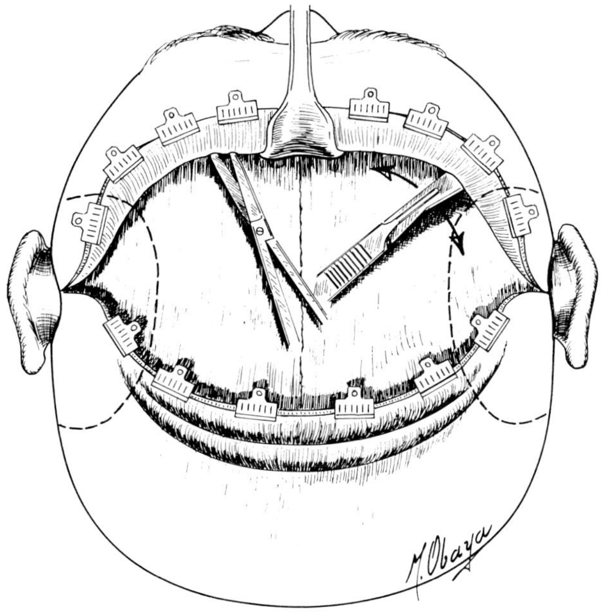

Figure 4-6

By bluntly dissecting in the midline over the glabella and cautiously spreading parallel to the fibers of the supratrochlear and supraorbital nerves (as the dissection is extended laterally) as shown in Figure 4-7, preservation of these neurovascular bundles is achieved.

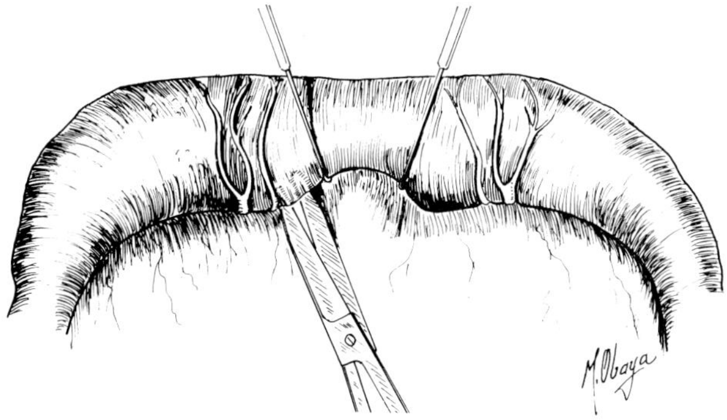

Figure 4-7

An alternative technique is to grasp the flap in one hand while the thumb elevates and subsequently peels the flap inferiorly as the fibrous connections to the periosteum are cut behind the thumb (Figure 4-8). This maneuver frees the brow from its periosteal attachments on the orbital rim. Once orbital fat is visualized, a satisfactory elevation has been achieved. As this elevation goes from lateral to medial, the supraorbital and supratrochlear nerves are identified and preserved.

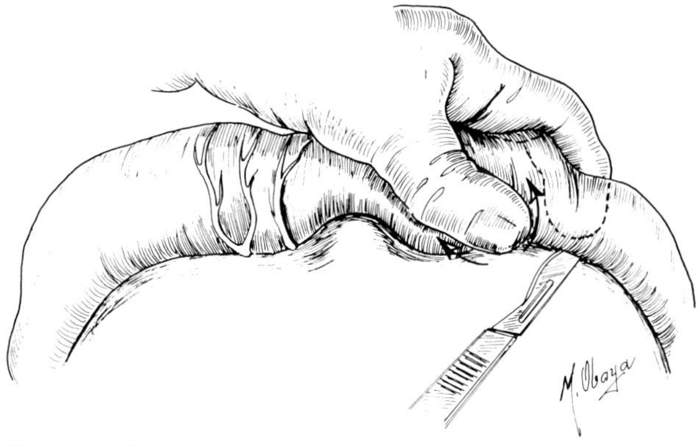

Figure 4-8

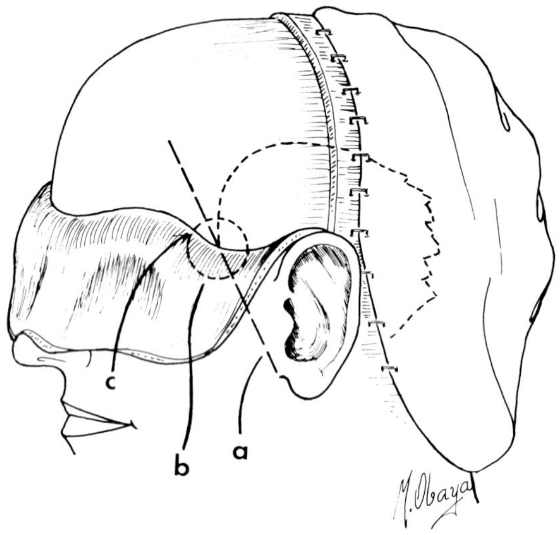

Figure 4-9

As shown in Figure 4-9, the forehead flap is bluntly undermined to the superior border of the zygomatic arch (b). Elevation more inferiorly at this level runs the risk of damaging the temporal branch of the facial nerve (a). The transition zone (c) over the zygomatic arch just anterior to the hairline finds the nerve coming from a deep to more superficial level.

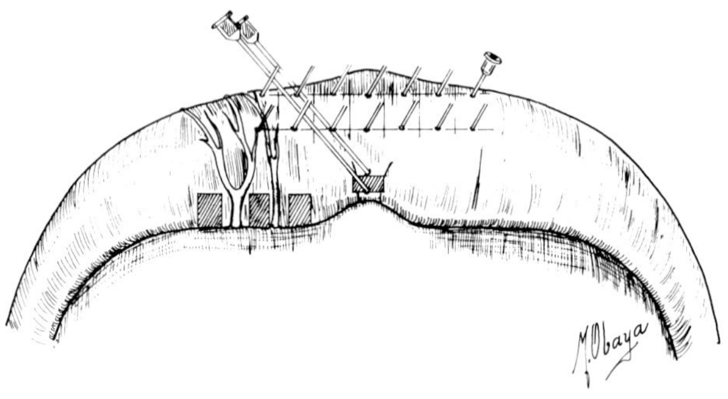

Figure 4-10

Muscle excision and scarification is now done to remove the vertical and horizontal rhytids (Figure 4-10). Placement of 25-gauge needles through the flap along each rhytid of concern is a safe technique for identification of the respective frontalis, corrugator, and procerus muscles. The corrugator muscle is cauterized or excised between the neurovascular bundles. The procerus is sectioned in the midline. The frontalis muscle is scarified with electrocoagulation or sharp sectioning. By connecting the needle point horizontally and vertically, the effective contraction of the frontalis muscle is reduced.

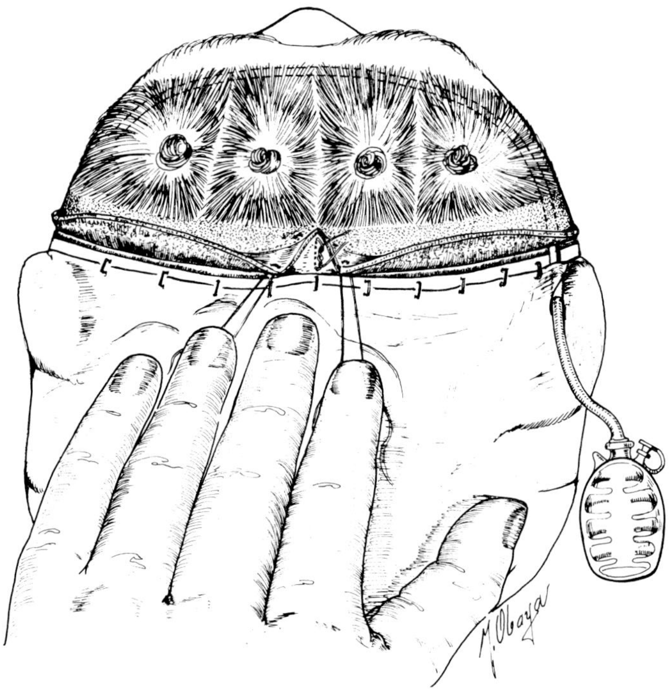

Figure 4-11

A flat Jackson-Pratt drain is placed along the supraorbital margin and brought out a separate stab wound (Figure 4-11). The forehead flap is repositioned and the midline (marked previously) is identified, and a skin splitting incision made. A 3-0 Dexon suture is placed subcutaneously at this point. (Remember to push forward on the posterior flap to effect an adequate excision of tissue). The excision of scalp is made parallel to the hair follicles to preserve the roots.

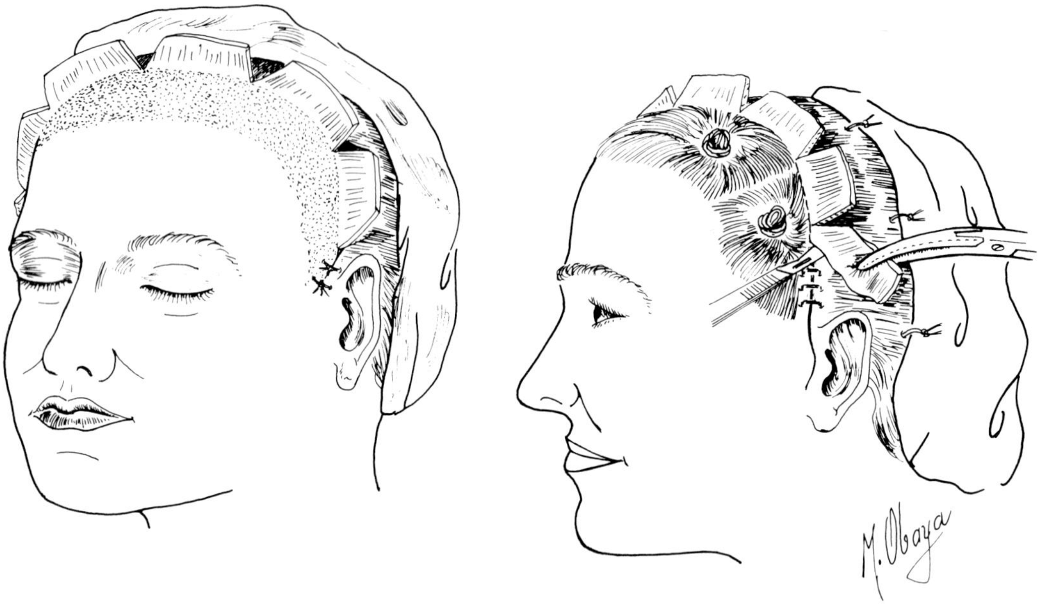

Figure 4-12

As the forehead flap is advanced anteroposteriorly, multiple skin splitting incisions are made and 3-0 Dexon subcutaneous sutures are placed through the galea (Figure 4-12). The redundant scalp is excised between these incisions and the wound closed with staples after hemostasis is obtained following removal of the paper clips. (The Dexon suture subcutaneously reduces the tension on the incision for at least 4 weeks, thereby reducing the possibility of a wide scar forming after the staples are removed.)

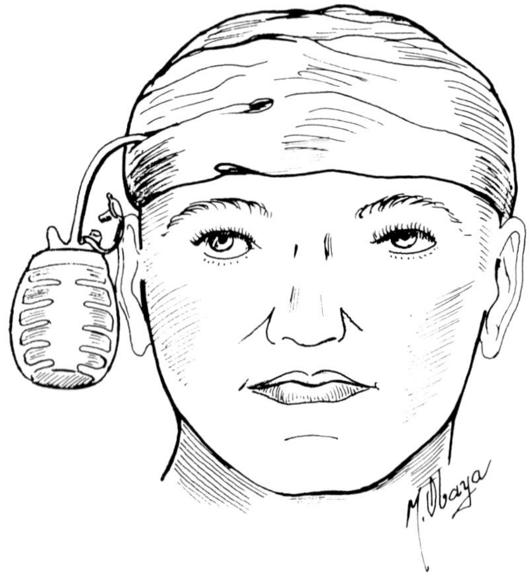

Figure 4-13

Antibiotic ointment is placed on the incision and a bulky dressing applied that is changed the next day (Figure 4-13). The drain is removed the first or second day after surgery.

Incisions

Several variations on the incision have been proposed when the forehead lift is done with the face-lift. By leaving an island of scalp between the incisions, the levels of undermining are kept separate (Figure 4-14). If any bleeding occurs postoperatively, it is "compartmentalized" and will not disrupt the other undermined areas.

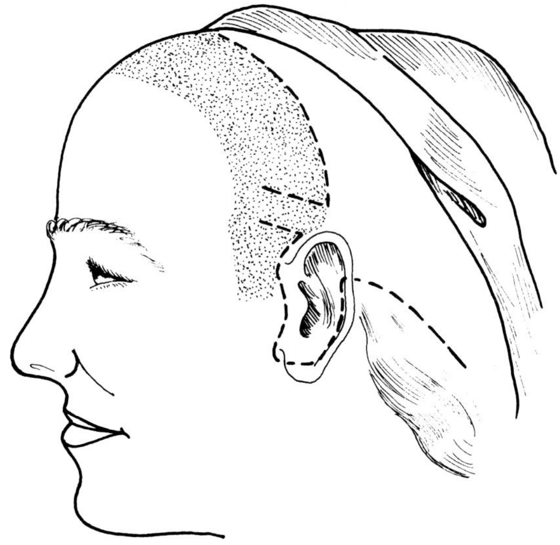

Figure 4-14

A limited temporal lift could conceivably be done through a three-fourths temporal incision as marked, but visualization, flap advancement, and long-term lasting results are compromised (Figure 4-15).

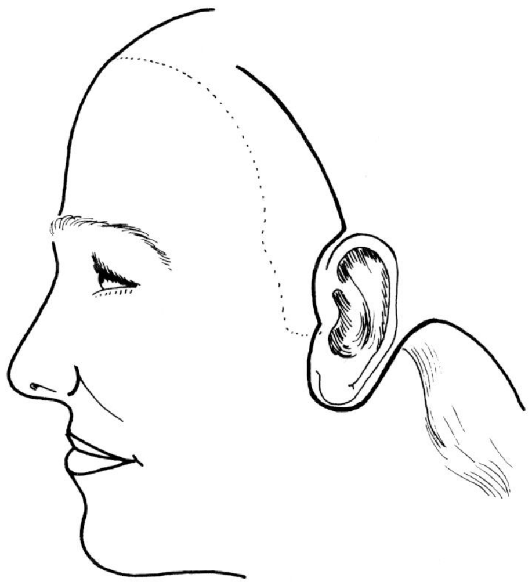

Figure 4-15

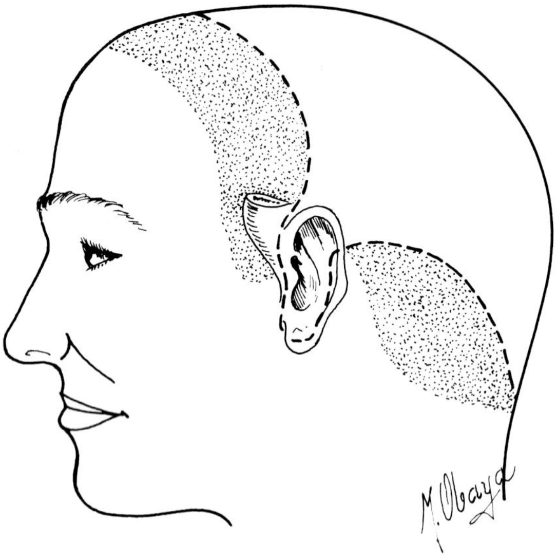

Figure 4-16

The facelift is performed first, leaving the redundant temporal skin flap "bunched up" at the root of the auricle (Figure 4-16). The excess is distributed when the forehead lift is done. The dissection of the. myeloplasty is in the subcutaneous layer on top of the subcutaneous musculoaponeurotic system (SMAS), while the forehead is undermined in the subaponeurotic layer. An island of tissue at the level of the zygomatic arch provides a transition zone from the forehead to the face for perservation of the temporal branch of the facial nerve.

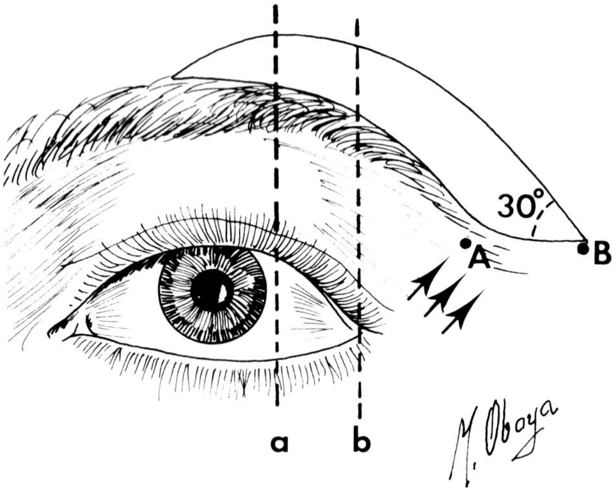

Figure 4-17

DIRECT BROW LIFT

With the patient in a sitting position (to appreciate the effect of gravity on the ptotic brow), the incision is marked over the lateral two-thirds of the eyebrow as shown in Figure 4-17. The high point of the brow is located between the lateral limbus (a) and the lateral canthus (b). Since the superior limb of the incision is the upper margin of the new eyebrow, it is marked on the forehead where the new browline is to lie. The lower incision is placed just inside the first line of hair follicles and runs laterally to meet the superior incision at a 30° angle. By extending the incision beyond the edge of the eyebrow (AB), the hooding of the lateral orbit will be corrected.

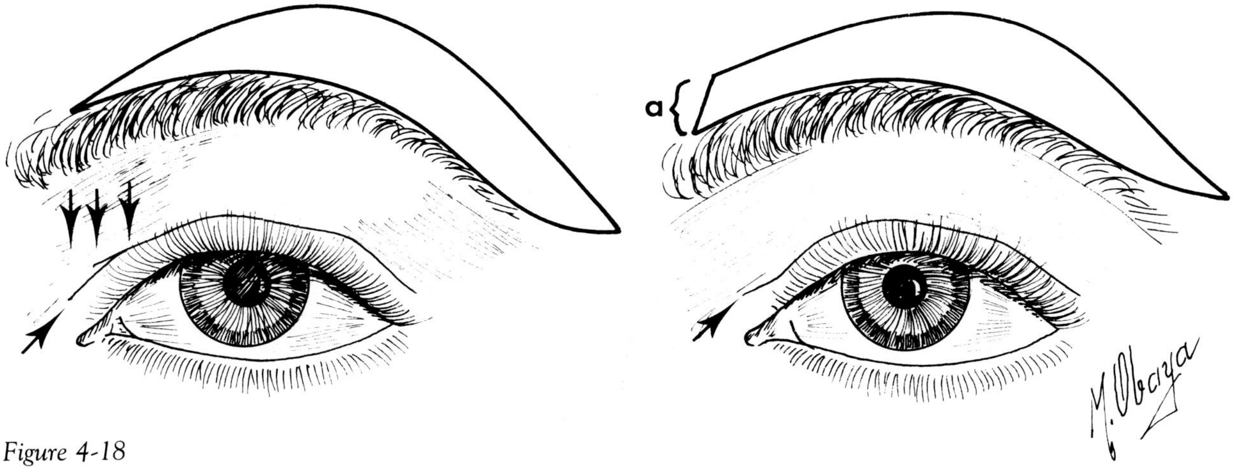

Figure 4-18

If the medial third of the eyebrow is ptotic, the incision is extended medially. Depending on the amount of elevation required, more skin (point a in Figure 4-18) may be excised medially, realizing that glabellar scarring becomes more of a problem as the amount of skin removed is increased.

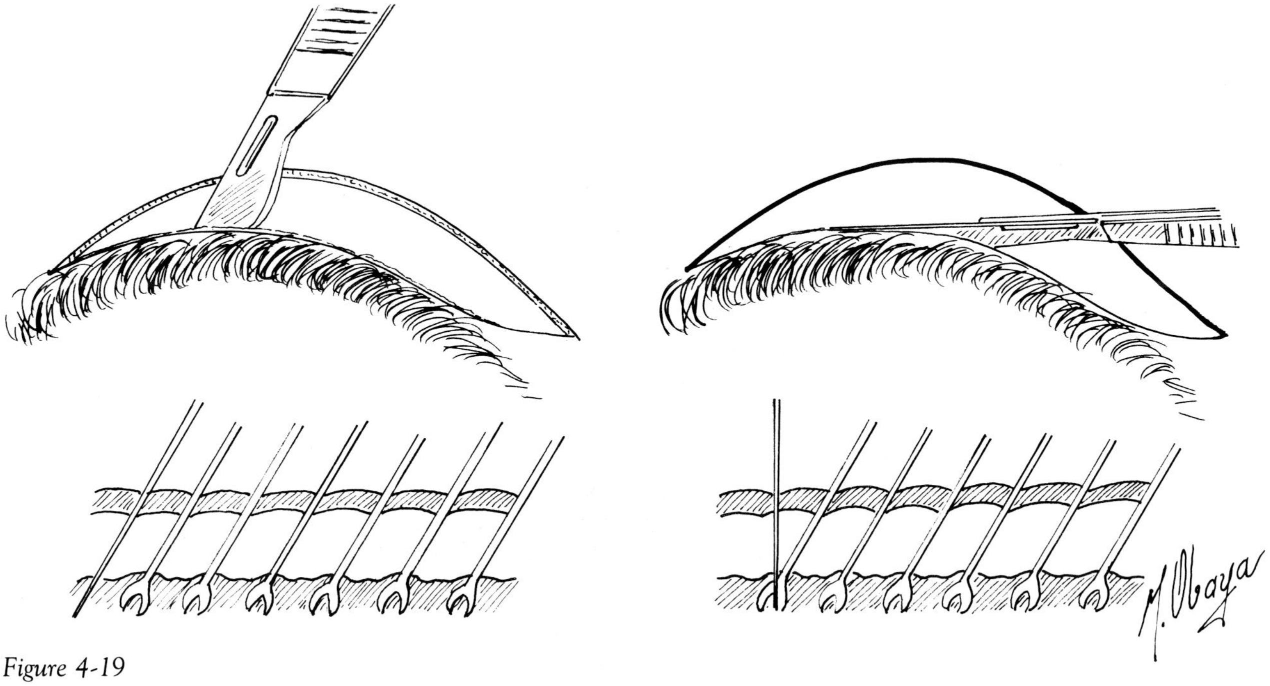

Figure 4-19

The inferior incision is beveled to run parallel to hair growth and prevent damage to the hair follicles. The upper incision is similarly beveled for closure (Figure 4-19).

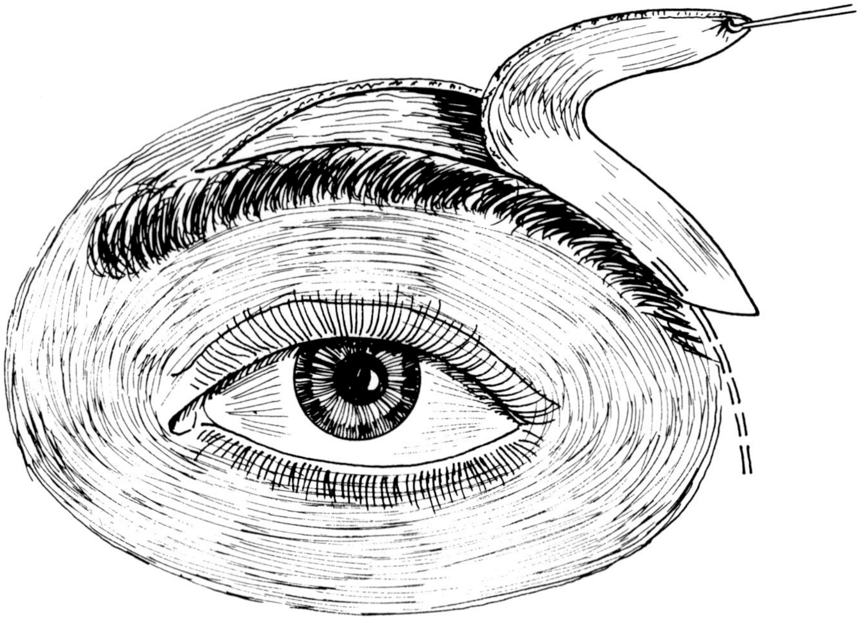

Figure 4-20

The skin is resected above the frontalis and orbicularis oculi muscles. The frontal branch of the facial nerve will not be injured if dissection is maintained superficial to these muscles (Figure 4-20).

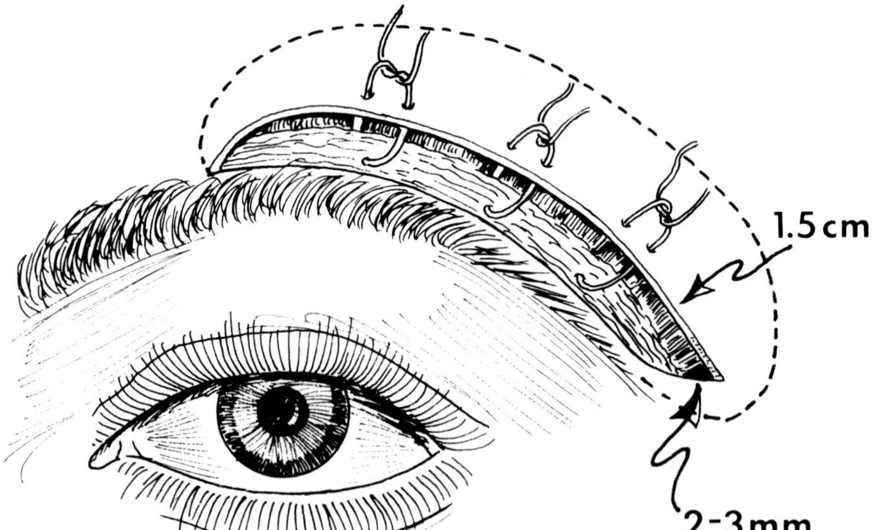

Figure 4-21

The upper skin margin is undermined 1.5 cm while the lower margin is separated from the orbicularis oculi by only 2–3 mm (Figure 4-21).

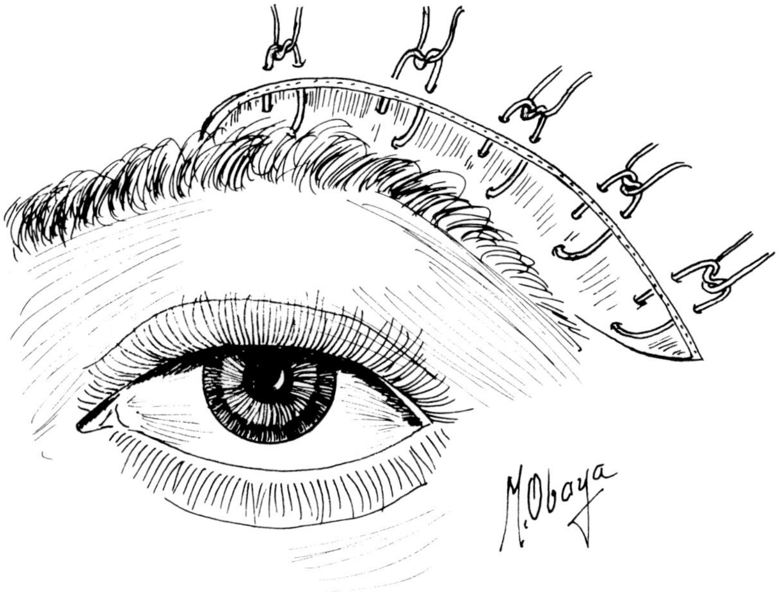

Figure 4-22

The first buried suture is placed at the high point of the brow. The remaining sutures (5-0 Supramed) are placed in such a manner that the wound edges are almost touching (Figure 4-22).

The wound is closed with interrupted vertical mattress sutures to accentuate the eversion of the skin edges. Steristrips and ointment are placed across the incision (Figure 4-23).

On postoperative day 3 or 4, the sutures are removed and the wound retaped. Makeup may be worn after 10 days. In approximately 15 percent of patients, spot dermabrading of the incision is necessary at 6 months to camouflage the postoperative scar.

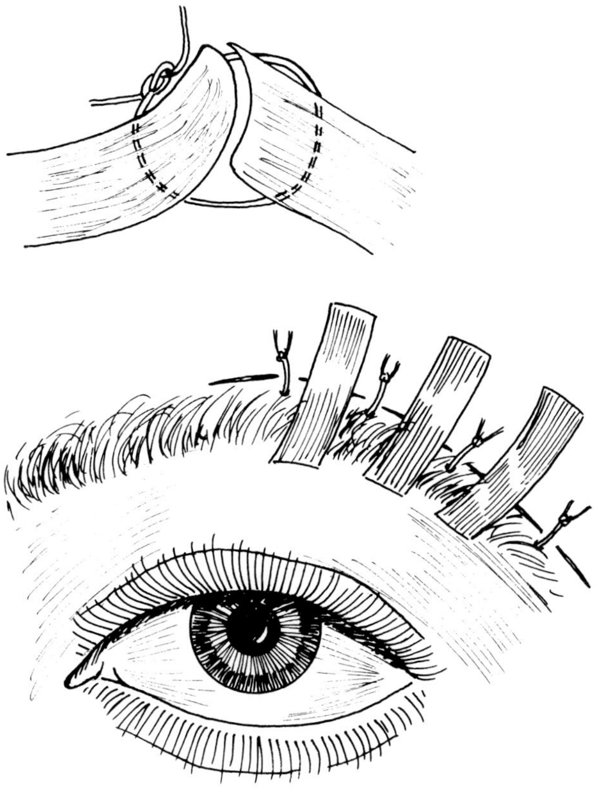

Figure 4-23

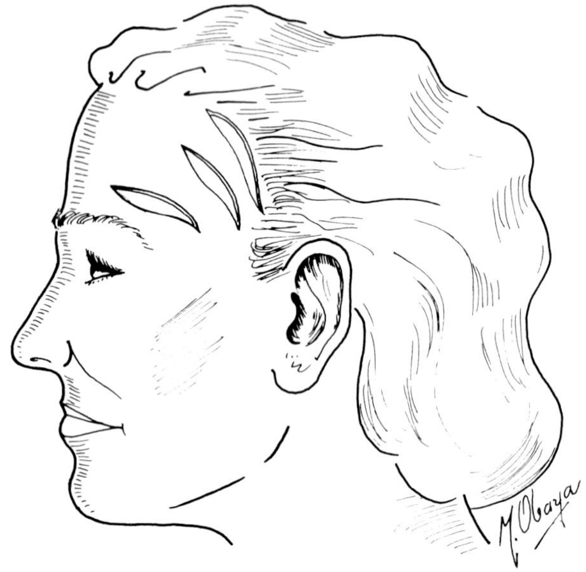
Figure 4-24

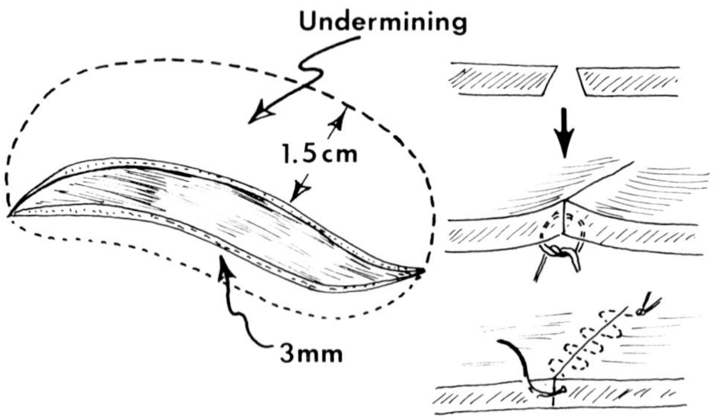

Figure 4-25

DIRECT BROW LIFT WITH MIDTEMPORAL OR HIGH TEMPORAL INCISIONS

When the patient has persistent deep skin rhytids in the lateral temporal area, simple skin excision is done using this natural crease for camouflaging (Figure 4-24). The superior limb of the incision is placed in the natural skin crease. An ellipse of skin is marked to conform to the relaxed skin tension lines of the forehead. A high hairline incision may also be used, but the scar may become visible as the hairline recedes or hair density decreases.

The wound edges are beveled to allow eversion in closure (Figure 4-25). The skin is excised lateral to the frontalis muscle as before. After undermining, the frontalis is plicated to elevate the ptotic brow. The edges are everted using 5-0 clear nylon and the wound closed with a running 6-0 black nylon.

The direct midforehead lift in selected individuals with prominent horizontal rhytids and a high hairline also provide a technique for brow lifting (Figure 4-26). Meticulous closure with eversion of the skin edges is essential for producing the most acceptable cosmetic scar postoperatively.

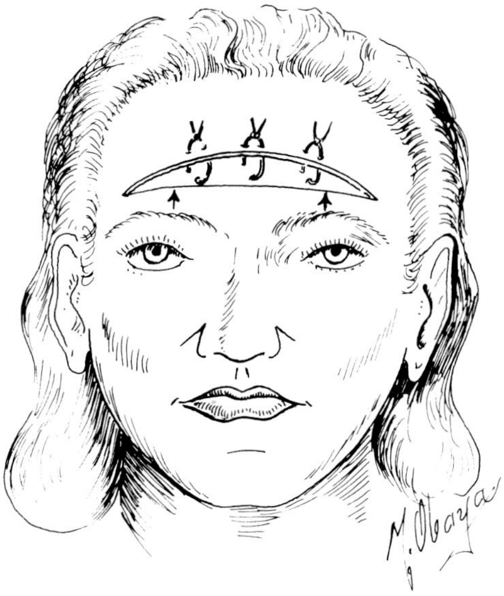

Figure 4-26

DISCUSSION

The coronal lift is contraindicated in patients with a high hairline, those whose subsequent hair loss will likely expose the incision (see male pattern baldness) and those with sparse hair growth. The different direct approaches to the forehead and brow leaves potentially visible scars. Meticulous closure notwithstanding, the patient must understand and accept this sequelae, or the surgeon will be bothered by a disgruntled patient.

The local excisions are much simpler operations for brow pexis compared to the versatile coronal lift, which can correct all forehead abnormalities. However, obtaining symmetry of both eyebrows and peculiar sculpturing of the lateral third of the brow from injudicious skin excision make the direct excision technique more susceptible to patient dissatisfaction.

Complications following forehead and brow rejuvenation surgery include sensory changes, such as temporary anesthesia of the forehead due to stretching of the supraorbital and supratrochlear nerves. This is to be expected, however, and will gradually resolve over 3–6 months. Permanent numbness in the vertex is not uncommon because the coronal incision divides the sensory nerves. Preoperative counseling prepares the patient for this sequelae in case it does not gradually resolve to the patient's expectations. Hyperesthesia and occipital pain in the immediate postoperative period is a common complaint that may require potent analgesics for 3–5 days. Motor nerve changes may also result. Transient weakness in the frontal branch may occur if the nerve is stretched. By limiting elevation of the flap to blunt dissection as the zygomatic arch is approached, cutting of the nerve will not occur. Similarly, crosshatching of the frontalis muscle between the pupils as illustrated in Figure 4-2 will also prevent injury to the frontal nerve.

Bleeding and edema are additional possible side effects. Occasional marked edema and ecchymoses of the periorbital area will develop postoperatively. Placement of closed suction drains and a firm bulky dressing will remove the serious fluid and tamponade any potential bleeding. If a concommitant blepharoplasty has been done, however, careful and close monitoring of the patient for increasing orbital pain, loss of vision, and other side effects must be treated with appropriate drainage procedures. For the most part, hematoma formation is extremely rare.

Scarring and hair loss may also occur. Gradual widening of the coronal incision as a result of overzealous scalp excision and closure of the wound under excessive tension is best treated with secondary excision and closure at least 12 months after surgery. Occasionally "follicular shock" with transient hair thinning gradually resolves with new hair growth. During this interval of several months, patient reassurance is necessary. Wide forehead scars from direct excision techniques may be dermabraided at 6 months and, if depressed, augmented with collagen subdermally.

REFERENCES

1. Johnson, M. Jr., Anderson, J. R., and Katz, R. B.: The Brow Lift—1978. *Arch. Otolaryngol.*, 105:124–126, 1979.
2. Kaye, B. L.: The Forehead Lift: A Useful Adjunct to Face Lift and Blepharoplasty. *Plast. Reconst. Surg.*, 60:161, 1977.
3. Liebman, E. P., Webster, R. C., Berger, A. S., *et al.*: The Frontalis Nerve in the Temporal Brow Lift. *Arch. Otolaryngol.*, 108:232–235, 1982.
4. Pitanguy, I.: Indications for and Treatment of Frontal and Glabellar Wrinkles in an Analysis of 3,404 Consecutive Cases of Rhytidectomy. *Plast. Reconst. Surg.*, 67:157–166, 1981.

5

Septorhinoplasty

Charles E. Clark

Certain key aspects of the art of rhinoplasty are outside the scope of a surgical atlas. However, they are key to a successful outcome and future patient referrals.

The personality of the patient must be evaluated and a good working patient–physician relationship developed. A psychological profile or consult is rarely indicated but is obtained when indicated. If good communication is not developed, both the patient and the physician are in for a long and unhappy experience—regardless of surgical results. A second opinion is recommended.

The most important nonsurgical time is that of preoperative analysis and continuing postoperative follow-up and review of slides. Four standard photographs are taken of all of the author's patients: a full face view, a base view, and right and left profiles. Occasionally a smiling profile and an oblique view are added. One set is in color slides, and the other set is in black and white 5 × 7-inch prints. Two prints of each view are made. These prints are studied, and then by placing them face down on a back-lighted surface (i.e., x-ray viewbox), it is possible to trace on the back of them and sketch potential changes. This is time well spent, for if one takes off too much hump with a pencil or overrotates a tip, it is much easier to repair with an eraser! It is an invaluable learning experience and greatly increases one's experience with each procedure.

The color slides are ideally retaken at 6 weeks, 3 months, and 1 year postoperative. Each time they are loaded in carousels, with the preoperative views in one and the postoperative views in a second. Then at leisure, and in privacy, they are simultaneously projected with the photocopied operative note in hand. This is the single greatest learning experience in rhinoplasty surgery.

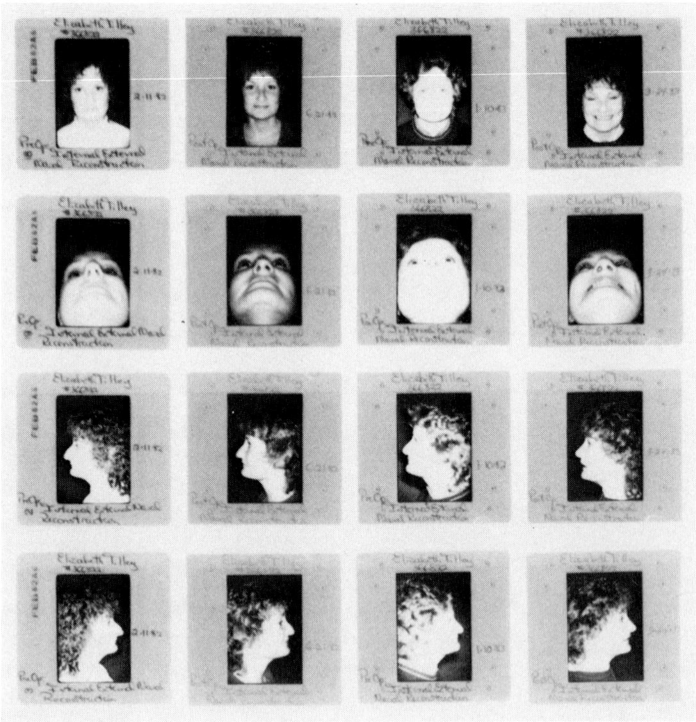

Figure 5-1A

Figure 5-1 A and B shows a set of standard photographs. The black-and-white prints (Figure 5-1B) are in duplicates to allow preoperative sketching of the same view. The plastic slide holder (Figure 5-1A) is well suited for slide storage in a ring binder.

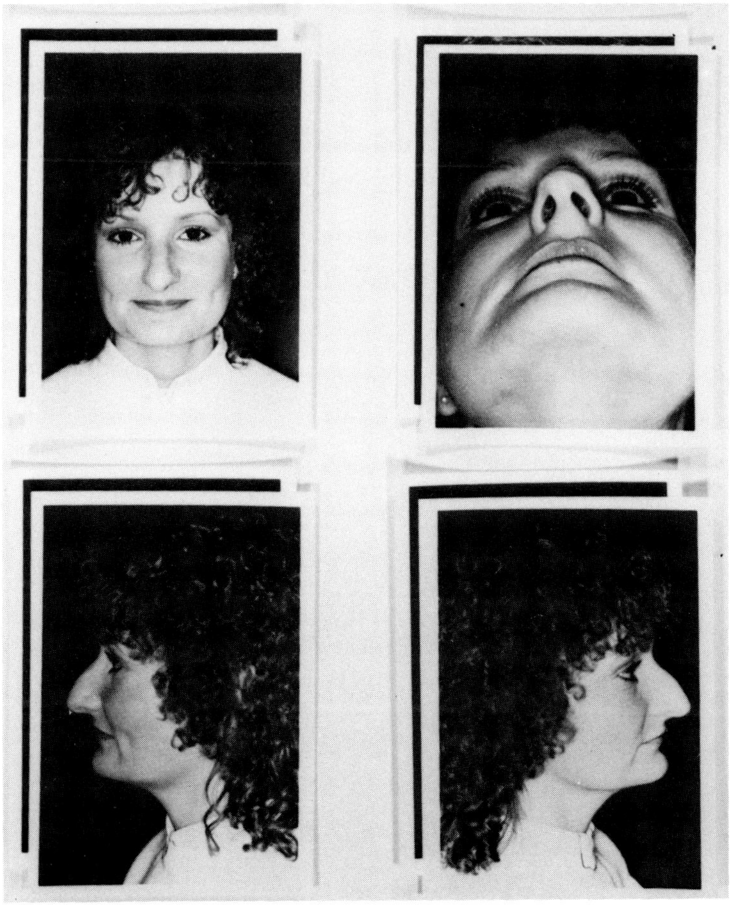

Figure 5-1B

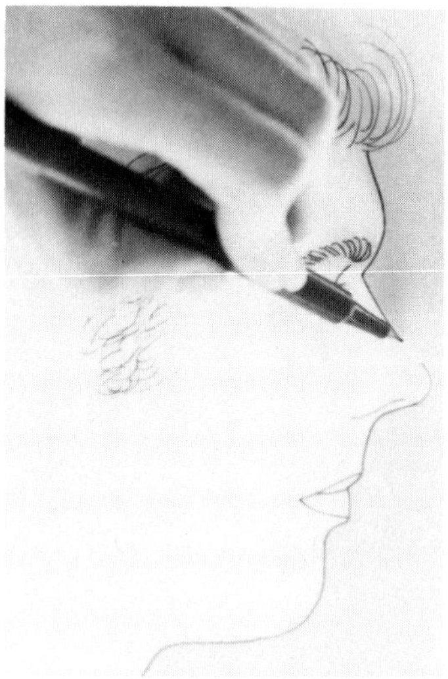

Figure 5-2

The prints should be developed on a paper that will allow pencil tracings and erasing. Waxed papers are poorly suited for this purpose. Another alternative is to use a high-quality vellum tracing paper. Figure 5-2 is a backlite 5 × 7-inch print being sketched.

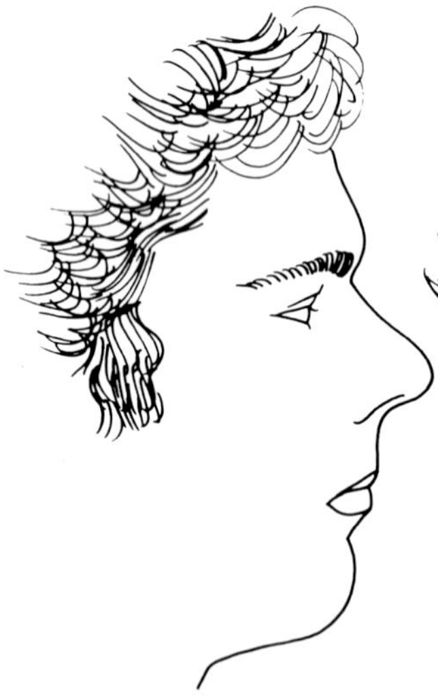

Figure 5-3

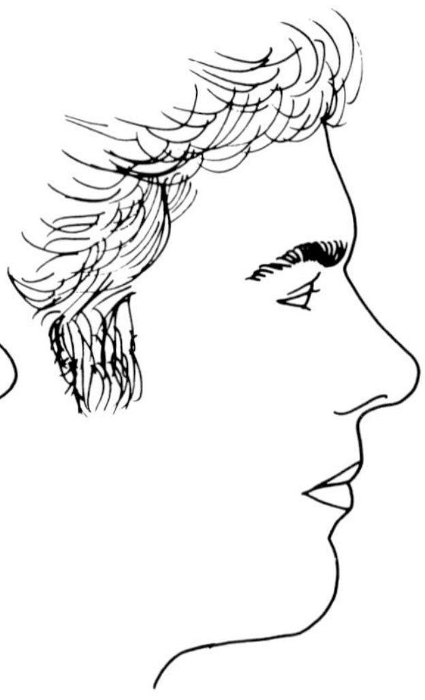

Figure 5-4

Figure 5-3 is the preoperative sketch, and Figure 5-4 is the sketch analysis to be discussed with the patient preoperatively. In this particular instance Figure 5-4 is also the 1-year postoperative tracing.

Figures 5-5–5-13 are examples of a stepwise evaluation of a preoperative plan. Figure 5-5 shows the preoperative profile.

Figures 5-6–5-13 show the proposed postoperative profiles, and the rhinoplasty shown in Figure 5-6 is used throughout this group of sketches. The postoperative alternatives are illustrated as follows:

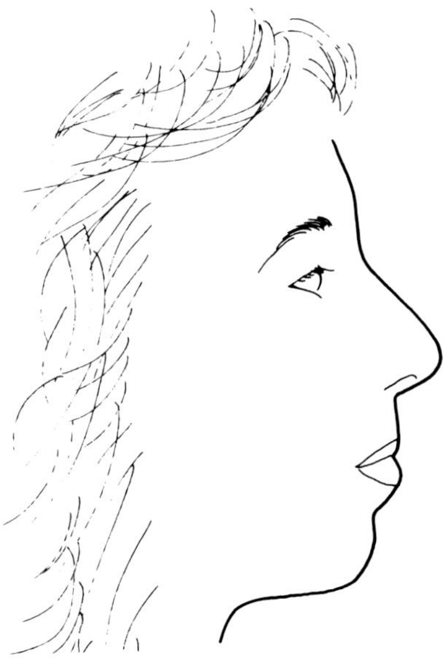

Figure 5-5

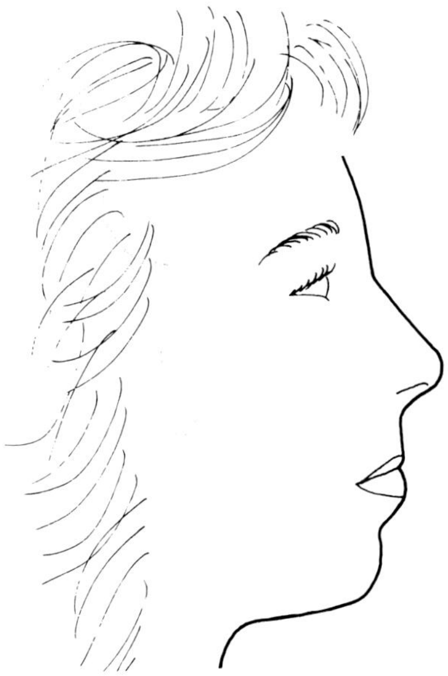

Figure 5-6

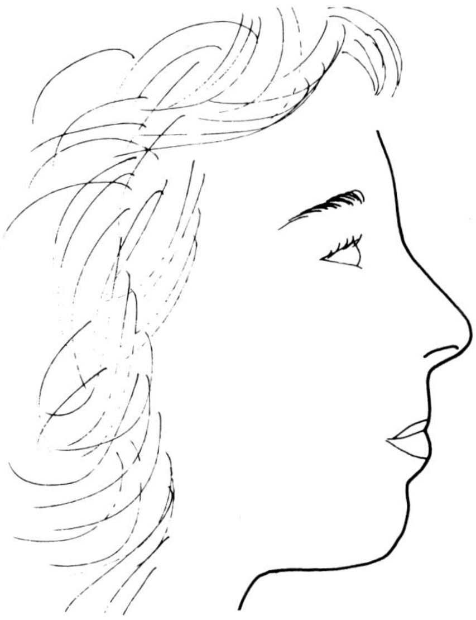

Figure 5-7

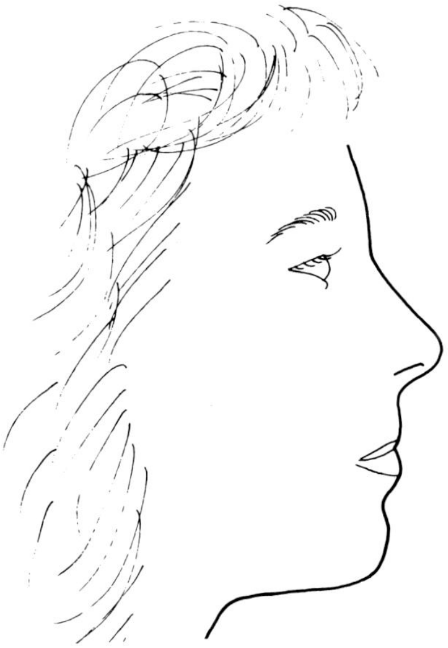

Figure 5-8

- Rhinoplasty with a small chin implant (Figure 5-7)
- Rhinoplasty with a larger chin implant (Figure 5-8)

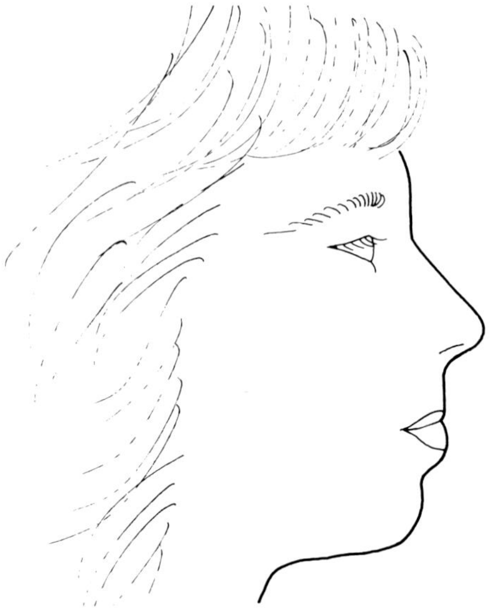

Figure 5-9

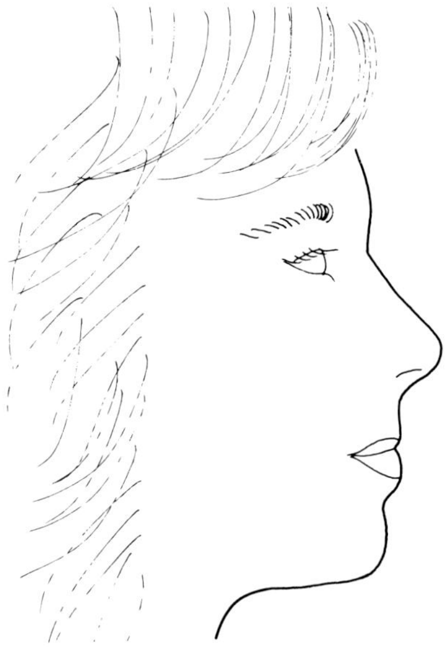

Figure 5-10

- Rhinoplasty with a deepened nasofrontal angle (Figure 5-9)
- Rhinoplasty with a deepened nasofrontal angle and a small chin implant (Figure 5-10)

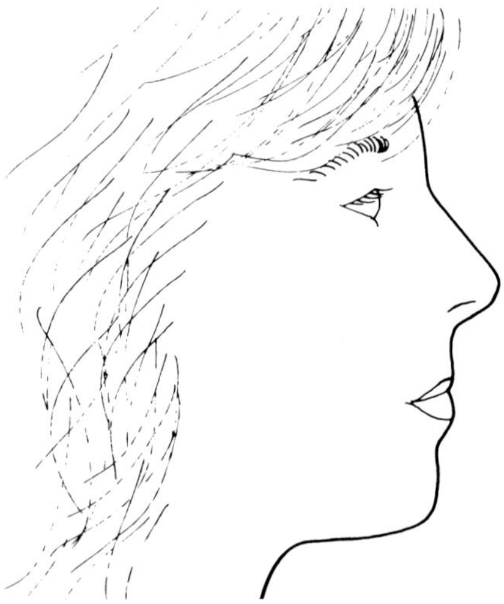

Figure 5-11

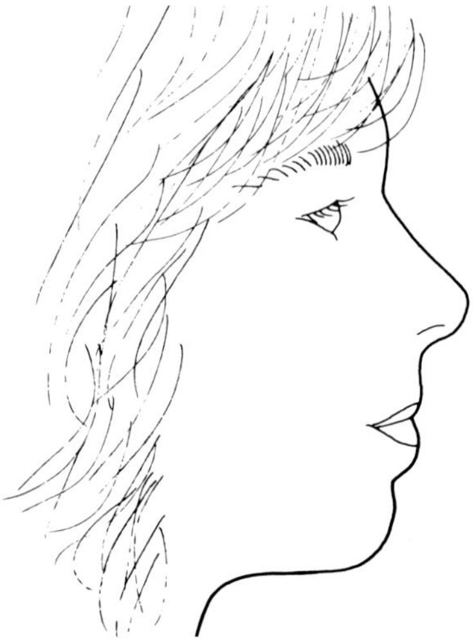

Figure 5-12

- Rhinoplasty with a larger chin implant and a new hairstyle with bangs (Figure 5-11)
- Rhinoplasty with a deepened nasofrontal angle, small chin implant, and a new hairstyle with bangs (Figure 5-12)

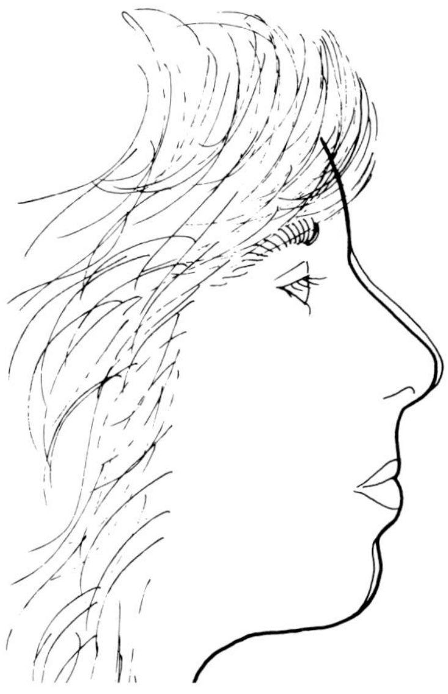

Figure 5-13

Observe the apparent change in the same basic rhinoplasty. The final illustration, Figure 5-13, is an overlaying of Figures 5-5 and 5-12 and shows the amount of surgery proposed. Note the relatively small reduction of the nose and nasofrontal angle needed with the small chin implant and hair styling change.

Detailed dictated operative notes are key for future review of results. These notes, combined with simultaneous projection of preoperative and postoperative slides, allow critical evaluation and future improvement. This on-going review provides the surgeon with invaluable insight into the rhinoplasty results. The projectors should be reversible so that constant comparison of the different views can be made at the time of review as each of many steps are compared. This will increase the surgeon's awareness of the changes between 6 weeks and 1 year or longer postoperative result. Figure 5-14 illustrates one method for setting up a review program.

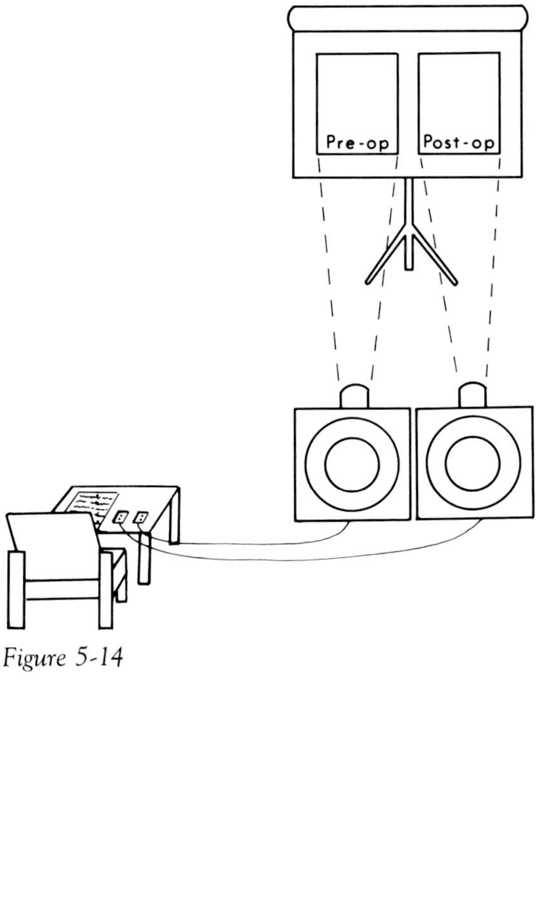

Figure 5-14

ANESTHESIA

Anesthesia starts with the surgeon's initial conversation with the patient, which should be relaxed and informative. When examining the patient, the surgeon's touch should be gentle, as this will set the tone for your future relationship. General discussions and photographs are taken the first visit. At the second visit, the black-and-white prints are reviewed as well as the sketches.

LOCAL

Local anesthesia is preferred, as it is safer and the patient's first postoperative day is much more comfortable. Also, there is generally less intraoperative bleeding.

Preoperative sedation for local anesthesia consists of:

- (Valium): 5–10 mg orally 90 minutes prior to surgery.
  - —Barbiturates [secobarbital sodium (Seconal), ethclorvynol (Placidyl), pentobarbital sodium (Nembutal)] may be used instead of Valium but has the disadvantage of causing a postoperative drug hangover in some patients.
  - —Barbiturates cause a greater degree of respiratory depression.
- Morphine: 5–10 mg (by weight) on call. Produces a euphoria not available with meperidine (Demerol).
- Promethazine (Phenergan): 25 mg (on call) is additive with morphine for analgesia and is a potent antiemetic.
- Glycopyrrolate (Robinul): 0.2–0.4 mg (by weight) on call is used in place of atropine or scopolamine as it does not cross the blood–brain barrier and prevents the hallucinatory or agitated effects sometimes seen with scopolamine.

Intraoperative sedation may also be given in certain cases. If the patient is still apprehensive after being greeted in the operating room or if after placing the cocaine pledgets internasally the patient is obviously still apprehensive, there are several intravenous (IV) medications available for further sedation.

- Valium: 2.5-mg increments up to 10 mg.
- Low-dose ketamine: 15–25 mg IV just prior to the infiltration of local will enhance analgesia and often provide amnesia of the infiltration. It also frequently alters the spacial relationships, so

that patients feel that they have been in the operating room for a very short time at the end of the case.

—The low dose is very important as it prevents hallucinations associated with higher doses.

—If the patient becomes agitated, 50 mg of Nembutal IV will work as a prompt sedative.

- Fentanyl 1–2 ml is a valuable alternative.

GENERAL

When not medically contraindicated, general anesthesia is a possible alternative for the extremely apprehensive patient. The topical and infiltrative anesthesia procedure is exactly the same as that described for the sedated patient. This is necessary to provide the needed visualization and hemostasis.

Topically Applied

For years cocaine has provided excellent anesthesia and vasoconstriction when applied topically to the mucous membranes of the nose. Multiple strengths have been used, and the "toxic dose" has been arbitrarily set at 250 mg to prevent seizures and reactions. Since the maximum dose is not known, careful monitoring during its use is mandatory.

A 5% cocaine solution in contact with the mucosa for 5 minutes will produce marked vasoconstriction and anesthesia. The following technique uses 4 ml of 5% cocaine well squeezed out on cotton pledgets. Four pledgets are formed. Bayonet forceps are used to place the cotton in the nose. Make sure that the first placement covers the anterior septum as well as the inferior turbinate. This is done so that subsequent instrumentation will be touching an already anesthetized portion of the septum. Then repeat this on the opposite side with the second pledget.

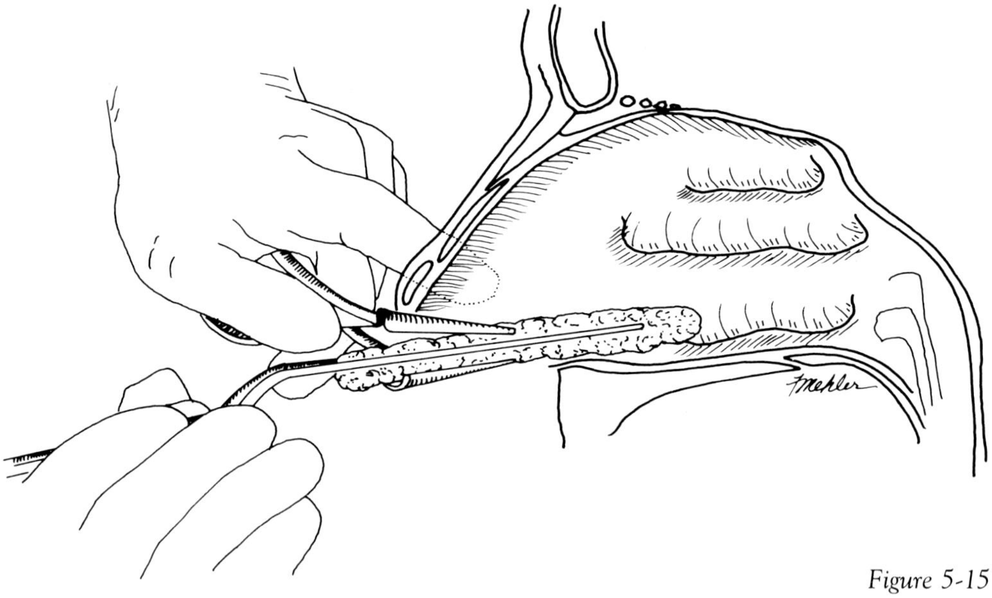

Figure 5-15

As shown in Figure 5-15, the bayonet forceps should have narrow blades and a very light spring action. All instruments should be as narrow as practical as this greatly increases the operator's field of vision.

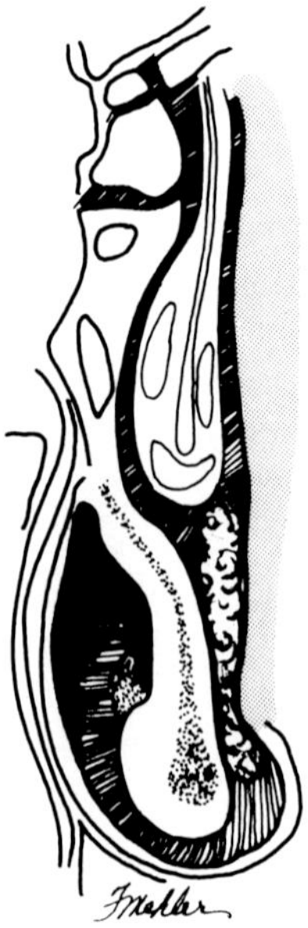

Figure 5-16

Figure 5-16 shows the first pledget placed between the inferior turbinate and the septum. Note the narrow space between the middle turbinate and the septum.

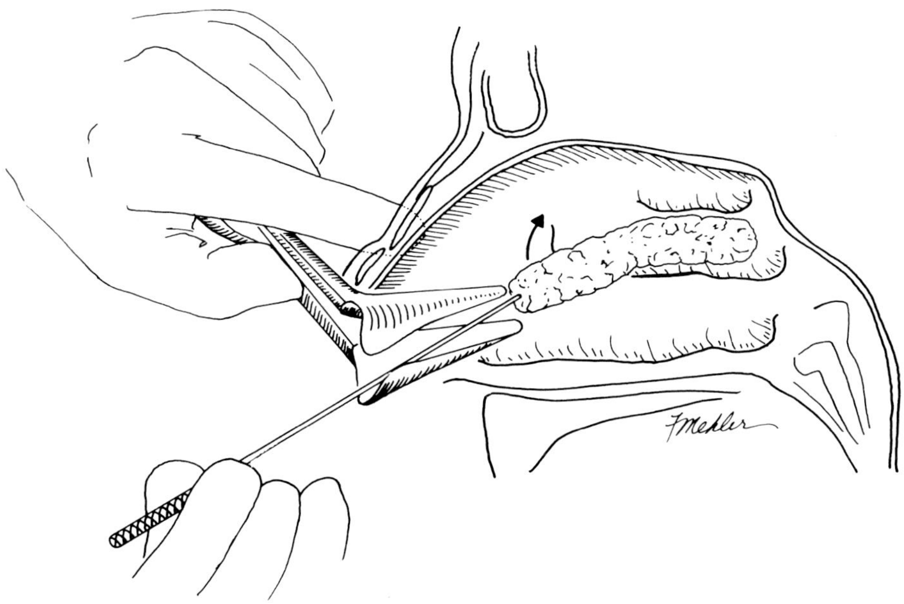

Figure 5-17

Next, remove the first pledget and gently place the third pledget between the middle turbinate and the septum. As this area is narrower and has more sensory innervation, this must be done very gently. A stiff wire often is more useful for placement as it requires less room than bayonet forceps. The wire applicator shown in Figure 5-17 is used for final placement in narrow areas. Now replace the first pledget more posteriorly and proceed to the opposite side and remove the second pledget, placing the fourth pledget again between the middle turbinate and the septum, and then replace the second pledget. These pledgets are then moved more posteriorly during the initial infiltration of the anterior septum and turbinate. This more posterior placement prevents any blood or extravasated infiltrative anesthesia from reaching the posterior pharynx. In addition, it allows a longer duration of contact of the posterior mucosa with the cocaine.

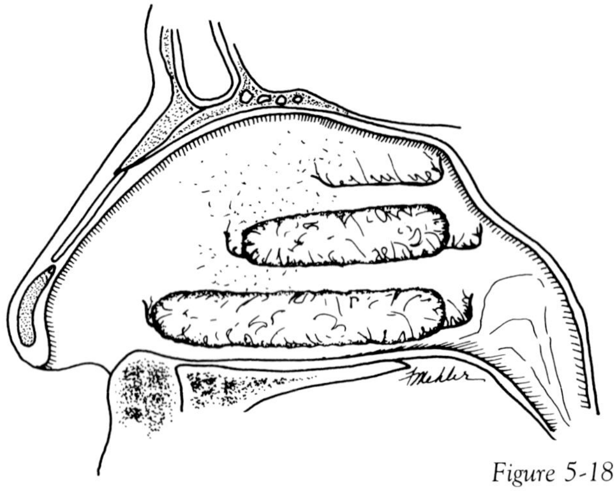

Figure 5-18

Figure 5-18 shows placement of pledgets at the time of the infiltration of the cartilaginous septum. This will be moved more posteriorly or removed as necessary for the infiltration of the posterior septum and lateral wall of the nose.

INFILTRATION OF LOCAL ANESTHESIA

Most of the pain associated with infiltration is due to the rapid distention of tissues. Infiltrate slowly; less distention will result in less discomfort. The two main goals are hemostasis and anesthesia. Clinically the greatest need for hemostasis and visualization is anteriorly. Use 2% lidocaine (Xylocaine) with 1 : 100,000 epinephrine (Adrenalin) anteriorly for infiltration of the septum, anterior portion of the turbinates, and the external nose. Use 1% bupivacaine (Marcaine) with 1 : 200,000 Adrenalin for the posterior septum, posterior portion of the inferior turbinate, middle turbinate, and sphenopalatine area. By using the Marcaine solution there is less Adrenalin used, and generally a much more comfortable patient in the immediate postoperative period, particularly if posterior septal work has been performed.

The skin and subcutaneous structures are infiltrated with 2% Xylocaine with 1 : 100,000 Adrenalin in such a manner that a field block is obtained. If small amounts are used and the local anesthesia is gently massaged in, it will diffuse and not distort the tissues. The anesthesia thus obtained is excellent, and the hemostasis is superior to a regional block.

In general, a field block provides excellent anesthesia and superior hemostasis. Excess infiltration can distend tissues, however, masking critical changes in important structures. Regional block requires injections far removed from the operative site and introduces the risk of hitting larger vessels and increasing the postoperative ecchymosis. Also, hemostasis is less than that obtained with field block.

No local anesthesia is injected along the line of planned lateral osteotomies at this time, as it will be performed toward the end of the procedure, and is not needed presently. Also, the risk of penetrating the angular artery and development of a hematoma or excessive ecchymosis is avoided.

Infiltration Technique

The initial injection is made through the mucoperichondrium, just posterior to its junction with the vestibular skin, with a 26-gauge needle on a dental syringe. This syringe gives dropwise control to reduce the chances of overinjection. Note that the bevel is placed so that the Xylocaine will dissect under the vestibular skin. Thus later, after the last of the mucous membrane injections, the membranous columella can be injected with much less discomfort.

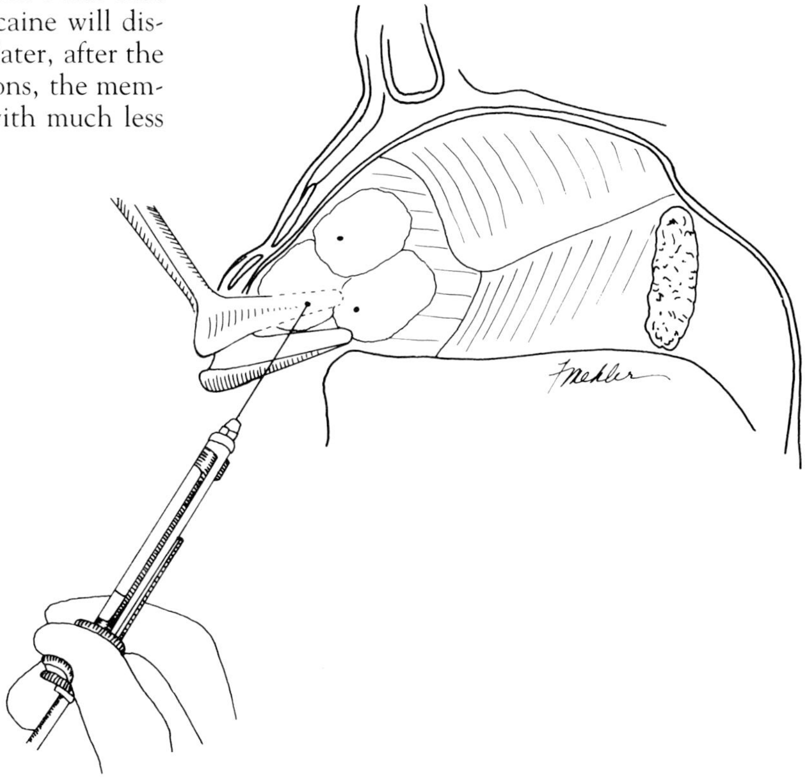

Figure 5-19

Make sure that some of the local anesthesia dissects anteriorly beneath the skin of the membranous columella at this time. Note the position of the posterior cotton pledget (Figure 5-19) to absorb any blood or extravasated local anesthesia and prevent the patient from coughing or expectorating. Subsequent mucous membrane injections are made at the posteriormost aspect of the previous injections; thus you work your way from anterior to posterior.

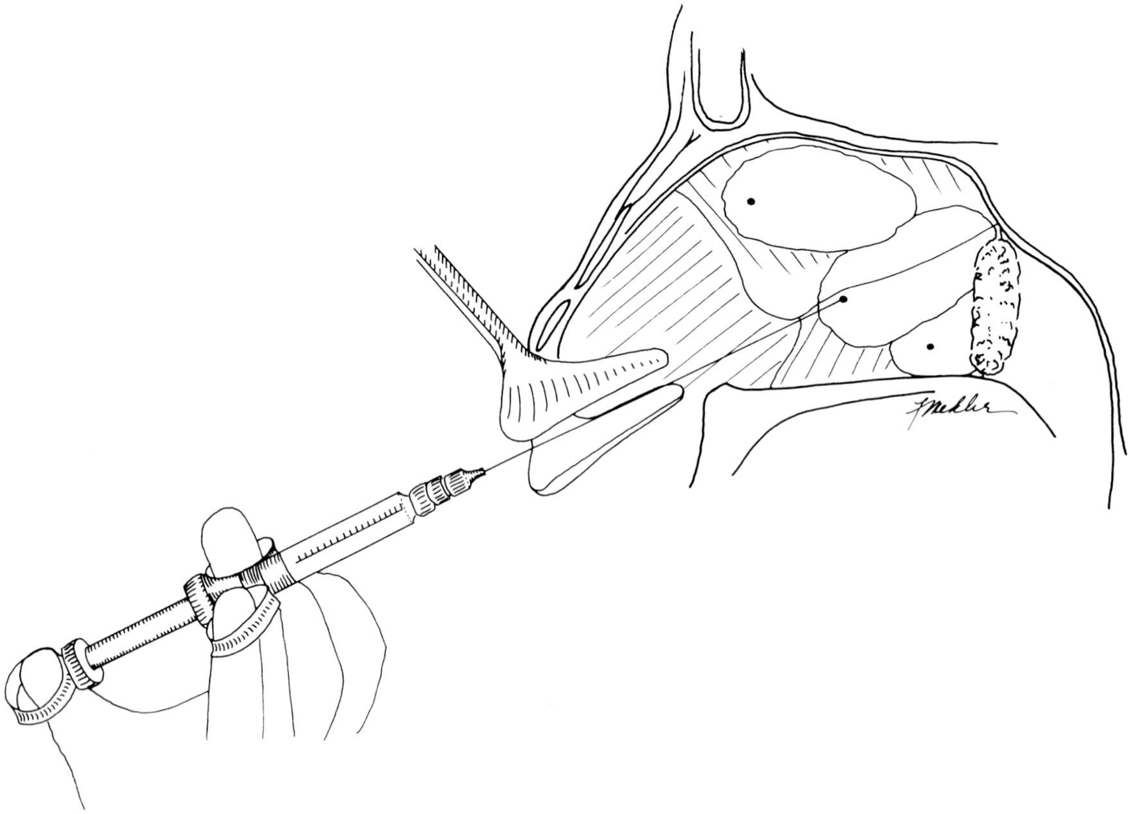

Figure 5-20

A 3½-inch 26-gauge spinal needle is used for this posterior injection of Marcaine (Figure 5-20). This allows excellent visualization and control of the infiltration.

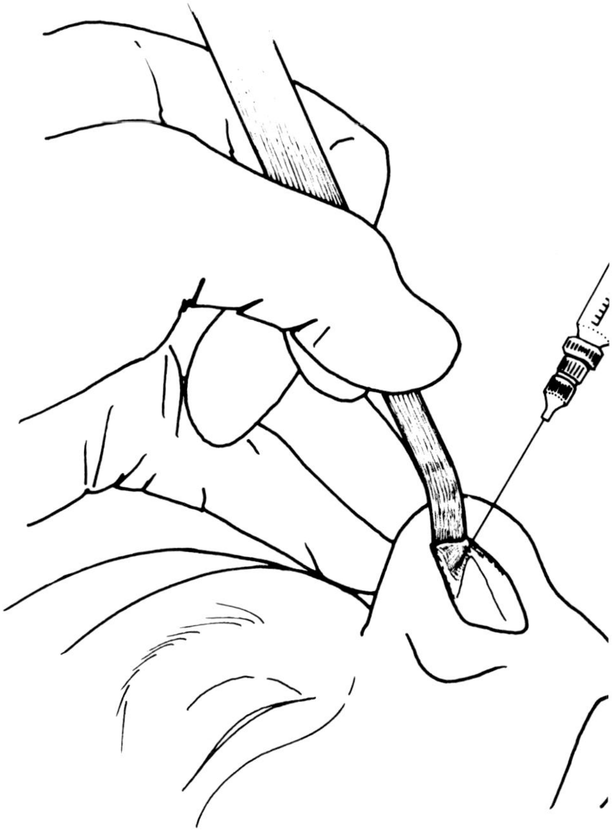

Figure 5-21A

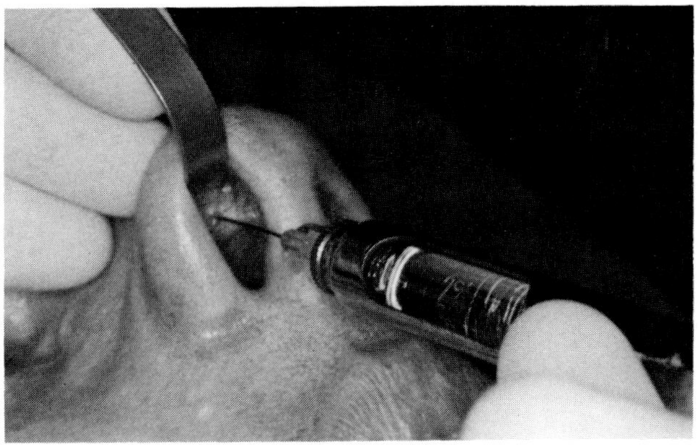

Figure 5-21B

The dental needle is passed through the intercartilaginous space, which is well visualized with a Park nasal retractor. It is then passed up to the glabella. The injection is then started during the withdrawal of the needle. Marked care must be exercised as it is removed that no excess local is injected as it will distort the landmarks for the intercartilaginous incision. Park's retraction provides the tension that exposes the intercartilaginous area best, allowing penetration of the needle just above the upper lateral cartilage (Figures 5-21A and B).

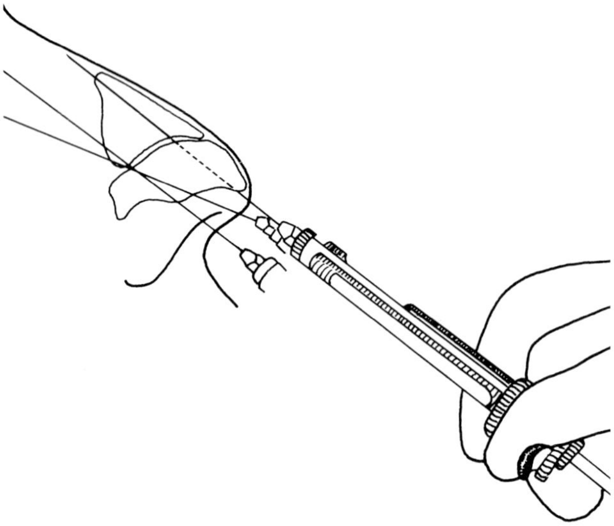

Figure 5-22

After passing through the intercartilaginous space, the needle is passed superiorly as far as needed (Figure 5-22). Then the local anesthesia is injected as the needle is withdrawn.

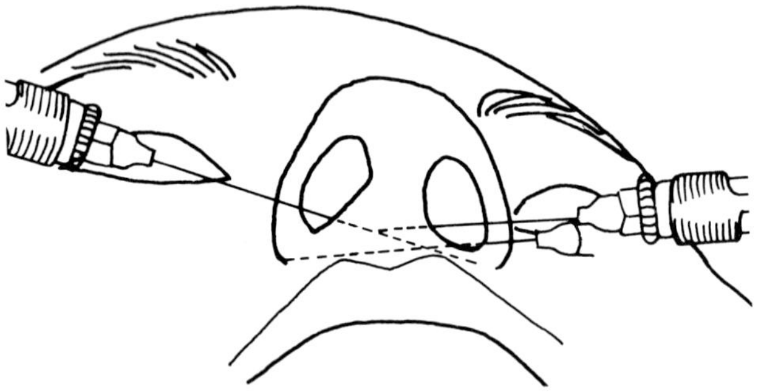

Figure 5-23

Injections are also made anterior to the anterior nasal spine, and laterally at the junction of the alae within the sill area, as illustrated in Figure 5-23. Initially the anesthetic is infiltrated at the base of the columella, and then the needle is advanced to the alar-facial groove and more anesthetic is infiltrated (Figure 5-23).

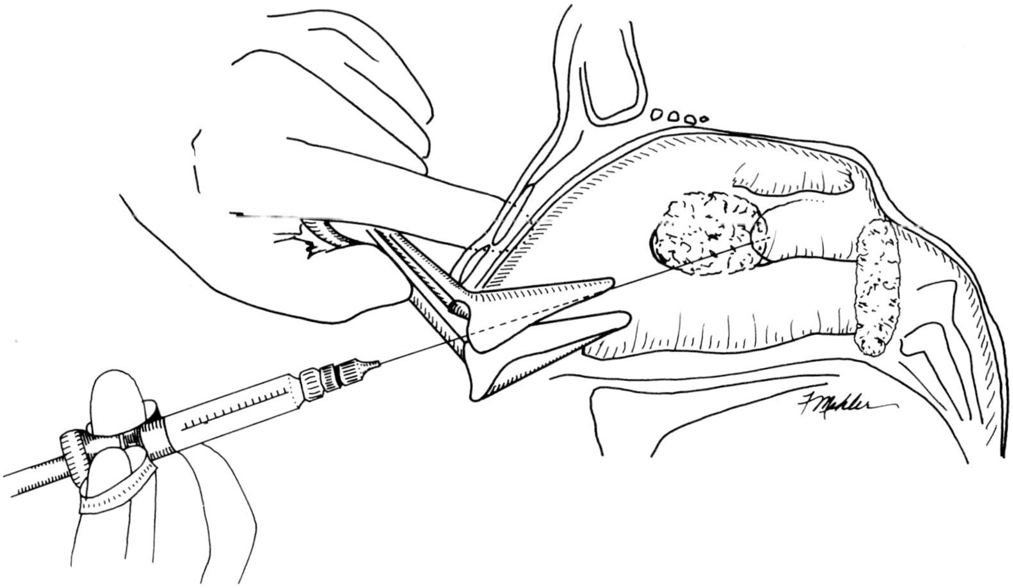

Figure 5-24

The middle turbinate and inferior turbinate are injected as well with the Marcaine if posterior septal work is to be done. The middle turbinate can be outfractured without fear of bleeding or subsequent mucocele formation. This outfracture provides better visualization and allows infiltration in the immediate area of the sphenopalatine ganglion. The large nasal speculum is used to perform the outfracturing. In Figure 5-24 note the cotton pledget placed posteriorly, absorbing any extravasated local or blood from the injections.

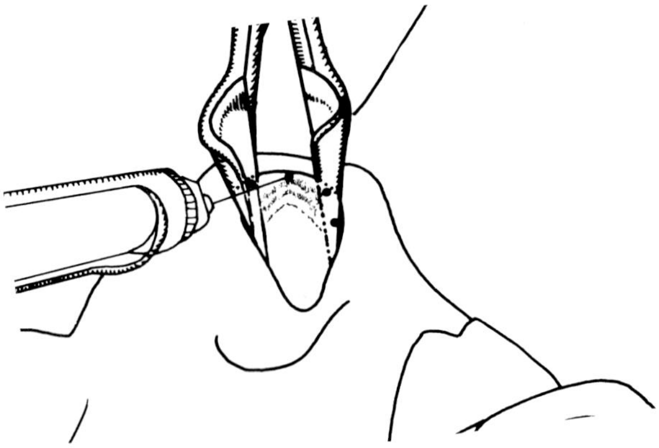

Figure 5-25A

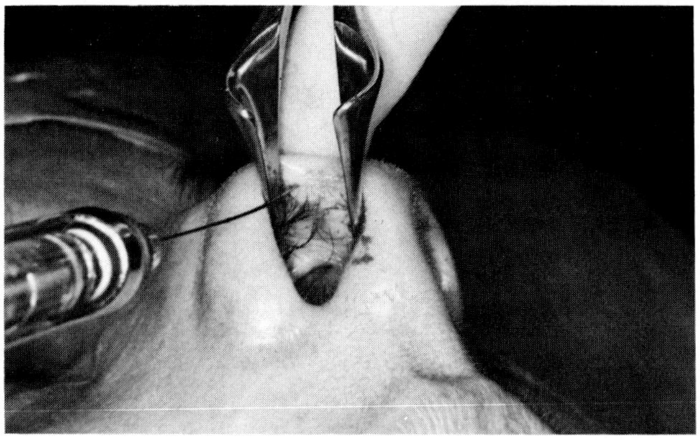

Figure 5-25B

The final injections are at the tip. These are made just caudal to the margin of the lower lateral cartilage. Again, minimal injection is the key to not obscuring important landmarks needed later for incisions. A nasal speculum can be used to provide exposure for infiltration of the dome area (Figures 5-25A and B).

TURBINATES

Turbinate hypertrophy is a common cause of nasal obstruction. It can be bony, mucosal, or a combination of both. The goal in altering the turbinates is to improve the airway without impairing turbinate function.

The etiology of turbinate hypertrophy can be allergic, vasomotor, compensatory, or the result of excess bony development.

Treatment consists of allergic referral, requiring lifetime therapy if successful; intratubinal steroid injection, which provides temporary relief; topical steroid spray, requiring lifetime therapy; electrocautery with partial destruction of the turbinal tissue, which affects only the mucosa; and cryosurgery with partial destruction of the turbinal tissue, which also affects only the mucosa. Additional treatment includes partial surgical resection of turbinate, which may result in significant postoperative bleeding; outfracture of turbinate bone, which is a temporary measure at best; and submucosal resection of the turbinate bone with partial loss of turbinal mucosal function secondary to fibrous healing.

TECHNIQUE

Submucosal resection is presented in detail, as it is the most effective procedure in the greater number of patients. Atrophic rhinitis does not occur following this procedure. The incidence of postoperative bleeding requiring additional packing or repacking is less than 1 percent. This is significantly less than that reported in the current literature for surgical resection (amputation), partial or complete. The disadvantage is that it requires more time to perform a proper submucous resection of the inferior turbinate.

If possible, the turbinate surgery is performed prior to septal rhinoplasty. This allows better visualization throughout the remaining case; however, at times it is necessary to perform the septal surgery first to gain adequate room to operate on the turbinate. If turbinate surgery is performed first, it is helpful to pack the posterior choana transnasally to prevent pooling of blood during the remaining procedure.

The inferior turbinate is bracketed with a medium-long speculum (Figure 5-26). Occasionally it is necessary to first medially fracture the turbinate to allow the proper placement of the speculum blades. Simply compressing the soft tissue without fracturing the turbinate will often be of value in defining the location of the bone within the tissue. This greatly facilitates the initial incision and location of the proper subperiosteal plane for elevation.

It is best to make this initial cut from inferior to superior as illustrated in Figure 5-27. This positioning allows better visualization and control of the No. 15 scalpel blade. A long, narrow scalpel handle also allows better visualization. It is not necessary for this incision to extend to the pyriform aperture, and it is best if it does not as the bleeding will greatly increase.

After the initial incision, a sharp-pointed instrument such as the pick end of the Woodson is used to help locate and elevate in the subperiosteal plane. A thin, narrow-bladed nasal speculum is an essential aid at this time. The blades not only provide exposure, but by retracting the developing flaps, they decrease the bleeding. Figure 5-28 emphasizes the vertical orientation of the blades, thus allowing maximum visualization.

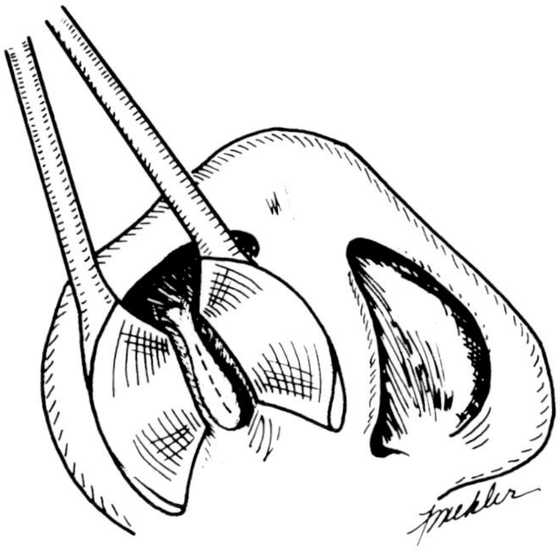

Figure 5-26

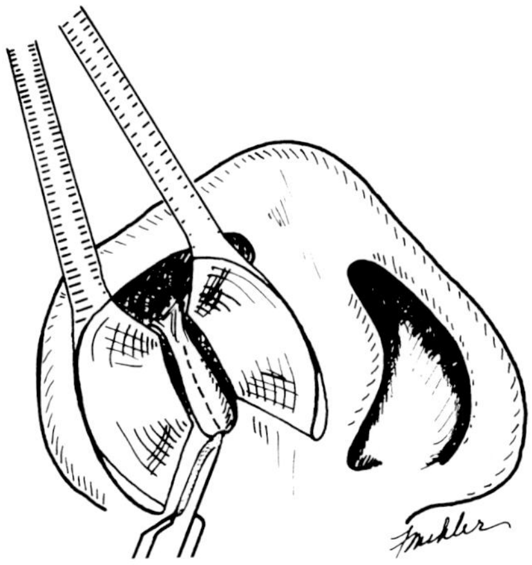

Figure 5-27

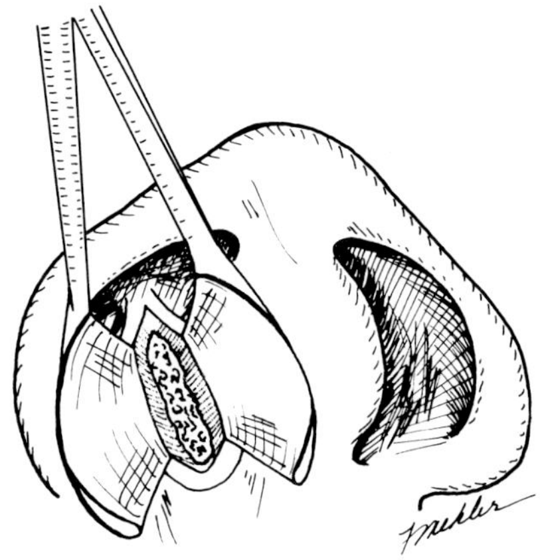

Figure 5-28

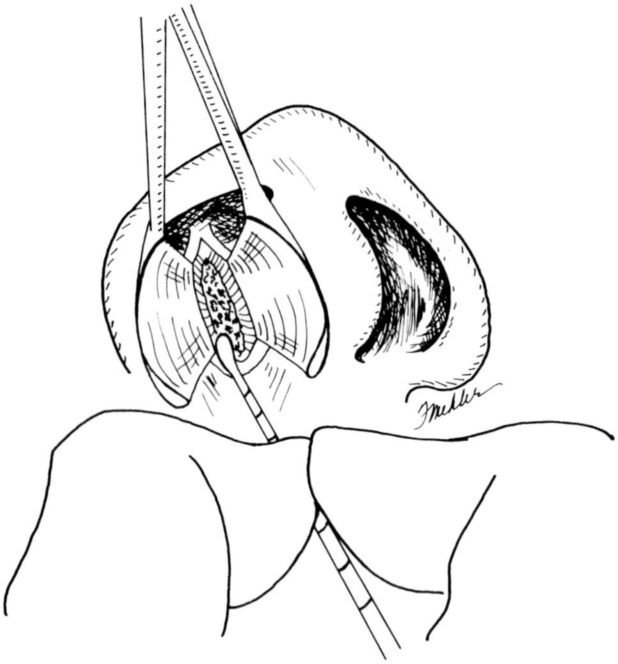

The surface of the turbinate bone is very irregular, making elevation difficult. The spade end of the modified Woodson No. 1 is well suited for anterior work, and the spade end of the Cottle elevator is best for more posterior work. It is essential to stay in the submucoperiosteal plane of dissection. Figure 5-29 shows the Cottle elevator approximately one-third of the way back.

Figure 5-29

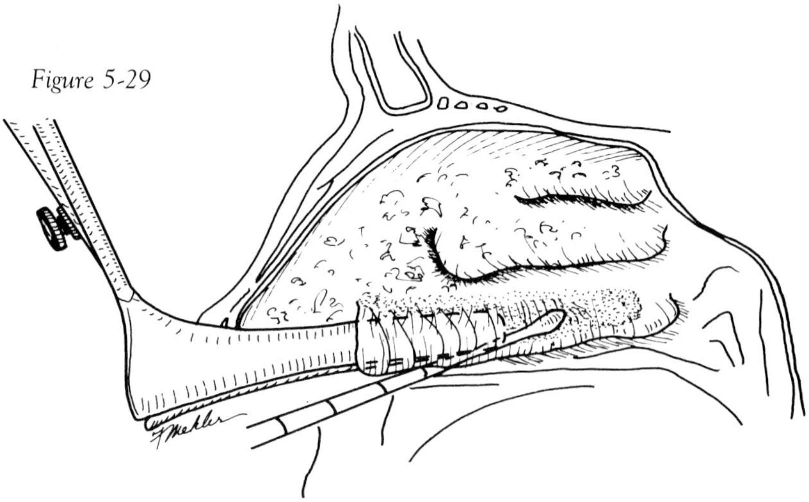

Figure 5-30

As the dissection continues more posteriorly, a longer nasal speculum is used to hold the flaps apart. The Cottle elevator is used to elevate and separate the mucoperichondrium from the turbinate bone. If, because of the curvature of the anterior turbinate bone, it prevents visualization of the more posterior portion, it is best to remove the anterior bone prior to more posterior work. If, during the elevation, the turbinate bone is fractured from its attachment to the lateral wall of the nose, the elevation becomes infinitely more difficult. Figure 5-30 illustrates more posterior work with a long, thin-bladed nasal speculum and a Cottle elevator.

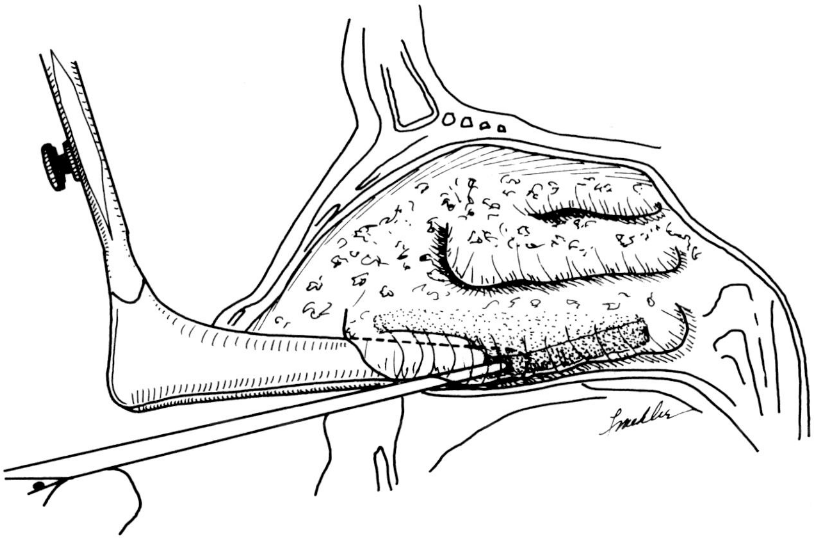

Figure 5-31

Small Takahashi forceps are used for bone removal. The long thin shaft allows visualization during the removal. The bone is generally removed in three to four segments. As illustrated in Figure 5-31, the forceps are used by grasping the bone and then twisting the segment. This obtains much larger pieces than simply biting one cup at a time.

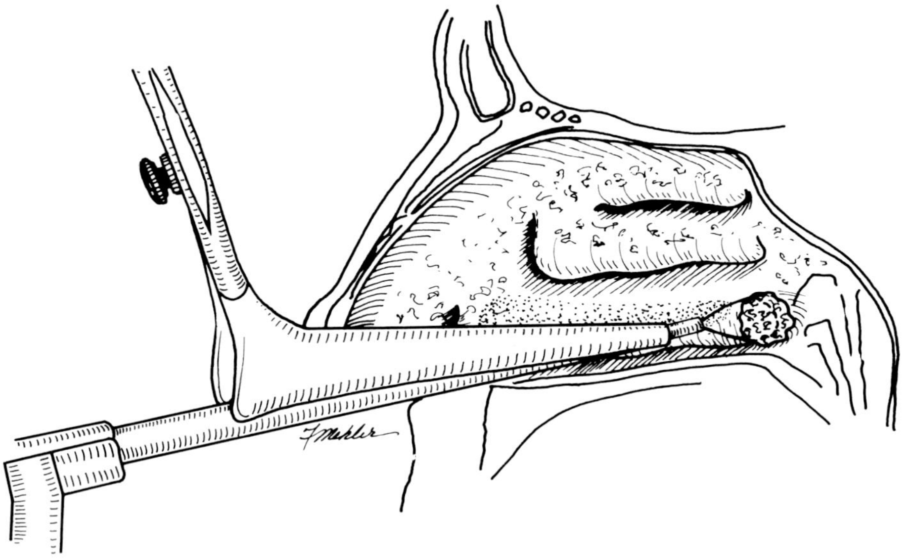

Figure 5-32

If there is polypoid degeneration of the posterior tip of the inferior turbinate, it is removed with a tonsil snare. The wire loop is placed around the degenerated tip, taking care not to include bone. Then slow tightening of the loop will crush the blood vessels and amputate the mulberry tip. It is then removed with a No. 8 French sucker tip. It helps to bend the wire loop approximately 30° laterally. This facilitates placement. Figure 5-32 shows the wire loop in place prior to tightening. Often it is necessary to temporarily remove the speculum for proper loop placement.

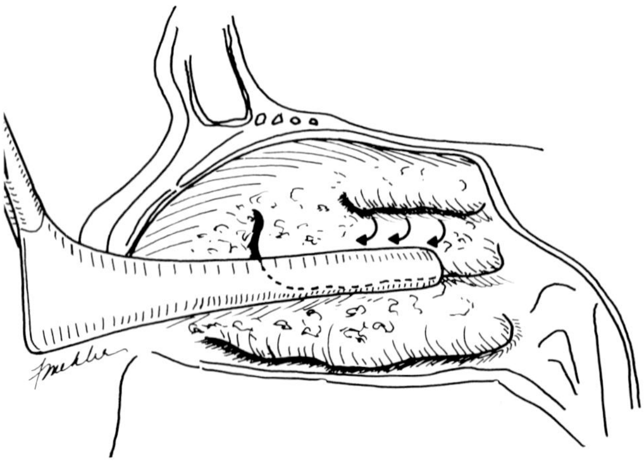

Figure 5-33

This is an ideal time to outfracture the middle turbinates if they are obstructive. This is an effective means of therapy and does not lead to mucocele formation. To reduce them submucosally will lead to late postoperative hemorrhage in a significant number of patients unless done microscopically. The large nasal speculum is a good instrument for outfracturing as illustrated in Figure 5-33.

The outfracturing of the middle turbinate, as contrasted to the inferior turbinate, is effective because it fractures and compresses the ethmoid cells within the turbinate (Figure 5-34A and B). The arrows in Figure 5-34B denote the amount of permanent reduction obtained.

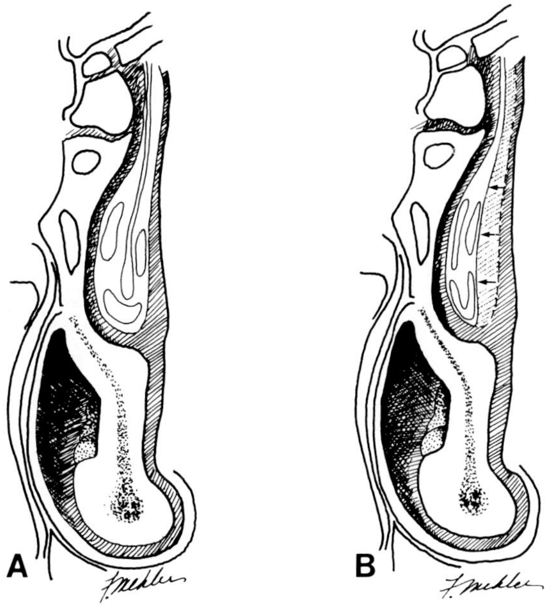

Figure 5-34

SEPTUM AND CAUDAL SEPTUM

Septal surgery generally is the key stone on which a rhinoplasty practice is built. The majority of new nasal patients will present with symptoms of nasal obstruction. As patient referral is the singlemost important new patient source, an excellent airway must be provided. In addition, much of septal surgery has a direct affect on the external nose. As in all nasal surgery, septal surgery is a stepwise procedure. The following technique allows a wide latitude and all steps are infrequently necessary.

The mucoperichondrial hemitransfixion incision is made within 2–3 mm of the caudal end of the septum. It has a gentle curve to it and can be extended laterally, paralleling the pyriform aperture for further exposure of the anterior nasal spine, maxillary crest, and floor of the nose as indicated. It should join the intra- or intercartilaginous incisions at an acute angle, as this facilitates subsequent accurate closure. If an open rhinoplasty incision is used, the septal surgery is performed transcolumellarly.

The incision is made over the septal cartilage, not in the membranous columella. This allows rapid development of the subperichondrial plane. It also limits the amount of scar contracture acting on the tip in the postoperative period. If it is made more than 4–5 mm behind the caudal end of the quadrangular cartilage, the flap is easily torn when retracted later on with the nasal speculum. Figure 5-35 shows the extension for exposure of the maxillary crest and floor of the nose.

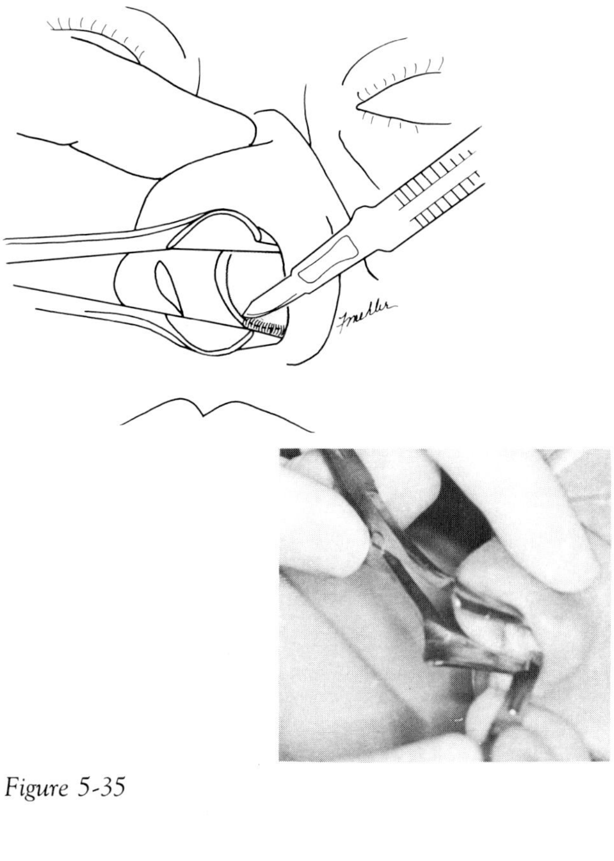

Figure 5-35

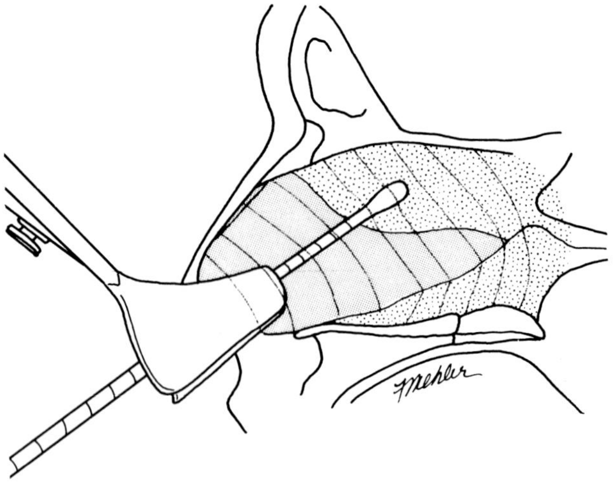

Figure 5-36

Elevation of the mucoperichondral flap is continued posteriorly to the perpendicular plate of the ethmoid and the vomer. In the same plane the mucoperiosteum over this bony septum is similarly elevated. This elevation is facilitated by using the blade of a medium-sized speculum to hold the septal cartilage toward one side and the mucoperiosteum under light tension on the opposite side. This then allows direct visualization for the elevation with the spade end of the Cottle elevator. If there is a significant bony spur impinging on the lateral wall of the nose, it is helpful to elevate the mucoperiosteum inferiorly and superiorly to the spur. Following this elevation, the two "tunnels" can be connected without tearing the flap. The spade end of the Cottle elevator is very useful for the posterior elevation. Its thin shaft allows good visualization of the thin spadelike end (see Figure 5-36).

Once the entire flap is elevated an incision is made through the cartilage just anterior to its junction with the perpendicular plate. The spade end of the Woodson is well suited for this incision. The cut is extended superiorly as needed to within 8 mm of the dorsum. To cut higher will interrupt the important dorsal hinge of cartilage attached to the upper laterals above and the perpendicular plate behind.

Figure 5-37 illustrates the initial incision extending down to the vomer.

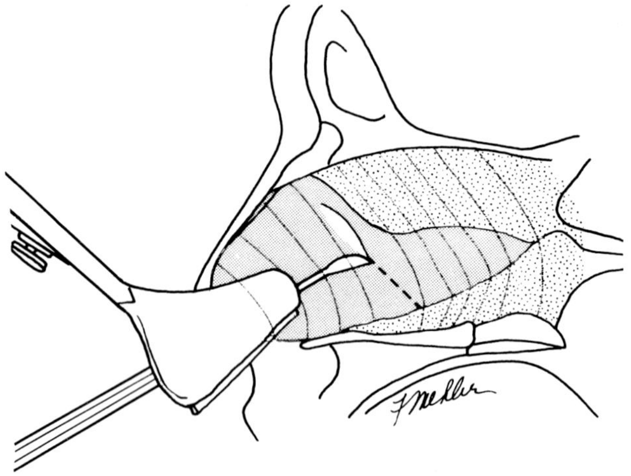

Figure 5-37

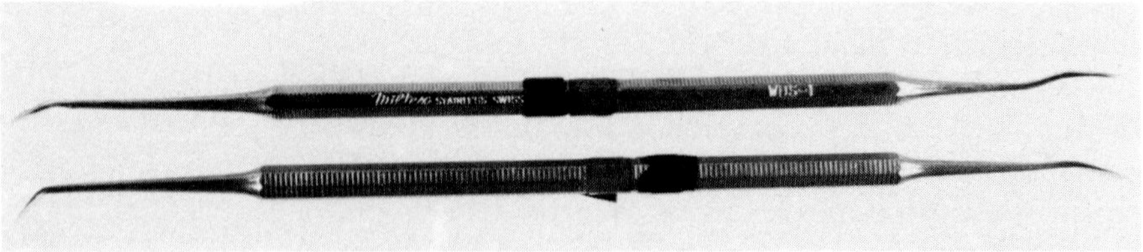

Figure 5-38

Figure 5-38 shows a Woodson No. 1 (above) and a modified Woodson (below). In particular note the change in the angulation of the spade end.

If the incision is extended superiorly far enough to weaken the dorsal hinge and subsequent septal surgery includes removal of inferior septal cartilage as well as posterior bony septum, a supratip depression (arrow) may result. (Figure 5-39.)

If the cartilaginous septum is functionally straight, the bony posterior work is continued as in the procedure illustrated by Figure 5-45 (later in this chapter). If the cartilaginous septal deformity prevents further surgery posteriorly, it is necessary to release the septal cartilage from its inferior attachment to the maxillary crest and vomer. A No. 64 Beaver blade is placed so that the cutting edge is positioned superiorly, and the rounded leading edge actually does the cutting. It is pushed onto the maxillary crest and vomer, and then posteriorly, thus cutting the excess cartilage that is subluxed out of the crest (Figure 5-40). This cut is started as the cartilage deviates from the crest and continues posteriorly until it joins the previous vertical cut. Figure 5-40 shows the cut approximately halfway completed. The dashed line represents the continuation to the existing vertical incision.

Then the periosteum that is attached to the vomer and maxillary crest is exposed by removal of the cartilaginous strip. The maxillary crest periosteum is then elevated under direct vision. Figure 5-41 shows the shortened septum being displaced by the nasal speculum, thus allowing the modified Woodson to elevate the periosteum attached to the vomer and crest on both sides. By shortened septum, reference is made to the inferior strip of cartilage that was removed in the preceding step. Thus it is shorter in a superior, inferior dimension.

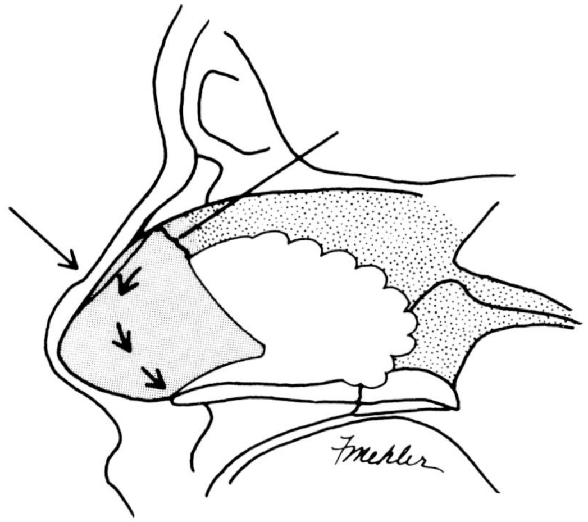

Figure 5-39

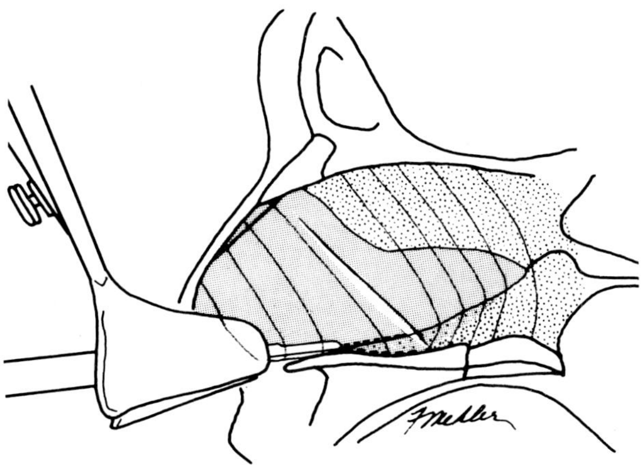

Figure 5-40

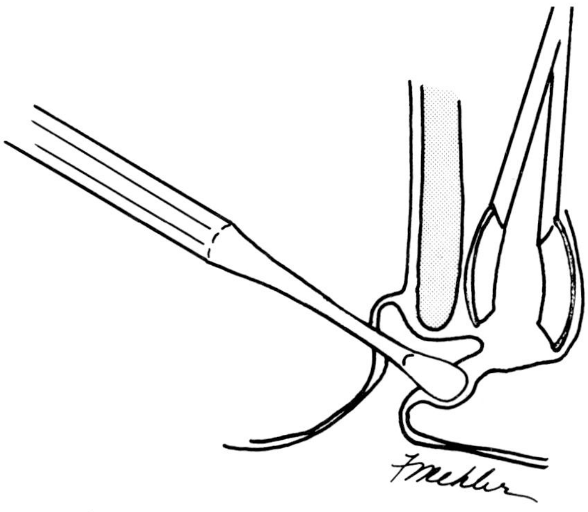

Figure 5-41

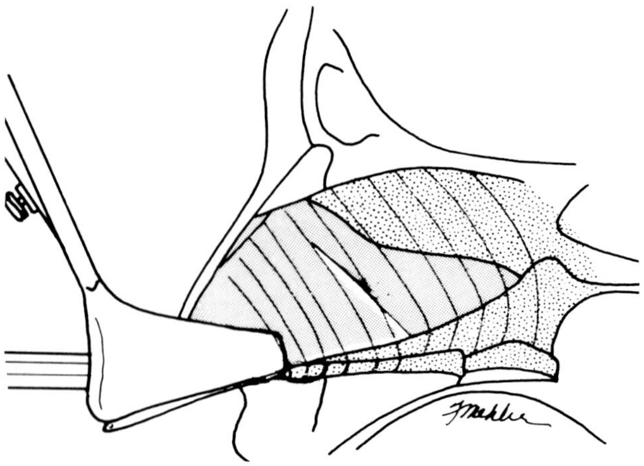

Figure 5-42

Figure 5-42 shows the remaining septal cartilage being displaced with the blade of the nasal speculum, and the periosteum on the right side of the maxillary crest and floor is elevated in a procedure similar to that illustrated in Figure 5-41.

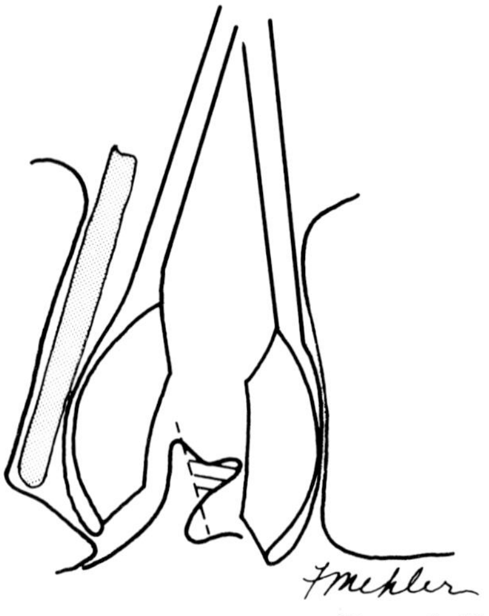

Figure 5-43

Following the periosteal elevation, the maxillary crest is bracketed with the nasal speculum and examined to ensure that it is not deviated. If it is, the deviated portion is resected with a straight chisel or Takahashi forceps. The chisel has the advantage of leaving some midline bone. The Takahashi forceps often break the bone off flush to the floor. In Figure 5-43 the dashed line represents the plane of the chisel, and the shaded bone to the right will be removed.

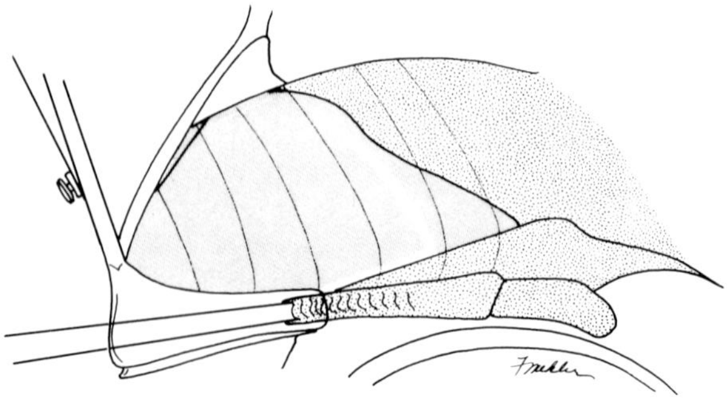

Figure 5-44

Figure 5-44 shows the chisel in place as it begins its cut.

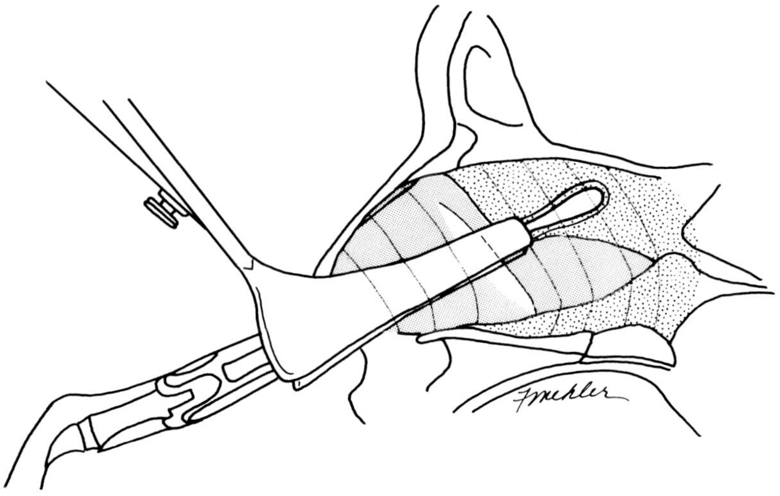

Figure 5-45

The long nasal speculum is then placed so that the perpendicular plate is between the blades, and the mucoperiosteum of both sides are retracted. Then an initial superior cut is made with the double-action Janzten-Middleton forceps. This will prevent accidental fracturing of the cribiform plate (Figure 5-45). Then the remaining deviated ethmoid and vomer are removed with the medium Takahashi forceps.

If there is a persistent deflection of the substance of the cartilage itself, vertical incisions can be made or ellipses of the fractured portion made and removed. The spade end of the Woodson is excellent for cutting the ellipses without damaging the mucoperichondrium on the opposite side. Portions of sharp angles or excessively wide cartilage may be sliver shaved at this time by use of a No. 11 or 15 scalpel. At times is is necessary to elevate the mucoperichondrium over a portion of the opposite side. Figure 5-46 shows two vertical ellipses that excised old fractured areas.

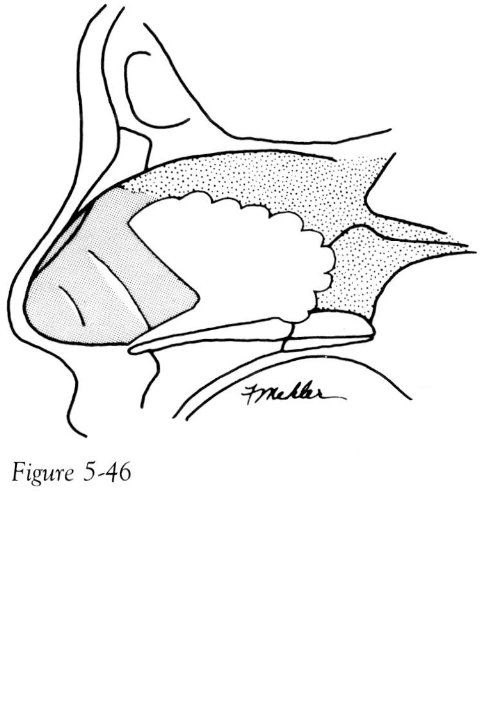

Figure 5-46

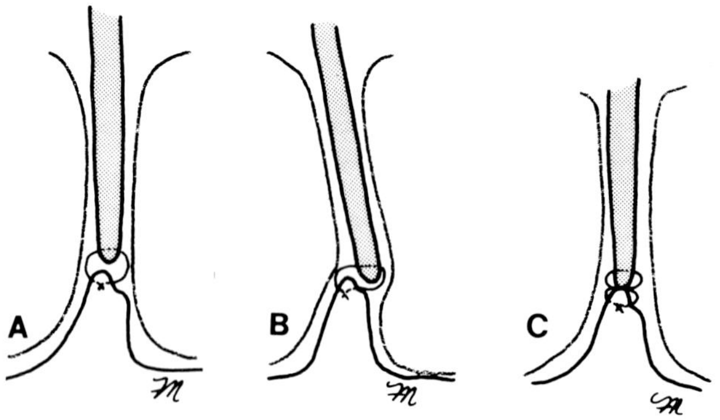

Figure 5-47

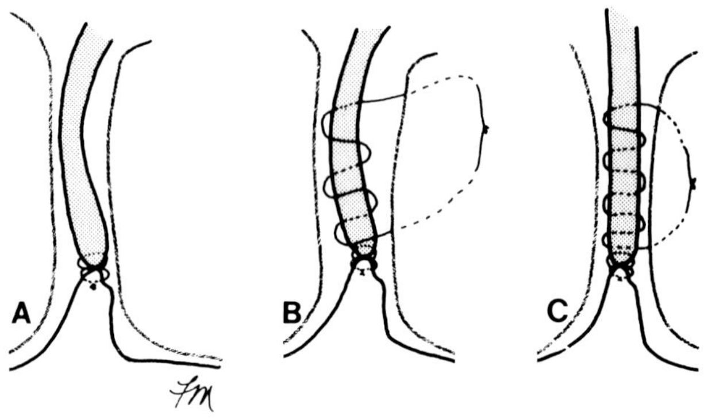

Figure 5-48

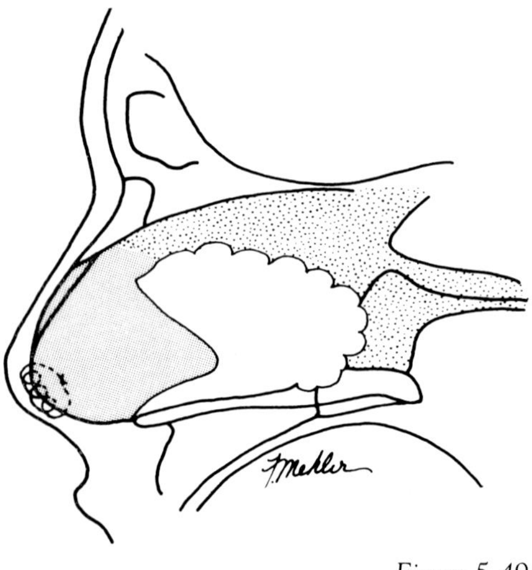

Figure 5-49

At the completion of a complicated septum the cartilage is often highly mobile. It is then anchored to the midline by placing a figure-8 suture through the inferior septal angle of the septum and the perichondrium of the anterior nasal spine. A simple suture will not suffice, as the cartilage can sublux in the postoperative period. Figure 5-47A shows a simple suture, and Figure 5-47B reveals how the cartilage can sublux to the side of the anterior nasal spine. Figure 5-47C shows that with a figure-8 4-0 clear prolene the septum cannot sublux.

In some cases the septum anterior to the nasal spine will persist in deviating in spite of being anchored to the nasal spine inferiorly. This can be corrected with a suture through the flap opposite the side of the deviation. This suture is placed through the flap, around the end of the septum several times in a simple overhand suture, and then back through the flap. It is then tied and pulls the septal cartilage to the midline. Figure 5-48A shows persisting cartilaginous bowing in spite of being midline both superiorly and inferiorly with the figure-8 suture. Figure 5-48B shows the 4-0 chromic suture being passed through the perichondrial flap as described above. Figure 5-48C shows the straightening of the cartilage after the suture is tightened and tied.

Figure 5-49 is a profile view of the same suture. Note that the placement through the perichondrial flap is posterior to the caudal border of the septum.

The septal cartilage is then sutured between the septal flaps with a running 4-0 chromic. This running suture is done anteriorly by using a Webster needle holder and a small speculum. It passes through the left perichondrium, septal cartilage, right perichondrium, back through the right perichondrium, septal cartilage, and left perichondrium, and then it is tied and the short end cut. Then the suture is run from the left nasal cavity to the right and back again, continuing posteriorly along the floor above the crest and then returning superiorly. Then the surgeon leaves the last loop long and ties to it. This running suture stabilizes the septal cartilage in its new relationship to the elevated flaps. It greatly reduces any chance for a septal hematoma, and it is used to approximate any inadvertent rents in the mucoperichondral or periosteal flap. Figure 5-50 shows a completed extensive septal plasty.

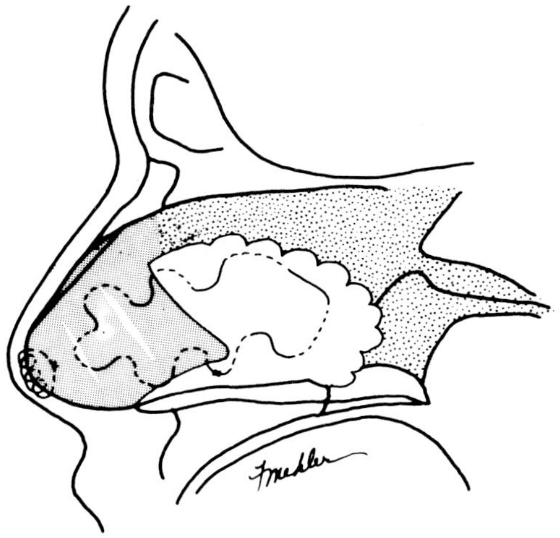

Figure 5-50

Splints made of Teflon are routinely sutured into place. They are sutured both anteriorly and posteriorly. A 4-0 green prolene works best for this as it is easiest to cut in the office at the time of splint removal. The splints prevent adhesions between the turbinate and septum. They prevent hematoma formation in that portion of the septum that they cover as they are sutured both anteriorly and posteriorly. Finally, they make postoperative nasal toilet more comfortable. Figure 5-51 shows the approximate size and placement of the splints as well as the sutures used. Care must be exercised to keep the splints from touching the anterior nasal spine area, or from coming forward too far and touching the membranous columella as this is uncomfortable.

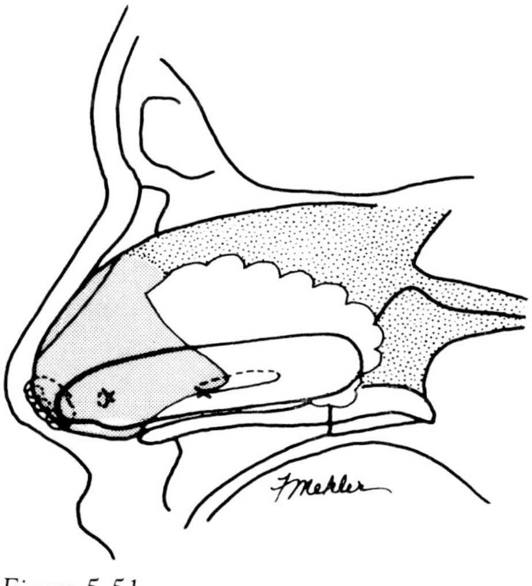

Figure 5-51

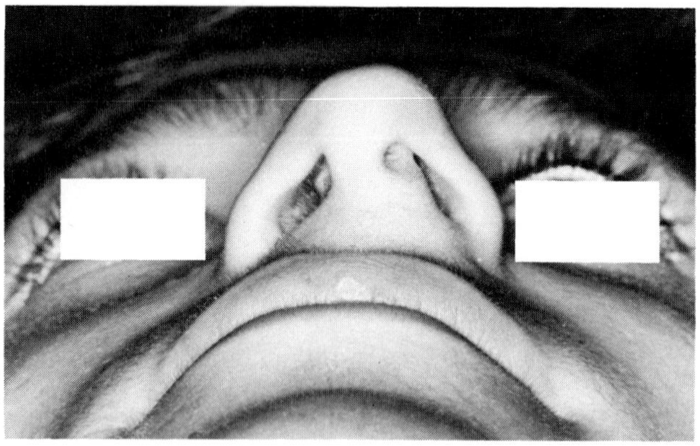

Figure 5-52

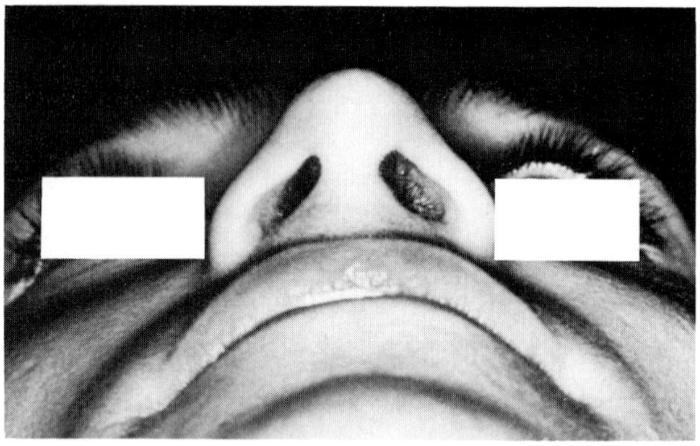

Figure 5-53

Figure 5-52 is a preoperative photograph. Figure 5-53 shows the same patient 1 year after the extensive septal surgery approach described above.

THE NASAL TIP

Safe effective changes in the nasal tip are small compared to that of the cartilaginous bony framework of the upper nose. Therefore, it is generally better to "set" the tip and then adjust the cartilaginous bony framework. Also, surgery of the tip produces much less intraoperative edema than the surgery of the cartilaginous bony framework. There is thus much less distortion when critical refinements are contemplated and performed. One obvious exception is when a high cartilaginous dorsum distorts the tip. The very fact that there are numerous approaches to the tip and many strong proponents for various techniques is positive proof that no technique is universally applicable to surgery of the nasal tip. The following techniques are presented for their predictability and safety. They still demand strict attention to detail and meticulous surgical technique.

A delineation of the nasal tip is shown in Figure 5-54. The term "crural arch" refers to the lower lateral cartilage in its entirety; the components are the lateral crura and the medial crura. The "tip defining point" refers to that point of the crural arch that is highest. Thus the tip should have two tip defining points; one on the right and one on the left, and they should be symmetrical. The "soft triangle" refers to the soft tissue forming the nostril rim immediately below the tip defining point.

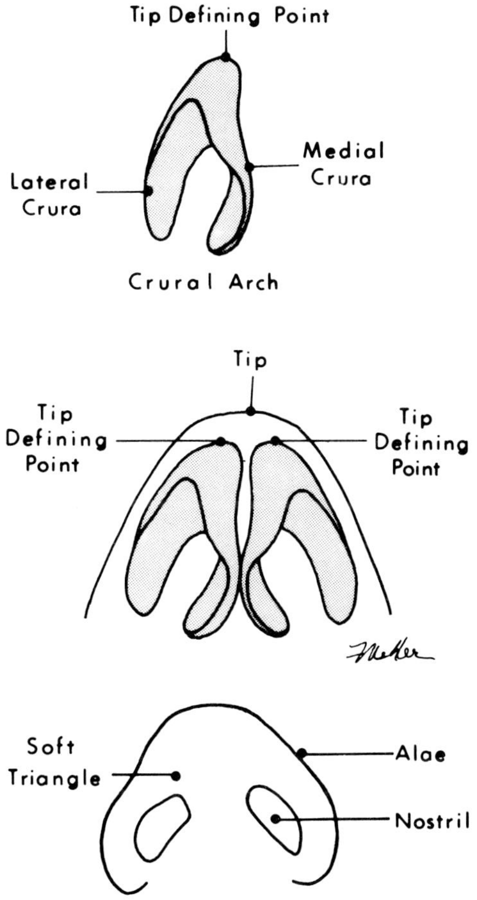

Figure 5-54

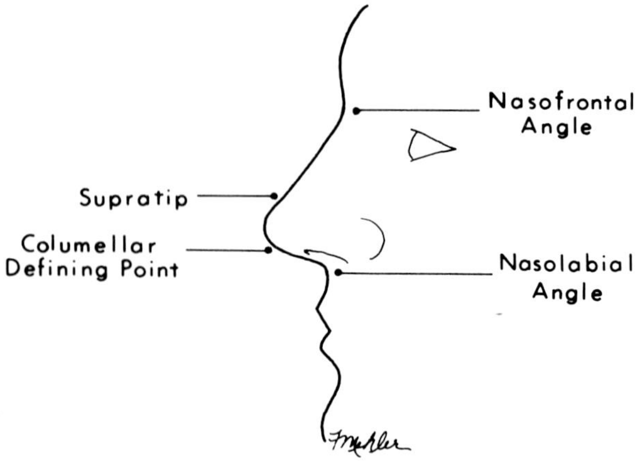

Figure 5-55

Figure 5-55 further defines the nasal tip. The supratip is the area inferior to the rhinion and superior to the cephalic border of the tip defining point; the infratip is the area inferior to the caudal border of the tip defining point and superior to the superior end of the columella. The columellar defining point is the anteriormost point of the columella in a profile view, commonly referred to as the "double brake." There are two columellar defining points (left and right), and they should be symmetrical. The nasolabial angle is the angle formed by the inferior end of the columella and the upper lip.

The general principles of nasal tip surgery are as follows:

1. Never violate the soft triangle. A notch will be the result as there is no cartilage within the soft triangle to support the two opposing skin surfaces during healing.
2. Always preserve vestibular lining for a meticulous closure. Failure to do this leads to healing by secondary intention. Resultant bands, webs, and scar contracture cause both internal and external complications (i.e., nasal obstruction, pinching).
3. Unless there is a preexisting tip asymmetry, both sides should be treated symmetrically. The incisions should have the same placement, length, and sutures for closure. The crural arch should have equal operative exposure. The crural arch is commonly asymmetrical; therefore, it is the remaining size, shape, and form that is critical, not the portion that has been removed.
4. Whenever possible, maintain an intact caudal border of the crural arch. The remaining lateral crura should be at least 5 mm wide, with rare exceptions.
5. The crural arch will buckle at its weakest point.

The major goals and precautions in tip surgery are refinement of tip form, superior tip rotation, inferior tip rotation, decreased tip projection, and increased tip projection. All these changes in the tip have the potential of changing other very important relationships.

Figures 5-56–5-58 contain base view tracing sketches of preoperative and postoperative patients. Figure 5-56 represents refining or narrowing of the tip.

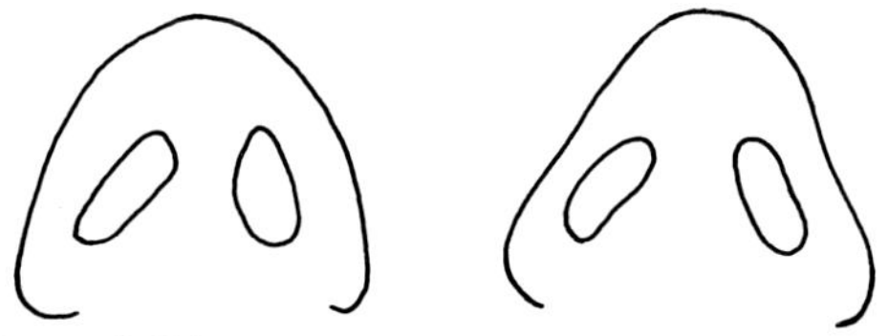

Figure 5-56

Figure 5-57 is an example of decreasing tip projection plus refinement.

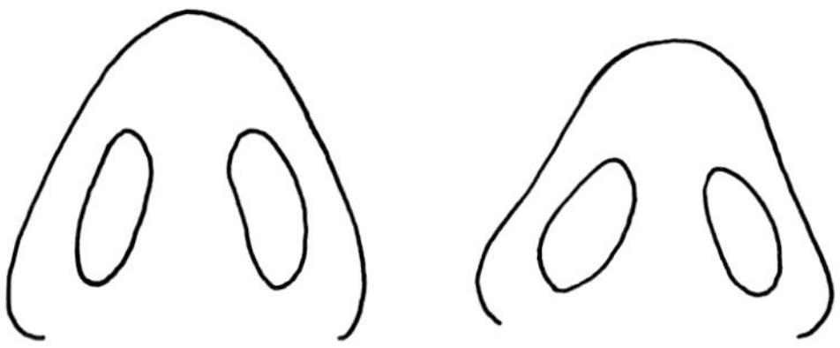

Figure 5-57

Figure 5-58 is refinement plus an increase in tip projection. Note the change in both nostril shape and orientation and alar shape.

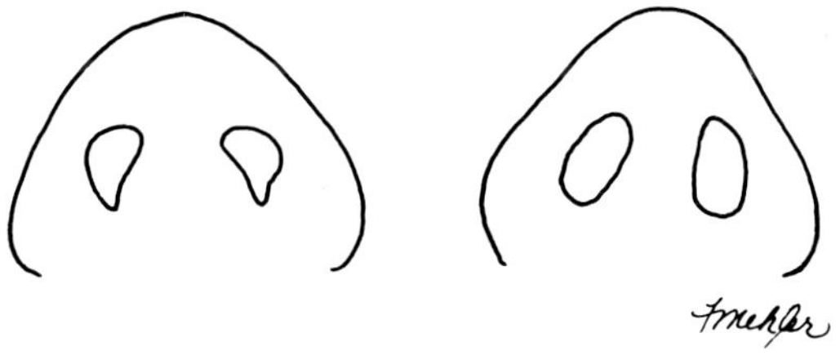

Figure 5-58

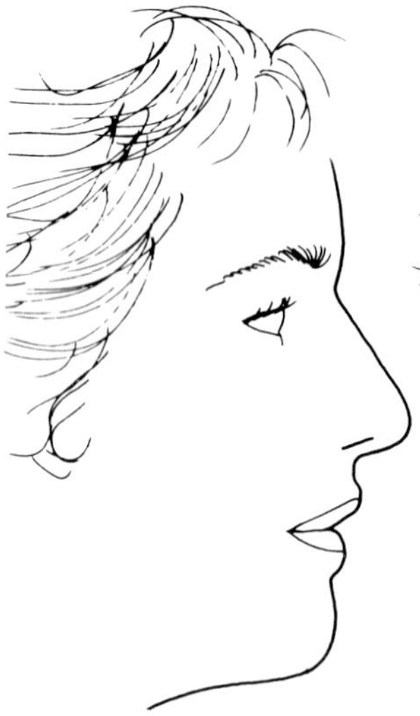

Figure 5-59A

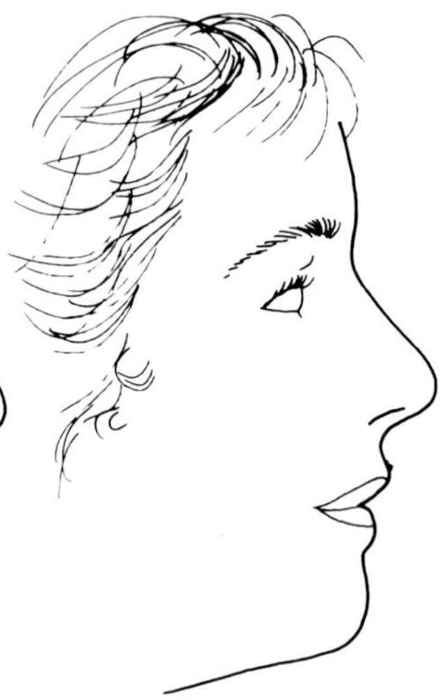

Figure 5-59B

Figure 5-59 demonstrates the desirable affect of superior rotation. Note the change in nasolabial angle and apparent increase in tip projection (Figure 5-59B).

Narrowing of the tip can lead to retraction of the nostril rim. Superior tip rotation can lead to excessive columellar show or create an unnatural columella defining point. Inferior tip rotation creates an apparent supratip fullness. Decreased tip projection quickly leads to an apparent flaring of the alae. Increased tip projection can quickly create a surgical tip. Awareness of these potential changes can enable one to compensate for or avoid them at the time of surgery.

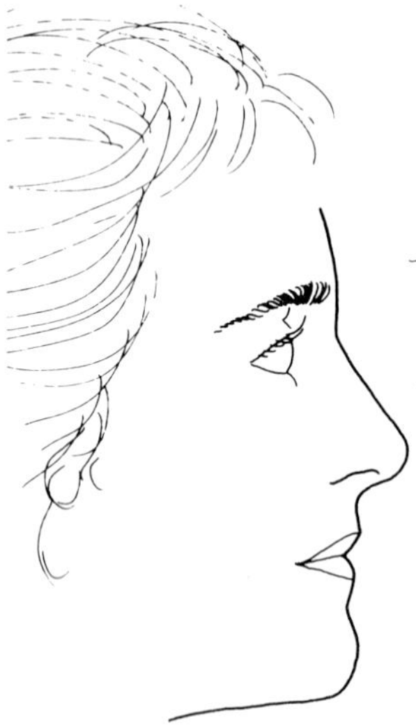

Figure 5-60A

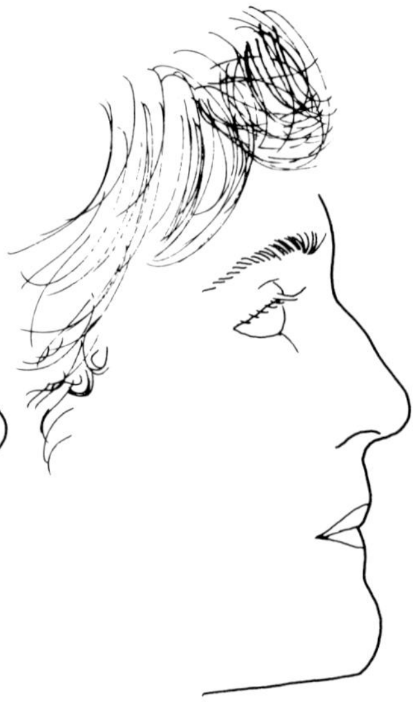

Figure 5-60B

Figure 5-60 shows how inferior tip rotation creates an apparent hump formation or supratip depression (Figure 5-60B).

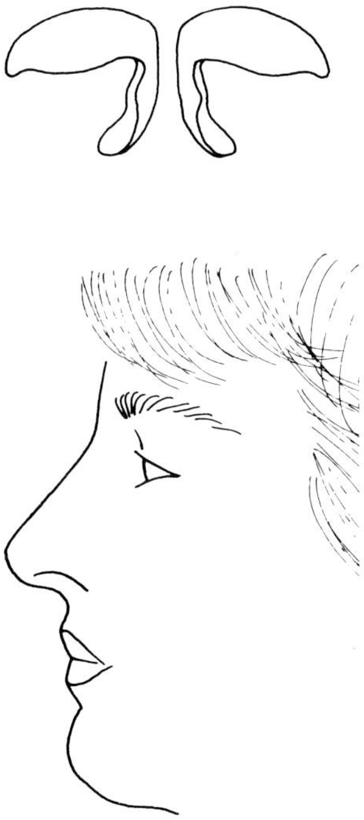

Figure 5-61A

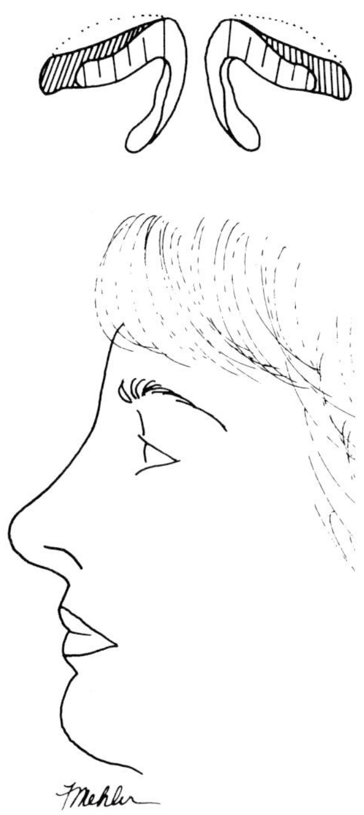

Figure 5-61B

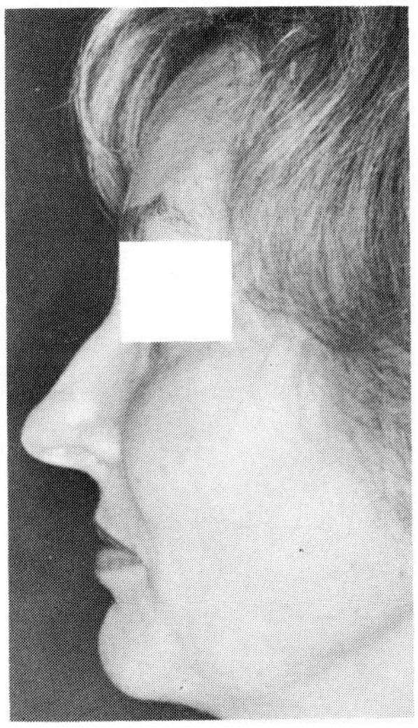

Figure 5-61C

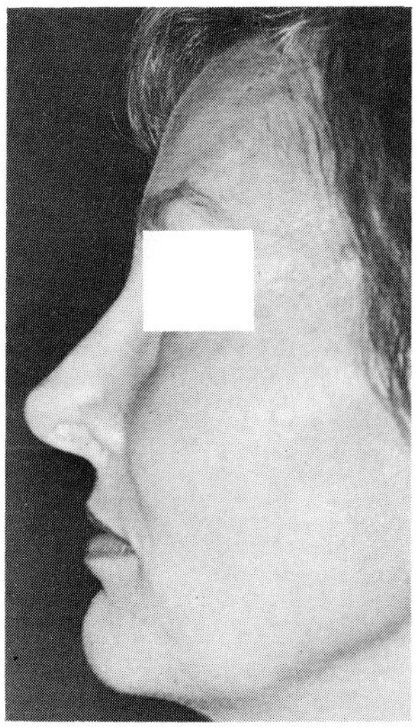

Figure 5-61D

Excessive columellar show may result from excessive resection of the lower lateral cartilage laterally with retraction of the alar rim (Figures 5-61A–D). The postoperative healing with cartilaginous support allowed contraction of the alar rim without notching. If the caudal border of the crural arch had been transected, notching would have occurred also. The shaded area in Figure 5-61B represents the excess removal. Figure 5-61A shows the preoperative sketch, and Figure 5-61C shows the preoperative photograph. The photograph in Figure 5-61D was taken 1 year postoperatively and illustrates considerable columellar show.

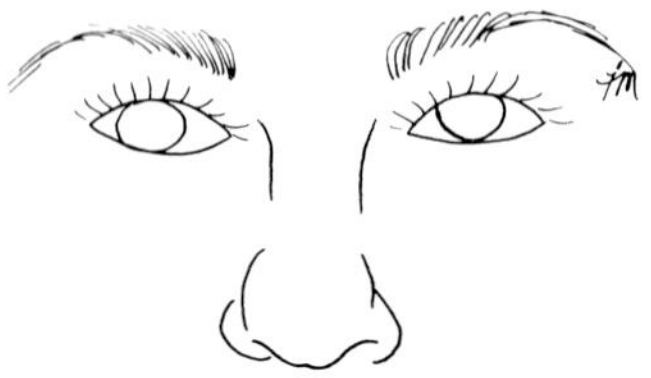

Figure 5-62A

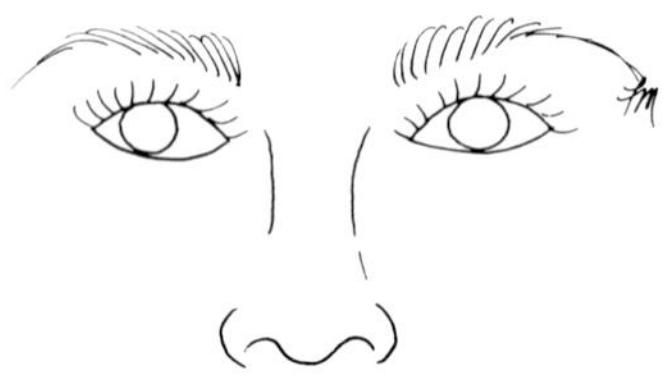

Figure 5-62B

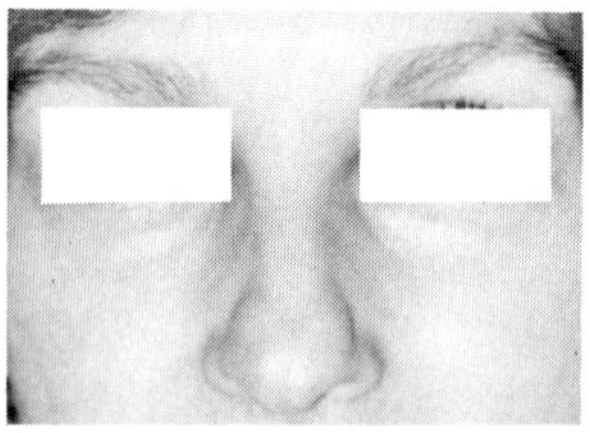

Figure 5-62C

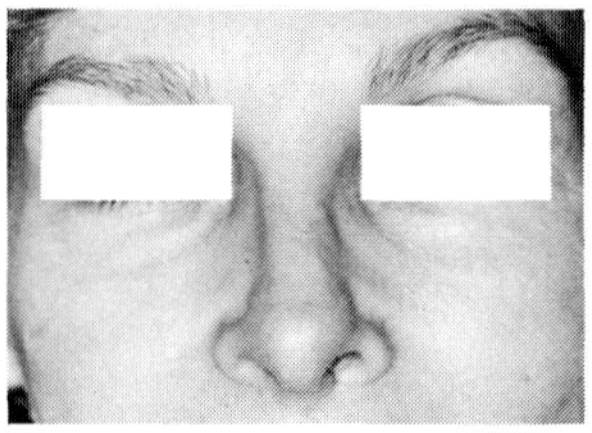

Figure 5-62D

Excessive narrowing of the tip and resection of the lateralmost portion of the lateral crura create retraction of the nostril rim. This is best treated by avoidance. Note the retraction without notching in Figures 5-62A–D. If the lateral crura had been transected, notching would have also occurred. The photographs are of the same patient as in Figures 5-61A–D.

Superior tip rotation can cause the amount of columellar show to increase. This is often desirable. If this becomes excessive or was preoperatively already excessive, however, it is best corrected following the tip surgery. Depending on the etiology, it can be compensated for by resecting a portion of the caudal septum, the membranous septum, the width of the medial crura, or any combination of the above. Figures 5-63A–D represents a combination of 2 mm from the caudal end of the septum and 2 mm from the caudal border of the medial crura. Note the change in the columellar defining point.

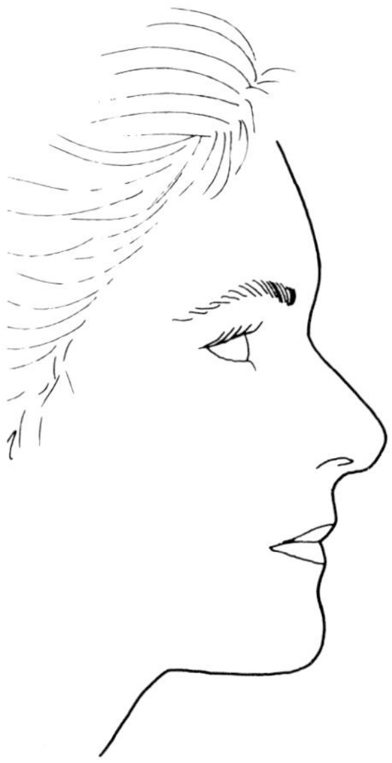

Figure 5-63A

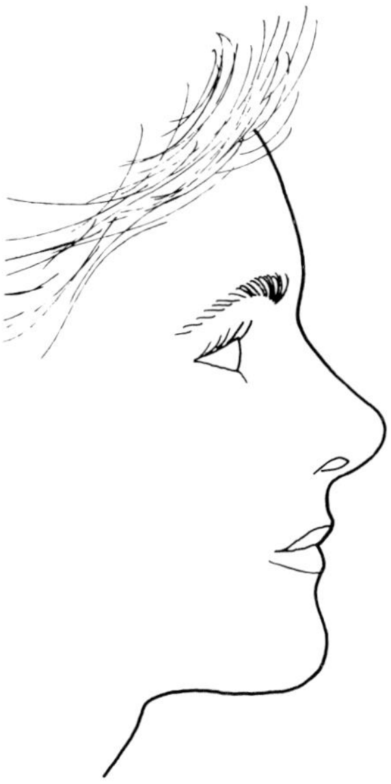

Figure 5-63B

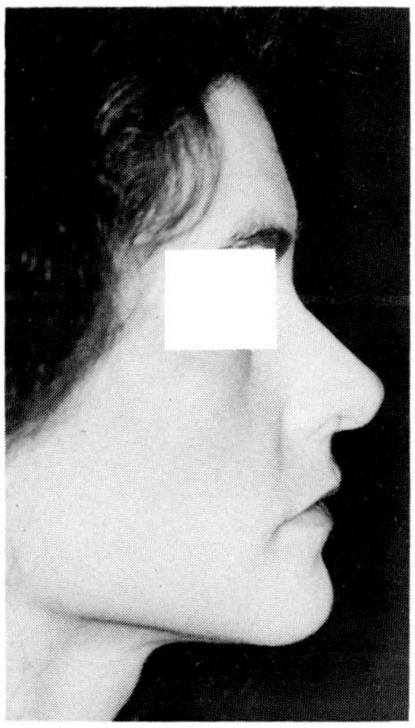

Figure 5-63C

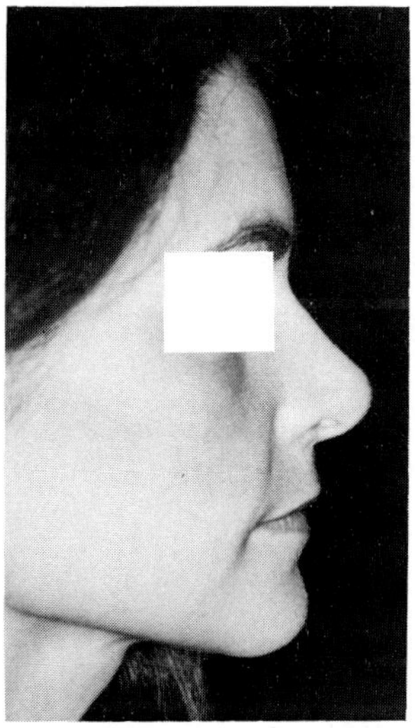

Figure 5-63D

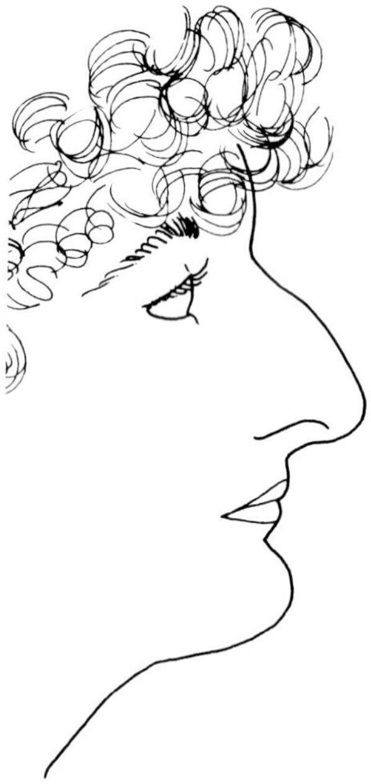

Figure 5-64A

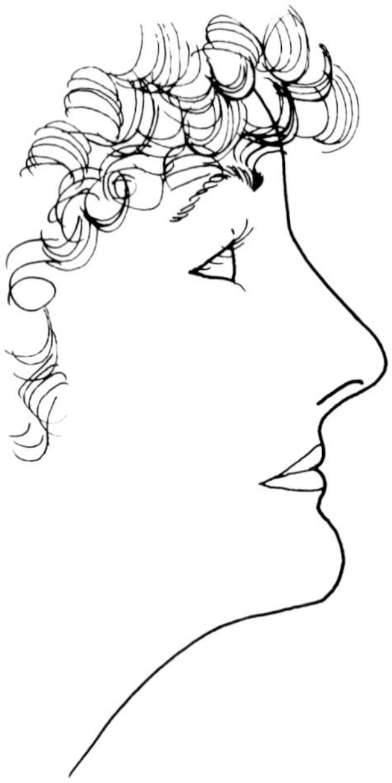

Figure 5-64B

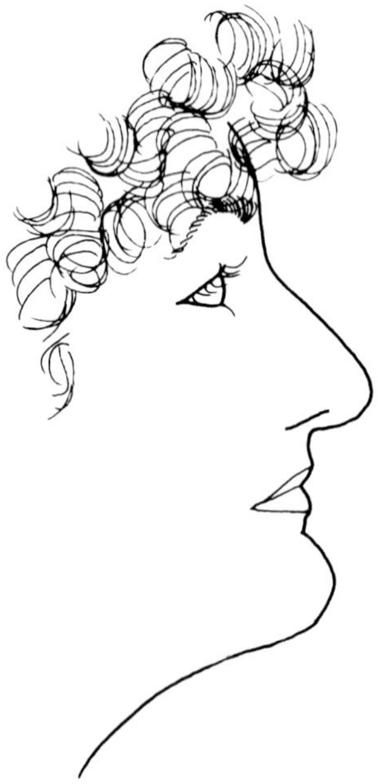

Figure 5-64C

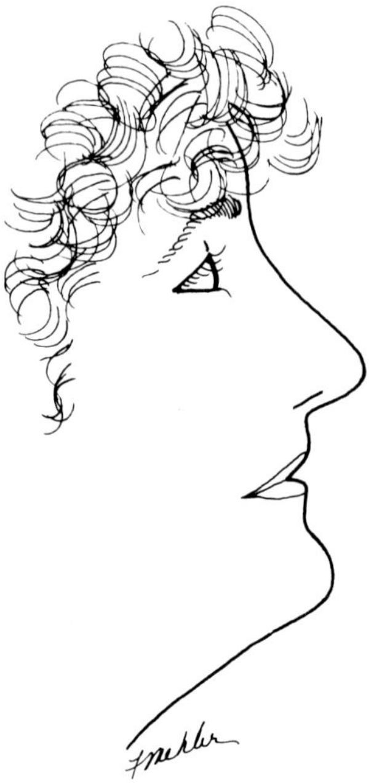

Figure 5-64D

Inferior tip rotation is nearly always undesirable. It commonly occurs in the postoperative period and is a frequent cause of the "polybeak" deformity. Some of the most common etiologies are a false sense of rotation at the time of the surgery due to the patient's recumbent head position, failure to resect some mucous membrane when resecting an excessively long caudal septum, failure to recognize and resect excessively long upper lateral cartilages, inadequate undermining of the soft tissues overlying the cartilaginous bony framework, and failure to recognize and compensate for the force of the scar contracture along the lines of the incisions. Figure 5-64 is an example of inferior tip rotation and its sequelae secondary to inadequate soft-tissue undermining to allow the extensive redraping necessary (sketch of same patient photographed in Figure 5-1). In Figure 5-64 the patient is shown preoperatively (A), intraoperatively (B), one year postoperatively (C), and at one year following revision (D).

Decreased tip projection causes widening of the base of the nose. This is best visualized on the base view. Figure 5-65 illustrates this preoperatively (A), intraoperatively (B), and also its correction with alar resections (C). (See Figure 5-156A–D later in this chapter).

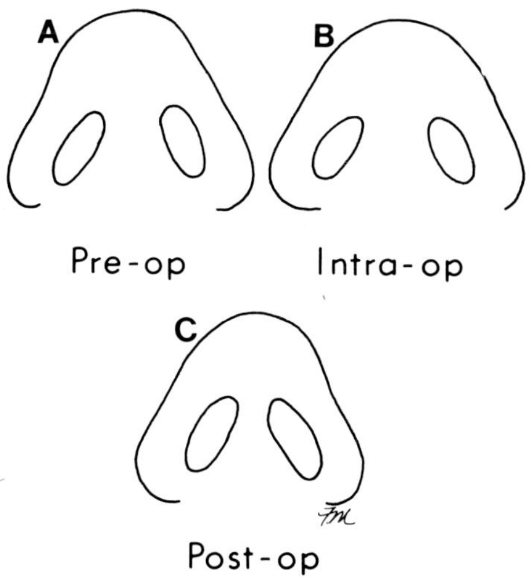

Figure 5-65

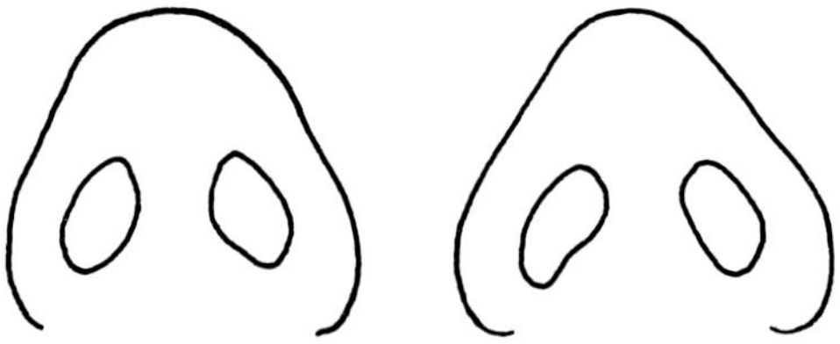

Figure 5-66A

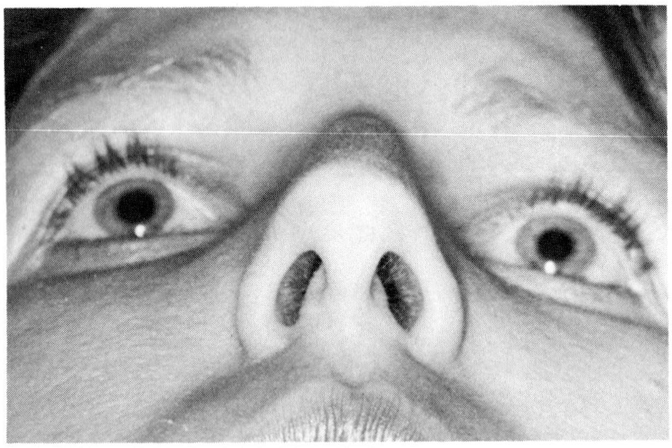

Figure 5-66B

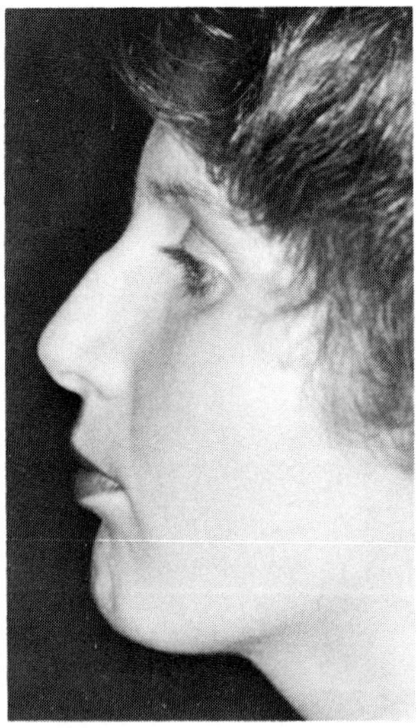

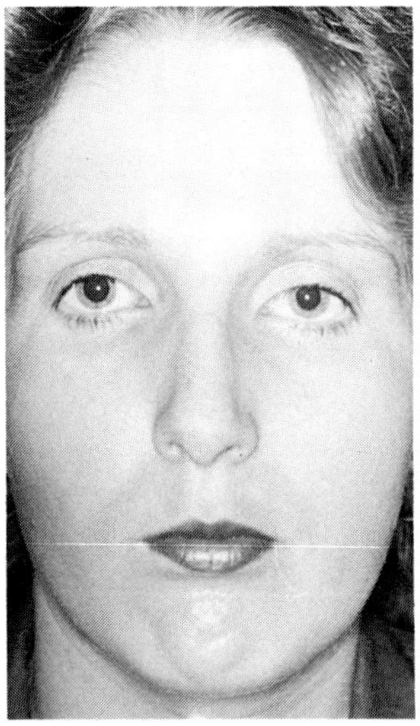

Figure 5-66C *Figure 5-66D*

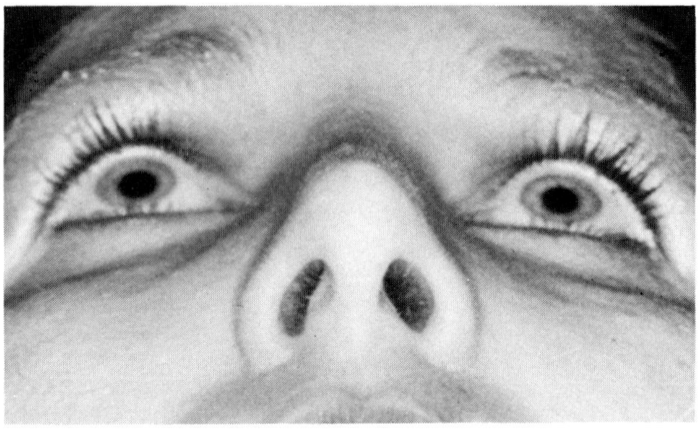

Figure 5-66E

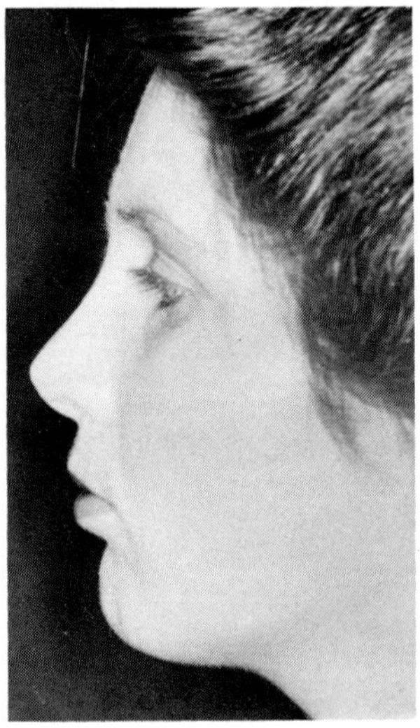

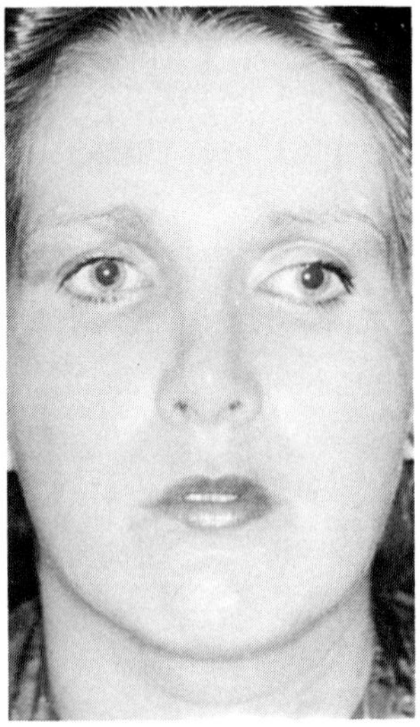

Figure 5-66F *Figure 5-66G*

A significant increase in tip projection through the use of free grafts, struts, or transecting the crura and suturing them together can cause an unnaturally pointed tip (Figure 5-66A). This is secondary to a "tent-pole" effect, and represents a tip with only one tip defining point. Figures 5-66B, C, and D are preoperative views with poor definition and lack of projection. Figures 5-66E, F, and G are postoperative views showing narrowing and increase in projection. Note the very surgical appearance of this nose. This is a tip with basically only one tip defining point.

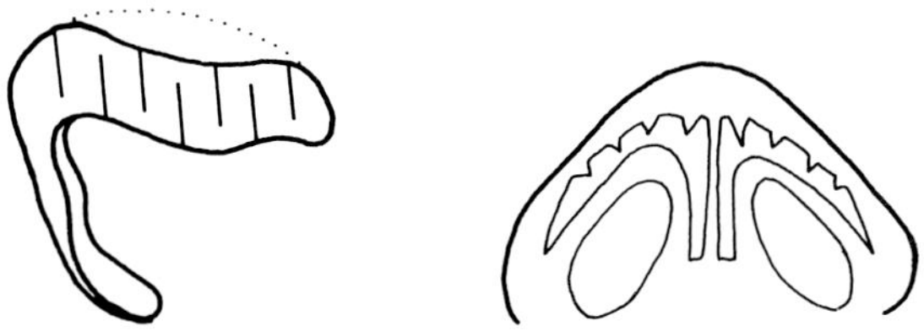

Figure 5-67A

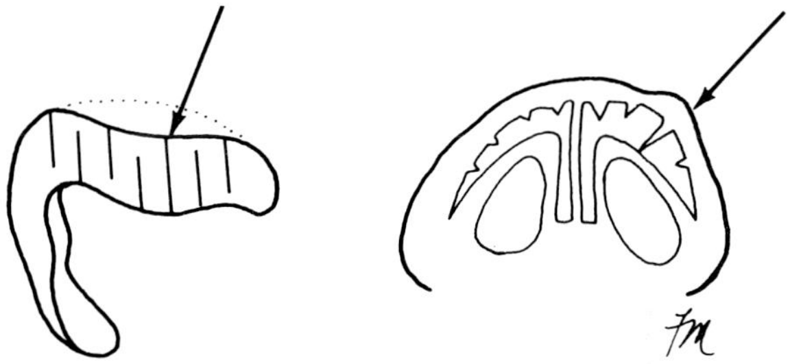

Figure 5-67B

If the scoring of the cartilages is unequal in depth or is weakened in any other manner (i.e. morsalization), the crural arch, if under tension, will buckle. Figure 5-67A represents the correct way. In Figure 5-67B the arrow points to area of greater weakening and subsequent buckle formation. Note that at 6 weeks the tip appeared symmetric (Figure 5-67C), but after 18 months the buckle was fully developed (Figures 5-67D and E). This is graphic representation of the poor value of photographs taken less than 1 year postoperatively. This defect first became visible at approximately 6 months.

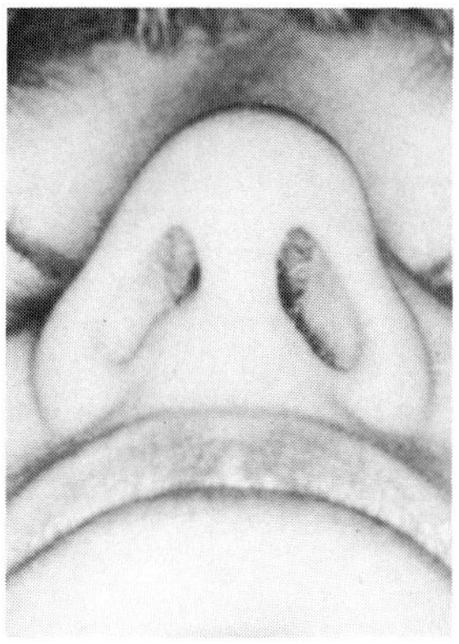

Figure 5-67C

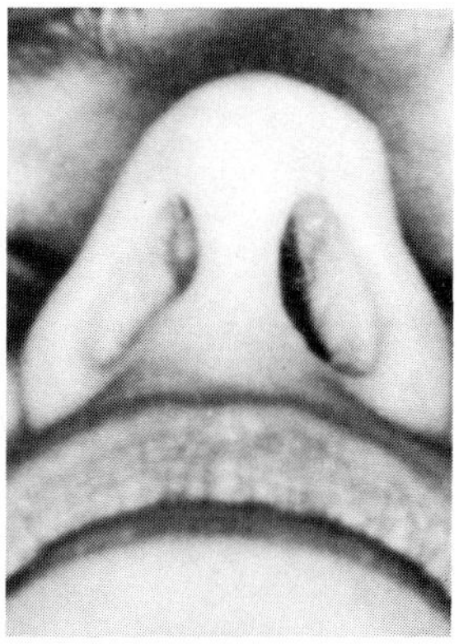

Figure 5-67D

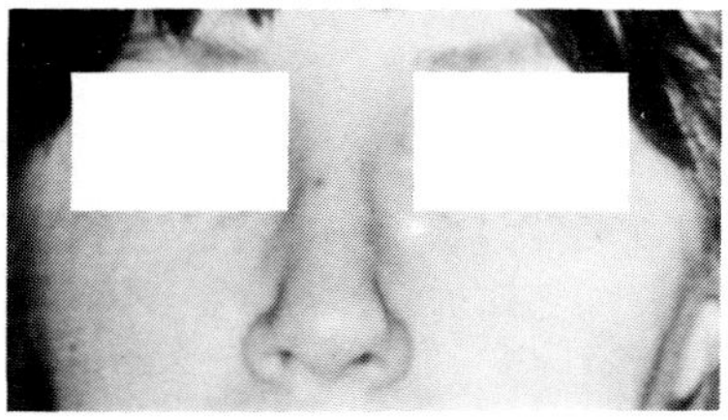

Figure 5-67E

TECHNIQUE

Full Delivery

Full or partial delivery of the crural arch is accomplished with two incisions. The first is an intercartilaginous incision, which joins a partial or complete transfixion incision. The second is a marginal incision. After dissecting the soft tissue off of the crural arch, it can then be delivered as a bipedicled chondrocutaneous flap. The major advantages are direct visualization, precise symmetrical surgery, and the ability to modify the cartilage that will remain to form the new tip. The major disadvantage is the resultant scar contracture along the incisions, which will act to decrease the tip projection in the postoperative period. This technique is routinely used for refining or narrowing a tip, superiorly rotating a tip, and mildly decreasing tip projection. If used in a tip with marginal or poor tip projection, it must be done with great care, remembering that the scar contracture will work against the desired projection and must be guarded against.

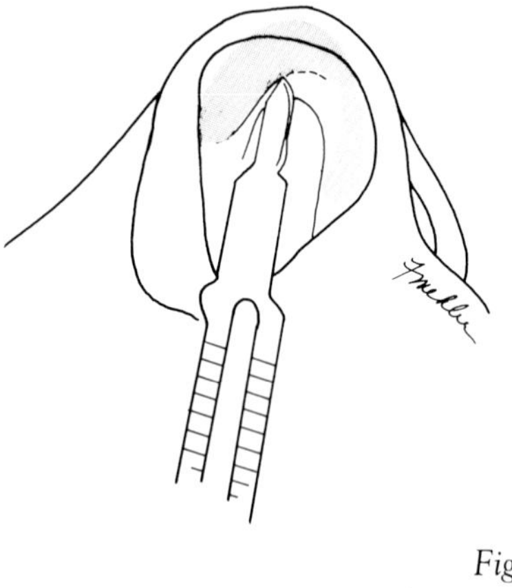

Figure 5-68A

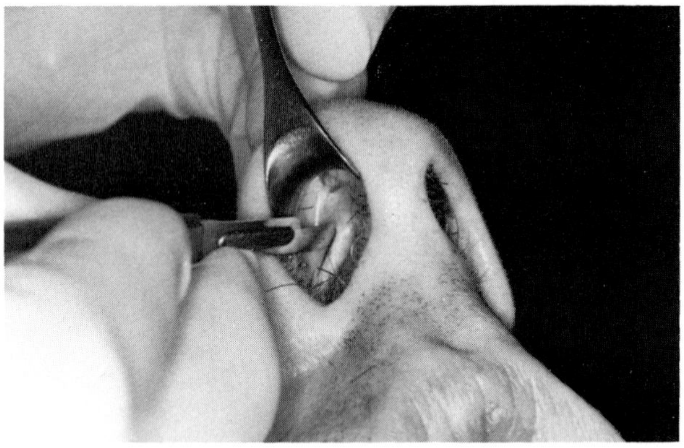

Figure 5-68B

The intercartilaginous incision is made between the scrolls of the upper and lower lateral cartilages (Figures 5-68A and B). It is placed along the caudal edge of the scroll of the upper lateral. It extends medially to parallel the anterior septal angle and joins a transfixion incision. An acute-angled mucosal cut at the anterior septal angle makes subsequent accurate approximation possible. The Parks or Goldman elevator is placed under slight tension to help separate the scrolls of the upper and lower cartilages to facilitate the incision.

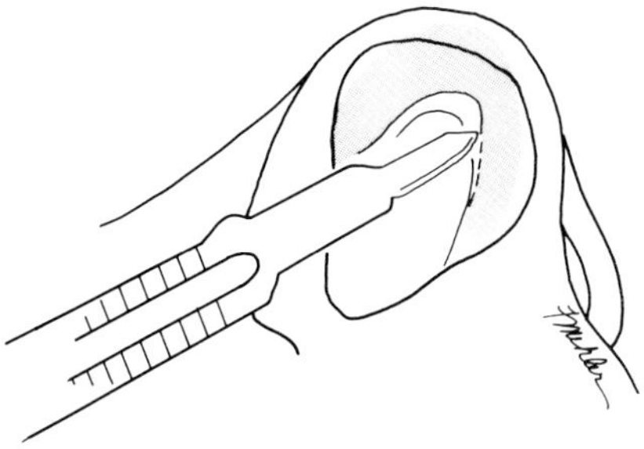

Figure 5-69A

The transfixion incision starts at an acute angle to the intercartilaginous incision and parallels the edge of the anterior septal angle (Figure 5-69A and B) This is extended along the caudal border of the septum as far as needed for exposure. Thus partial or complete transfixion refers to the length of the incision paralleling the caudal border of the septum. The term "hemitransfixion incision" refers to an incision on either the right or left side.

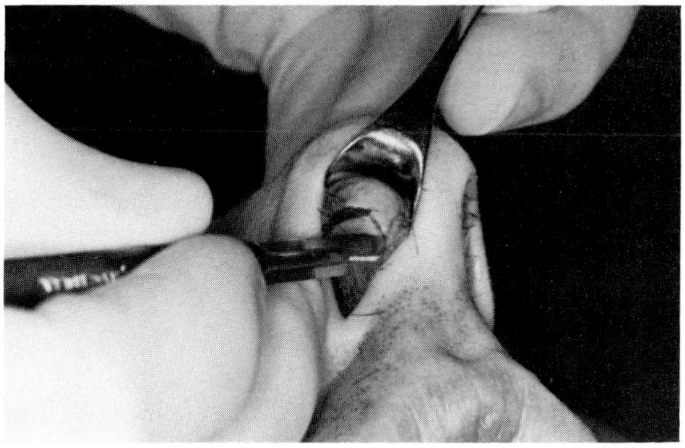

Figure 5-69B

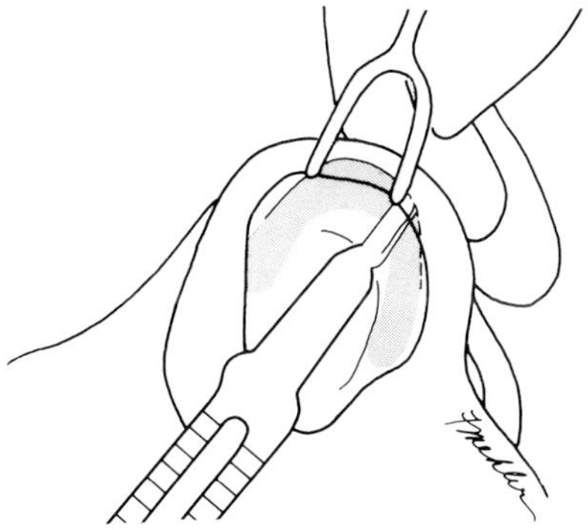

Figure 5-70A

The marginal incision parallels the caudal margin of the lower lateral cartilage (Figures 5-70A and B). This incision is made along the caudal border of the medial crura. Before the incision is made, the free border must be identified through the vestibular skin. This is facilitated by the use of a double sharp skin hook and everting the tip with the middle finger. The edge frequently is at the vibrissae line. Palpation with the handle of the scalpel is also valuable.

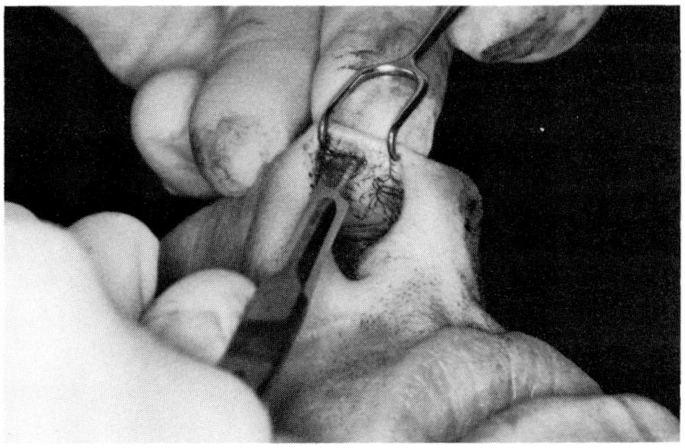

Figure 5-70B

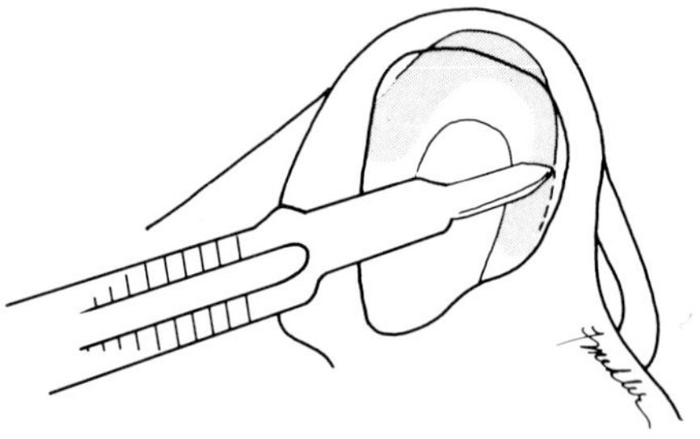

Figure 5-71A

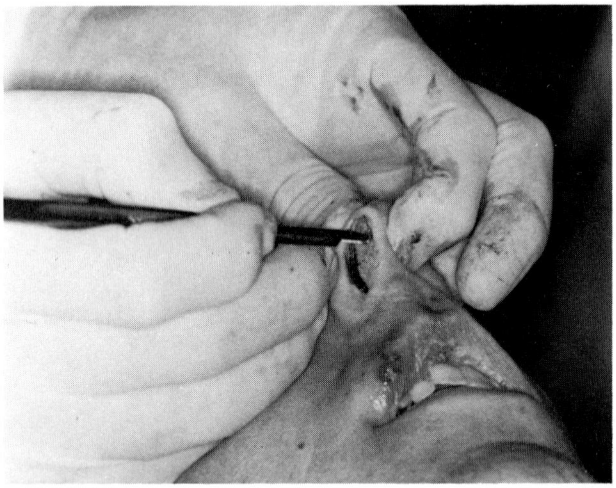

Figure 5-71B

Again the length of the incision is determined by the exposure required. The term "extended marginal incision" refers to extending the marginal incision along the length of the medial crura to its foot (Figure 5-71A and B). This extention allows complete dissection and delivery of both the medial and lateral crura.

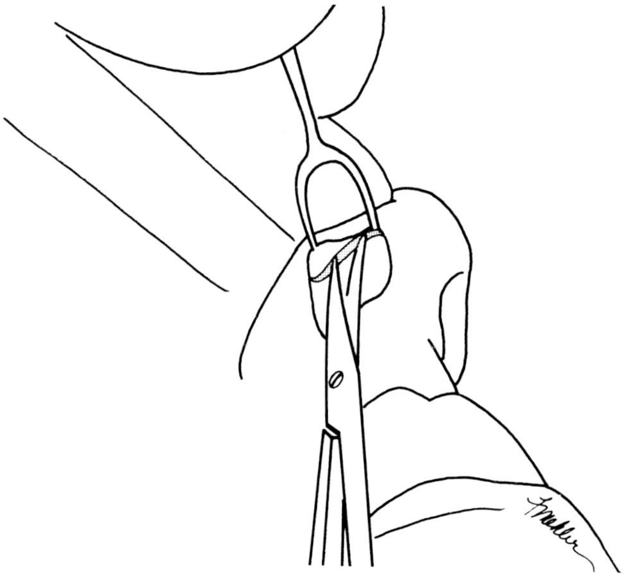

Figure 5-72A

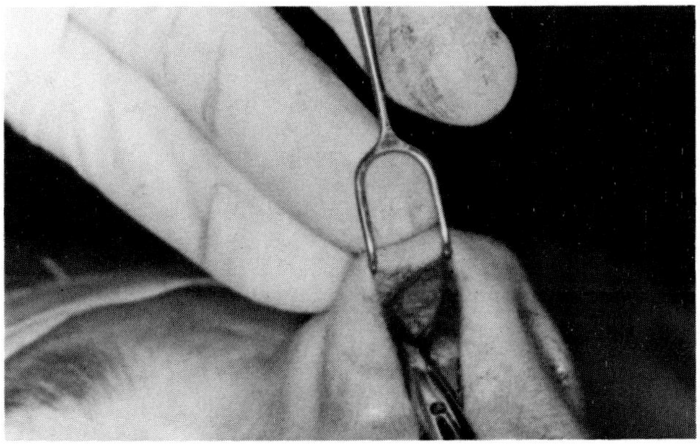

Figure 5-72B

Soft-tissue dissection is facilitated by retracting the alar rim with a double-pronged skin hook (Figure 5-72A and B). The Shea vein scissors are well suited for developing the desired perichondral plane which is relatively avascular. This plane of dissection is begun over the midportion of the lateral crural arch.

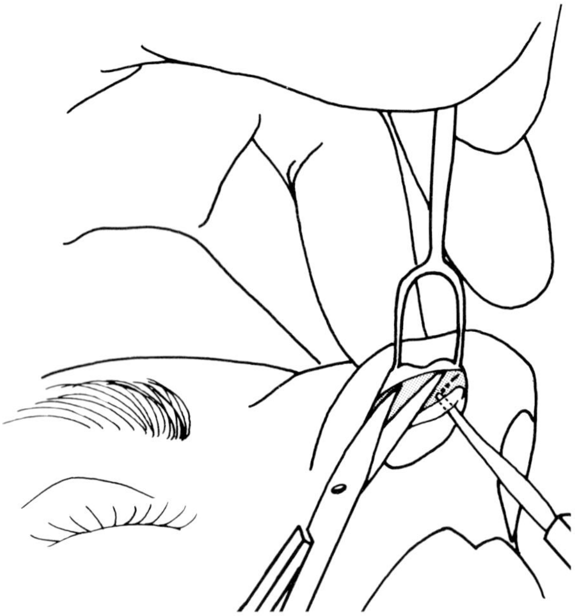

Figure 5-73A

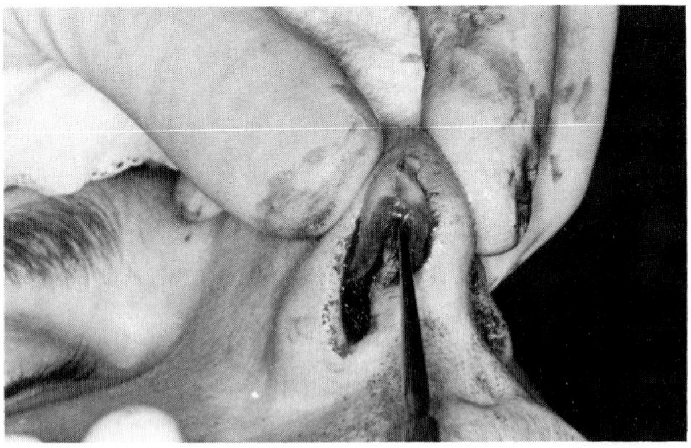

Figure 5-73B

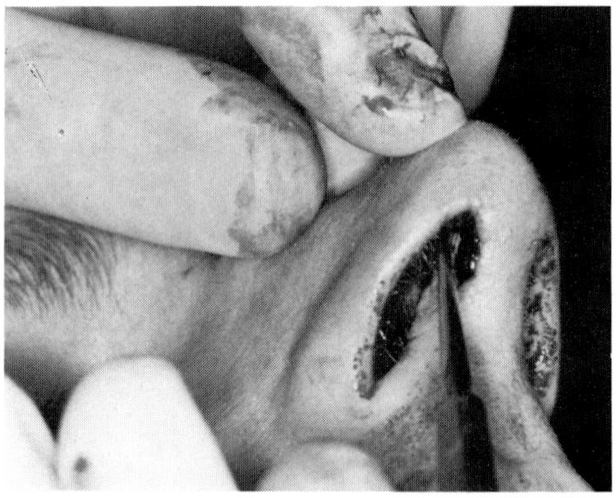

Figure 5-73C

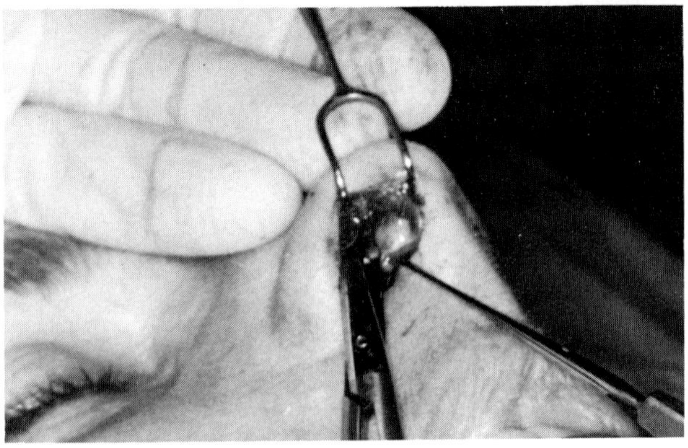

Figure 5-73D

Dissection of the scroll of the crural arch and the medial crura is facilitated by applying slight traction with a right-angled hook. The right angled hook is placed from below, up through the tip defining point (Figure 5-73A and B). This also serves as a useful reference point and can be marked with a marking pen when the hook is removed. Figure 5-73C shows the placement by palpation of the right angled hook through the tip defining point. Figure 5-73D shows the hook delivering the crural arch while dissecting with the Shea vein scissors.

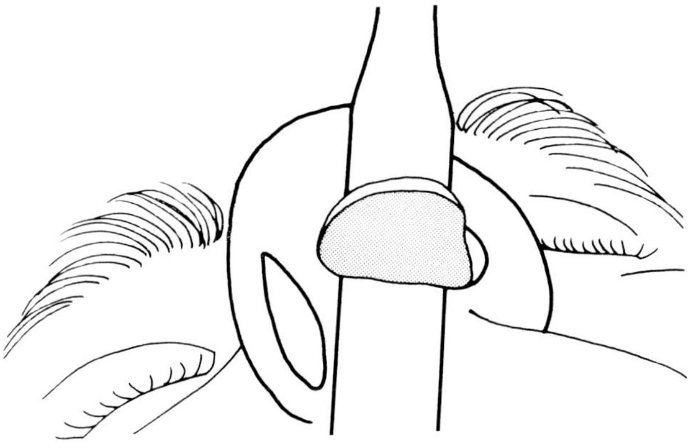

Figure 5-74A

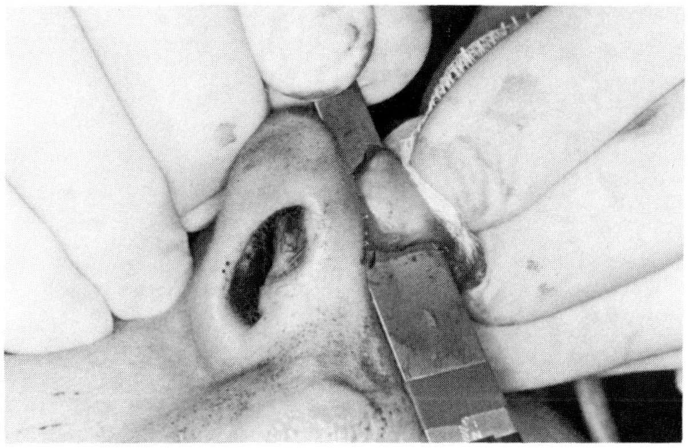

Figure 5-74B

The crural arch is then delivered and supported from below with a Park retractor (Figure 5-74A and B). The remaining soft tissue is then wiped off of the cartilage with a dry sponge. The Park retractor provides a firm base for the crural arch, easing subsequent incisions and excisions.

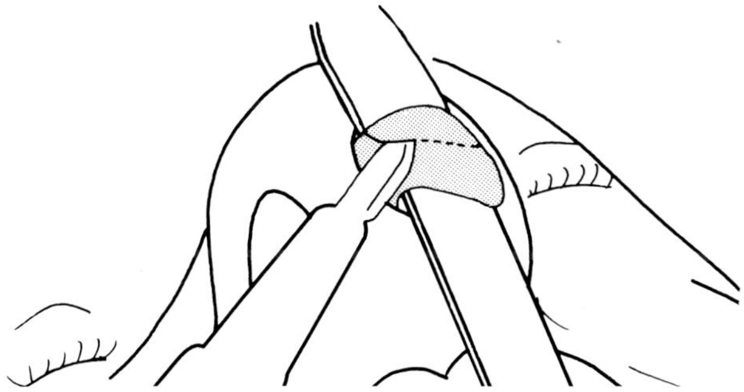

Figure 5-75A

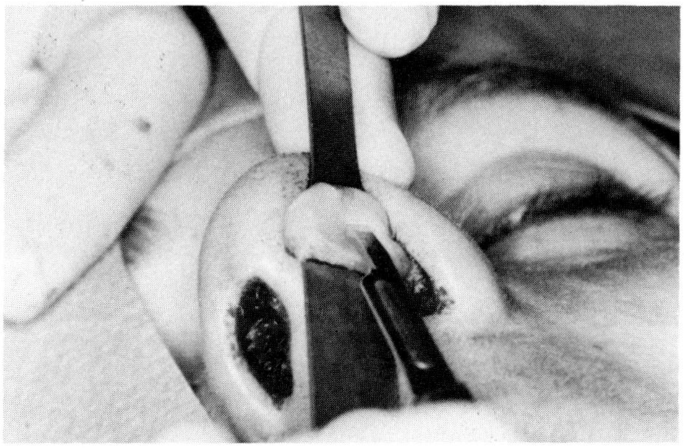

Figure 5-75B

The degree of narrowing and the amount of superior tip rotation desired determines the shape and size of the cephalic portion of the lateral crura to be excised. Excessive removal will result in too narrow a tip. This is then incised (Figure 5-75A and B) using a #15 blade on a beveled angle to prevent a palpable step in the future. This incision is through the cartilage, but not the vestibular skin.

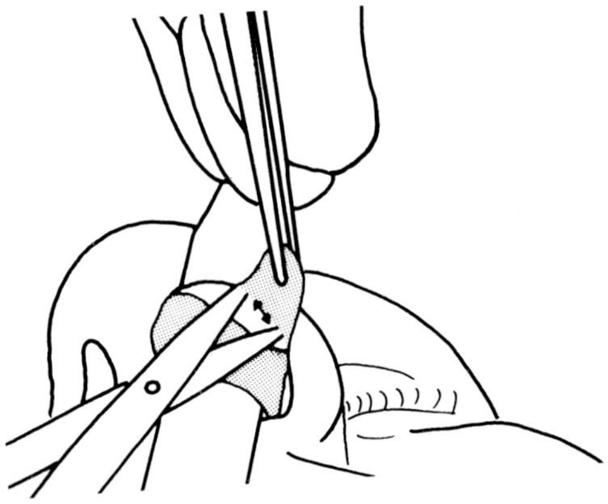

Figure 5-76A

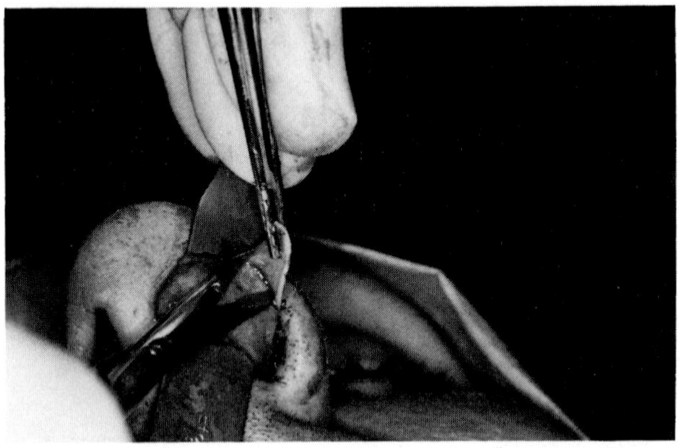

Figure 5-76B

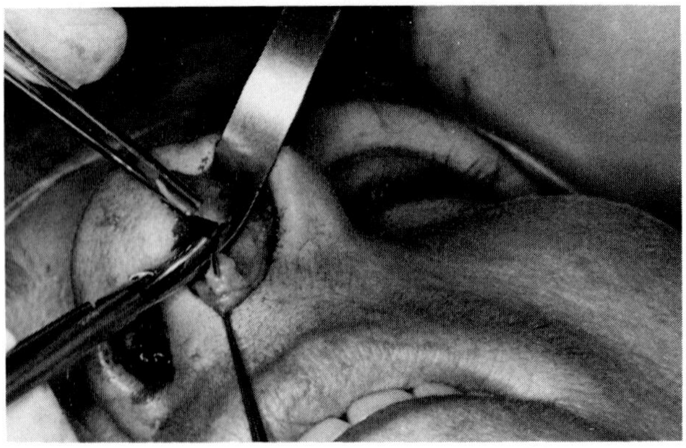

Figure 5-76C

Then with multitooth pickups (to avoid tearing the cartilage) the cartilage is dissected free from the underlying vestibular skin with the dissecting scissors (Figure 5-76A–C). To remove the lateralmost portion of the lateral crura, the right-angled hook is again used for slight medial traction (Figure 5-76C).

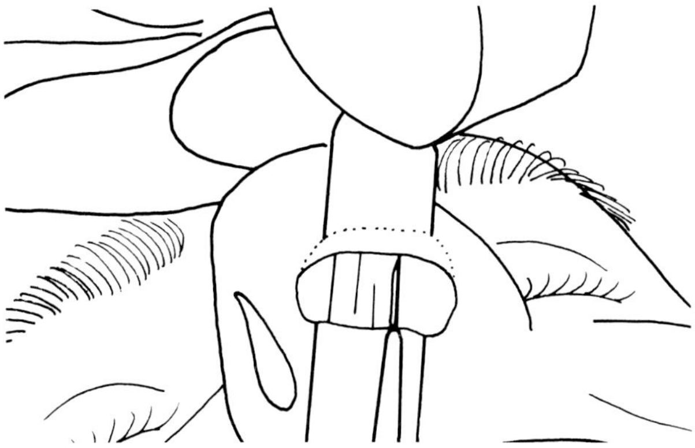

Figure 5-77A

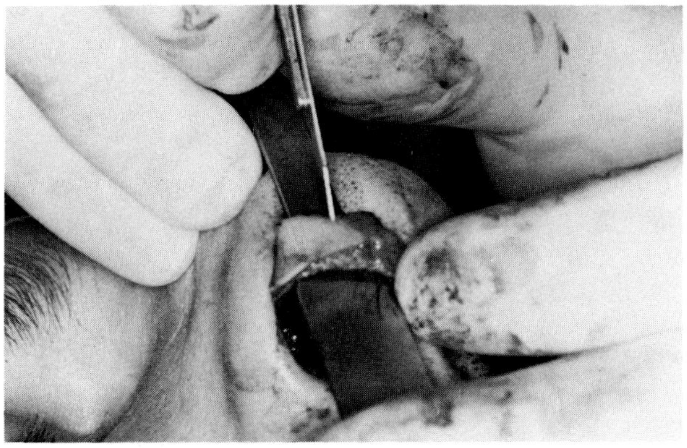

Figure 5-77B

After excision of the cephalic portion of the lateral crural arch, the remaining cartilage can be further refined. Further weakening of the remaining crural arch will soften the tip contours. If the weakening is excessive, however, the crural arch will buckle (see Figure 5-67). Morselization is too difficult to control and not exact enough. Vertical incision at 2–3 mm apart offer excellent results. The incisions are made with the belly of a No. 15 blade. They are 2–3 mm apart, and their depth is varied according to the thickness of the cartilage. The greater the break of the spring of the arch desired, the deeper the incision. The deepest and only complete incision should coincide with the new tip defining point. Selective alternating incisions, as championed by Jack H. Sheen offer even greater control and margin for error[6] (see Figure 5-77A and B).

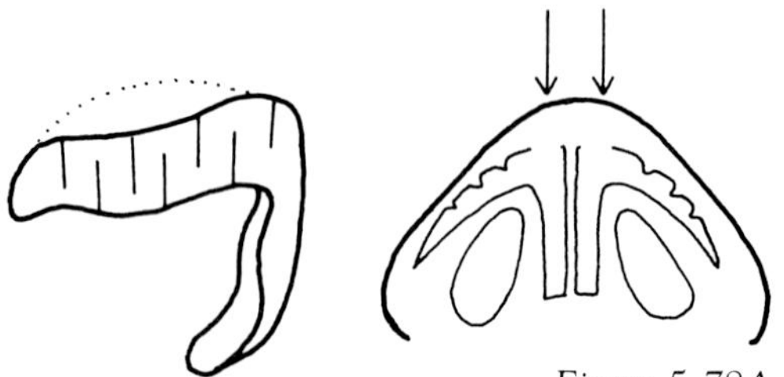

Figure 5-78A

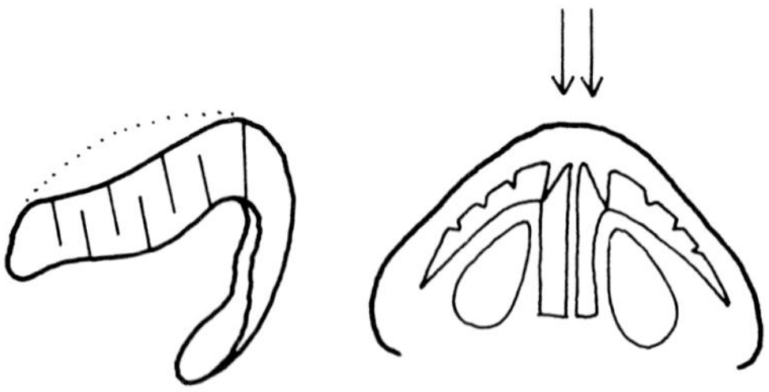

Figure 5-78B

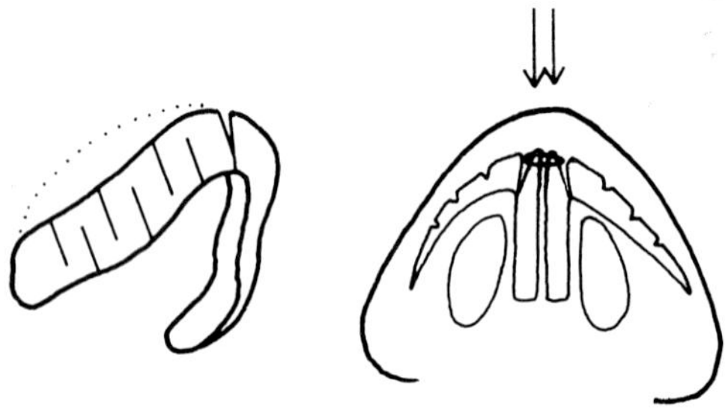

Figure 5-78C

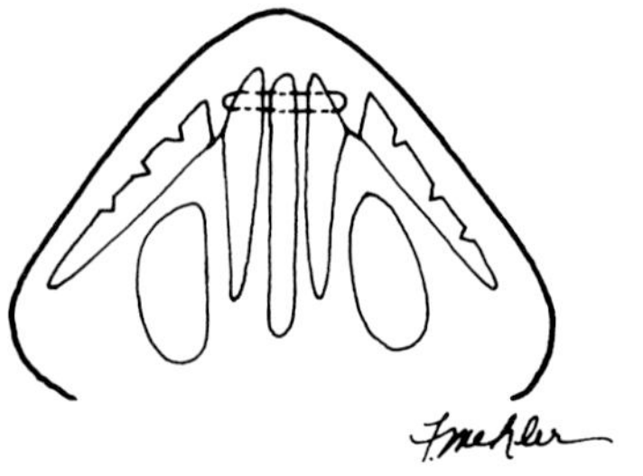

Figure 5-78D

After the preliminary surgery (Figure 5-78A) the tip defining point can be sharpened and narrowed with the use of a deep vertical incision (Figure 5-78B). Further narrowing and increase in projection can be obtained by suturing the medial crura together as in Figure 5-78C. Even greater projection can be obtained with the use of a strut between the medial crura as in Figure 5-78D. Note that the medial crura are approximated over the strut. This suturing of the crura over the strut lessens the possibility of a pointed tip. In the stepwise narrowing of a tip and increasing the tip projection, if the complete vertical incision is placed lateral to the original tip defining point, the projection will be increased by creating a new tip defining point. Note the closer approximation of the tip defining points (arrows) in Figure 5-78A–C. Also refer back to the photographs in Figure 5-66. This patient was treated in the same manner as represented in Figure 5-78C and obtained a poor result.

Increased tip projection and superior rotation is also produced with the use of plumping grafts. Multiple 2–3-mm pieces of bone and cartilage from the septum are placed in a soft-tissue pocket inferior to the feet of the medial crura and anterior superior to the nasal spine. A suture is commonly placed to approximate the medial crura to prevent the grafts from migrating superiorly (see Figure 5-79 shows the cartilage and bone grafts in place. These are routinely soaked in an antibiotic solution first.

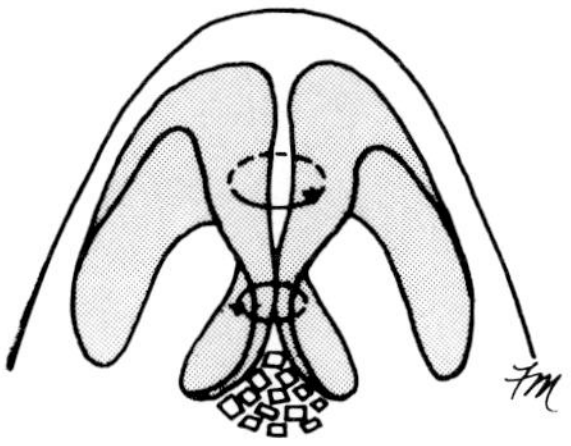

Figure 5-79

Figure 5-80 represents a lateral view showing the effect on the nasolabial angle.

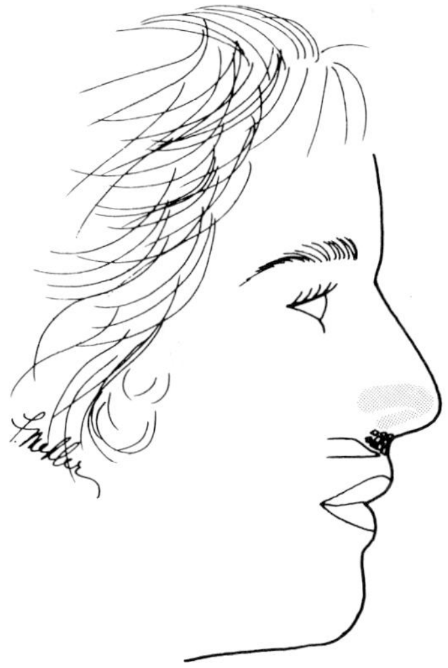

Figure 5-80

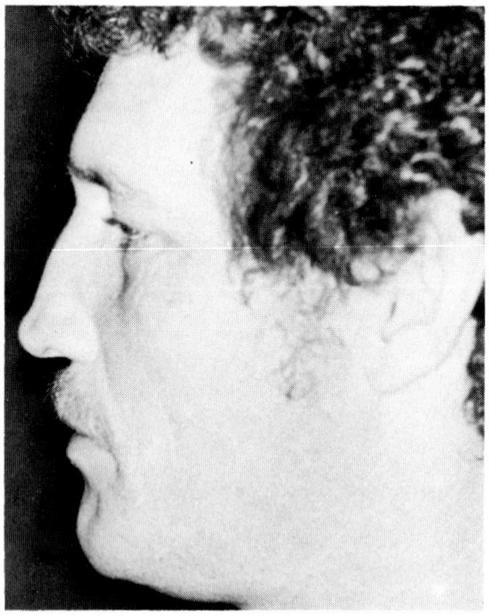

Figure 5-81

Figure 5-81 is a preoperative view.

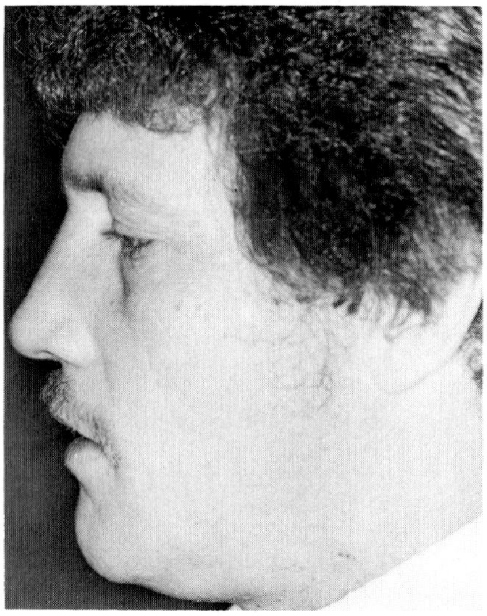

Figure 5-82

Figure 5-82 is a postoperative view using this method combined with a strut.

Inherent in the full delivery technique is some decrease in tip projection secondary to the normal fibrous healing in the planes of exposure. In a tip that is slightly overprojecting, this is a valuable way of decreasing tip projection. If greater reduction in projection is needed, weakening of the crural arch or resection of a portion of the crural arch is indicated. The crural arch is fully delivered with the use of an extended marginal incision. The surgery of the lateral arch is performed as in the full delivery technique, and then the crural arch is placed back into position, and the excess projection is evaluated.

Then they are redelivered, and 4–6 mm below the tip defining point an incision is made transecting the medial crura. Then a small segment of medial crura is resected. The relative decrease in projection is much greater than the size of the segment resected. Overresection must be guarded against. The vestibular skin may be preserved in a small resection and excised in larger resections. The closure must be meticulous.

Transection is done with preservation of the vestibular skin (Figure 5-83A–C). Figure 5-83B shows the initial incisions placed 3 mm apart. Figure 5-83C shows the excision with the preservation, in this case, of the vestibular skin.

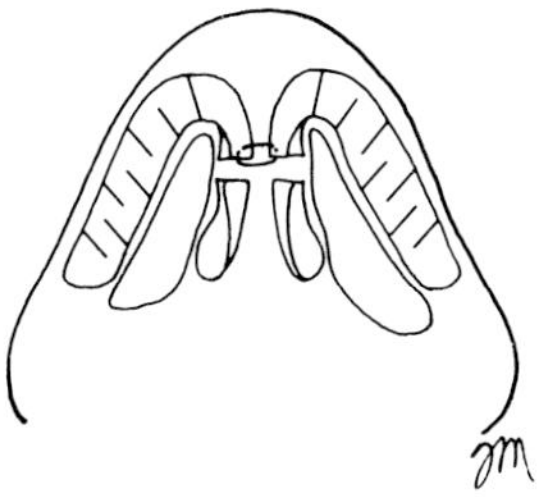

Figure 5-83A

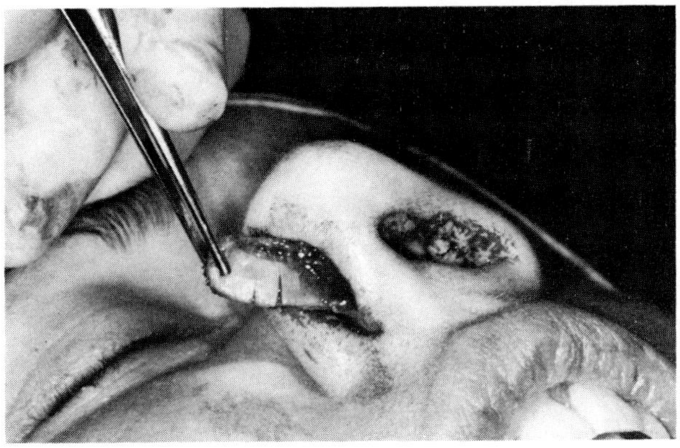

Figure 5-83B

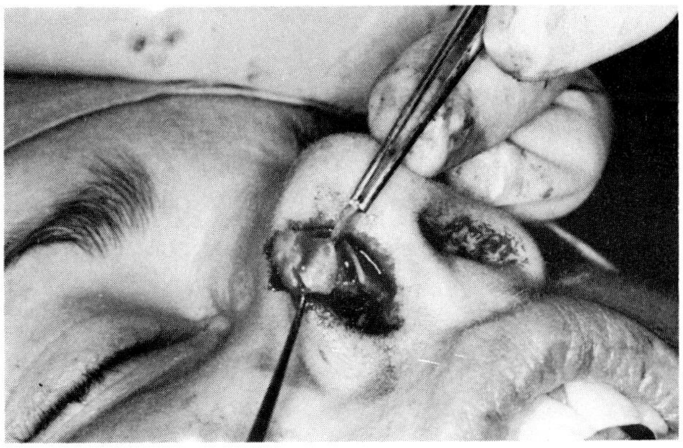

Figure 5-83C

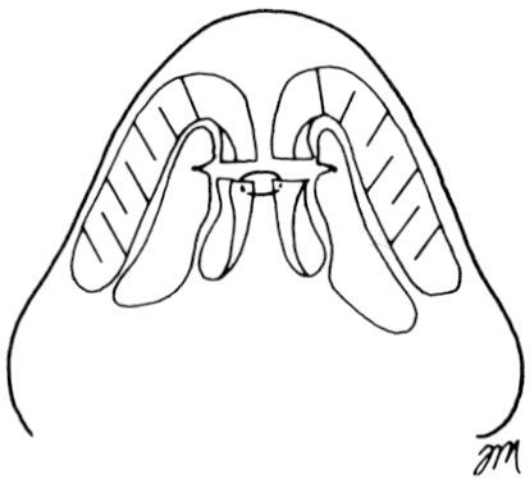

Figure 5-84A

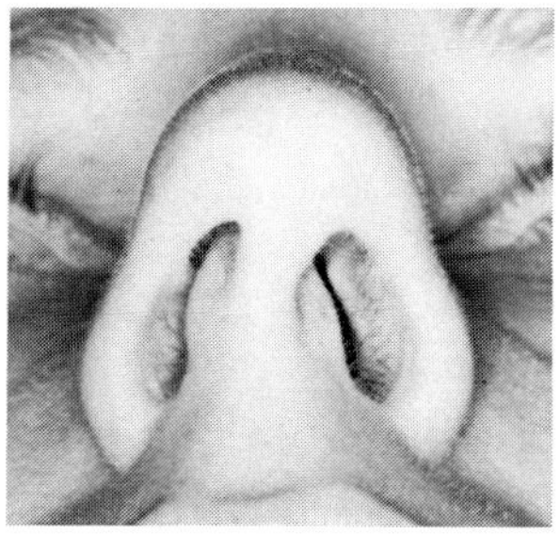

Figure 5-84B

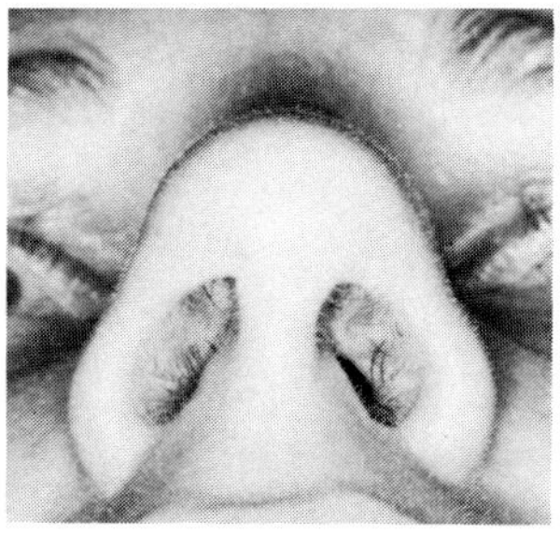

Figure 5-84C

When resecting vestibular skin it is helpful if the amount resected is less than the amount of cartilage excised. This allows better reapproximation. The suture may be of vestibular skin only or also include the underlying cartilage, depending on which provides the best approximation. If the medial crura flair or twist, they should be sutured together as shown in Figure 5-84A. Illustrations 5-84B and 5-84C are, respectively, preoperative and 18-months postoperative photographs of a tip treated in this manner. See also Figures 5-98A–D for profile views of the same patient.

Cartilage Splitting

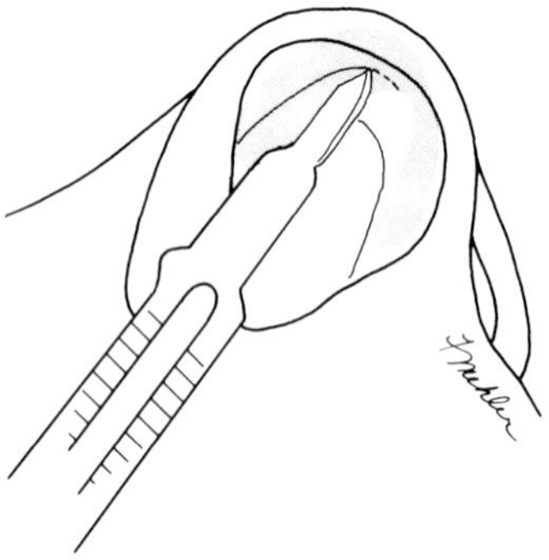

Figure 5-85A

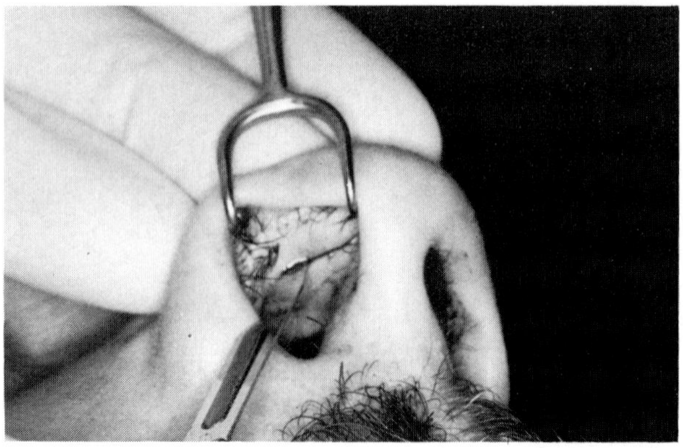

Figure 5-85B

The cartilage splitting technique is accomplished through an intracartilaginous incision that is joined to a partial or complete transfixion incision. This incision is placed in such a manner that it transects or splits the lateral crural cartilage at the position that will become the new cephalic border of the lower lateral cartilage after removal of the cephalic portion (Figure 5-85A and B). The major advantage is that there is less scar tissue formation as so little of the crural arch is actually exposed. This technique also allows good small soft-tissue pockets to be developed for placement of struts, battens, or tip grafts. The chief disadvantage is that the remaining crural arch of the new tip cannot be easily modified. In addition, many types of preoperative tip asymmetries cannot be corrected by this procedure. This technique is best suited to a preoperatively symmetric tip whose projection must be maintained or increased. The initial incision does not completely split the cartilage as this facilitates dissection of the vestibular skin from the cartilage to be resected. After elevation of the vestibular skin the cartilage is completely transected and dissected free from the soft tissue.

Open Flap

The open rhinoplasty is accomplished with a partially extended marginal incision, which is joined with a transcolumellar incision. The transcolumellar incision is made just inferior to the columellar defining point. The major advantage of the open rhinoplasty approach lies in the unparalleled and undistorted exposure. In particular, identification and correction of asymmetries of the upper laterals and bony dorsum are enhanced. Placement of a large graft is more accurate, and they may be easily sutured into position. Struts may also be trimmed and sutured without distortion. As advocated by W. K. Wright (personal communication), the use of mastoid periosteum as a graft material and the open rhinoplasty for exposure provides an excellent combination for repairing septal perforations. The disadvantage is the transcolumellar incision, which when meticulously performed and closed is not a significant problem (see Figure 5-95). Also, transection of the columella makes correction of the columella and nasolabial angle more difficult to evaluate at the time of the correction. The open rhinoplasty is particularly well suited for a crooked nose, septal perforation repairs, and revisions of previous rhinoplasties where the pathology is uncertain.

A marking pen is helpful for making an accurate incision, particularly if the columella is twisted (Figure 5-86A and B).

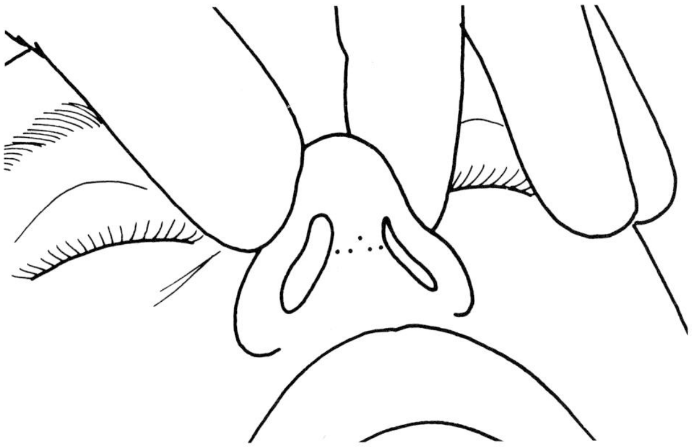

Figure 5-86A

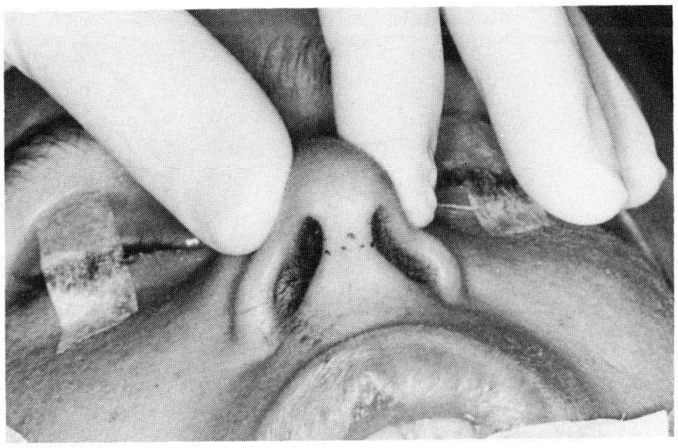

Figure 5-86B

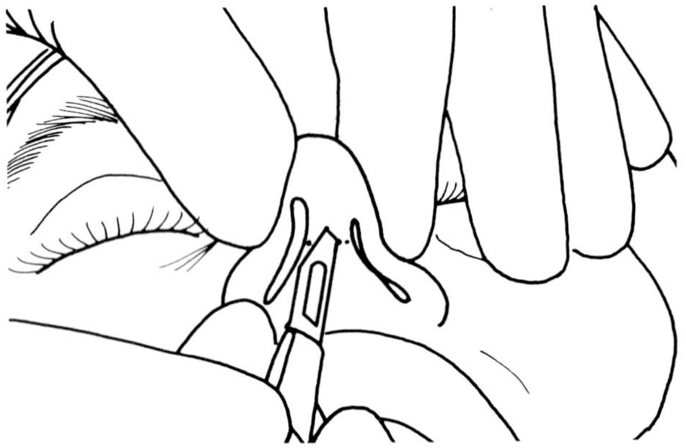

Figure 5-87A

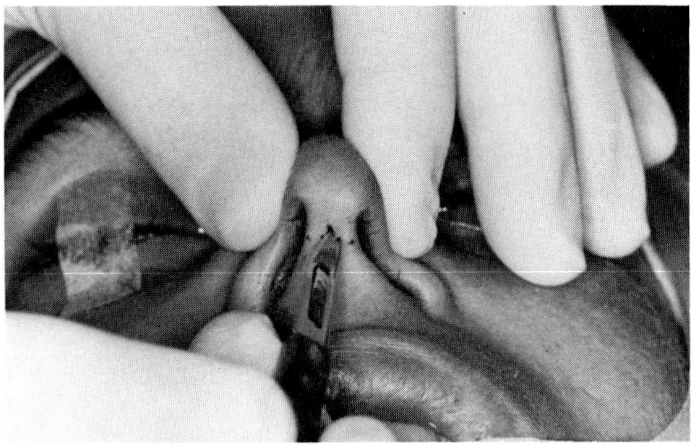

Figure 5-87B

Use of a No. 11 Bard-Parker blade in a slow stabbing motion gives a very accurate vertical leg (Figure 5-87A and B).

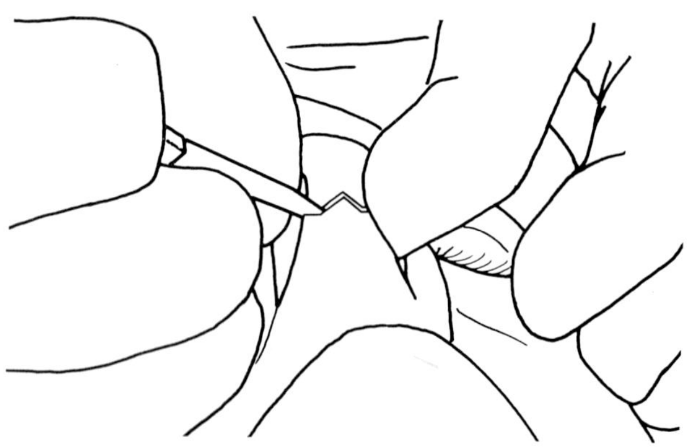

Figure 5-88A

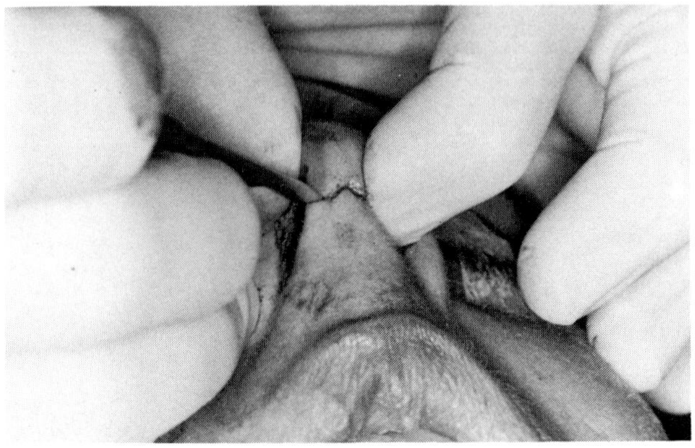

Figure 5-88B

A No. 15 Bard-Parker blade makes the horizontal limbs (Figure 5-88A and B). The left hand exerts firm pressure in a pinching manner to provide hemostasis. The incision must be through the skin, but not cut the underlying medial crura.

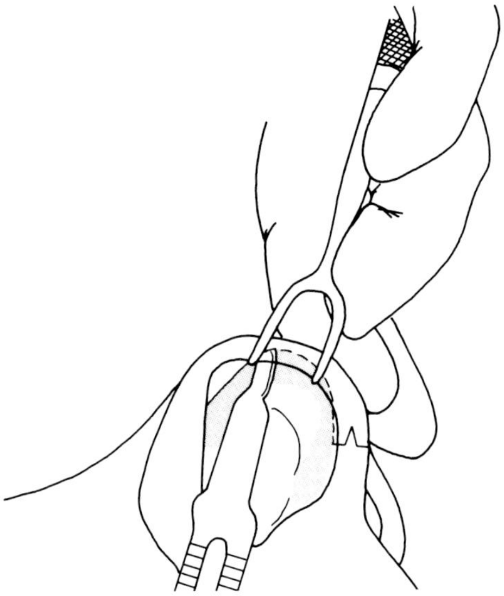

Figure 5-89A

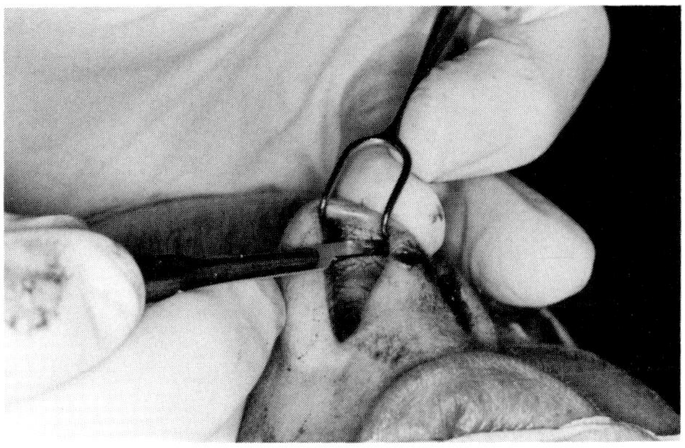

Figure 5-89B

The standard marginal incision is made and connected to the transcolumellar incision (Figure 5-89A–C).

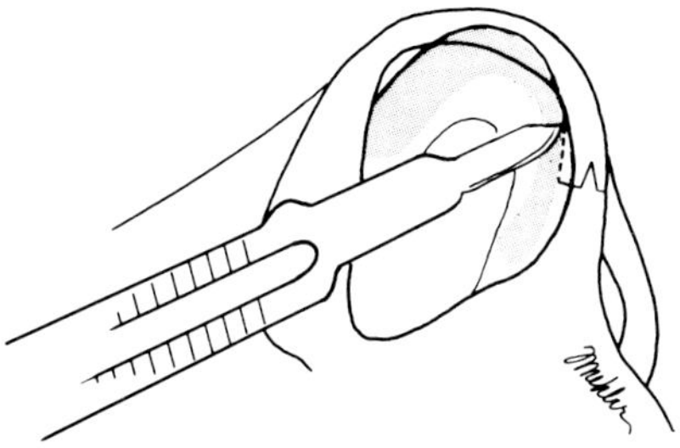

Figure 5-89C

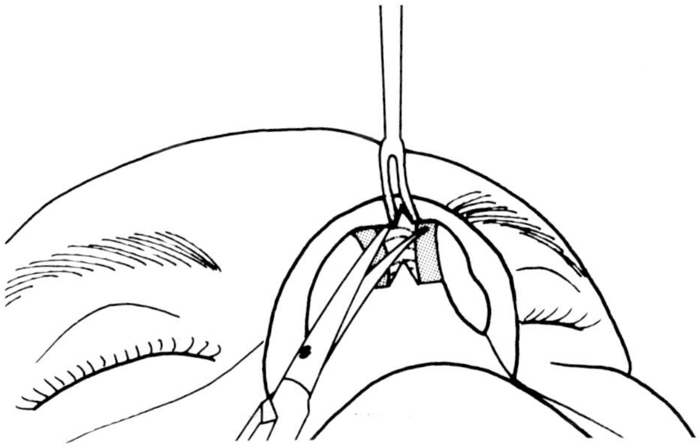

Figure 5-90A

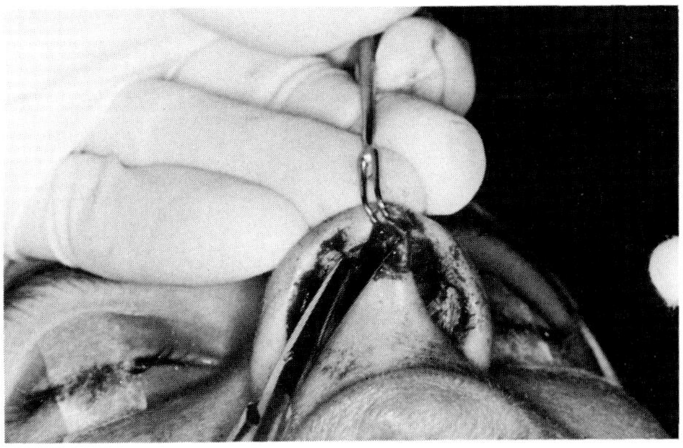

Figure 5-90B

The skin and soft tissue are then dissected free from the lower lateral cartilages (Figure 5-90A and B). A small two-pronged hook and dissecting scissors are used.

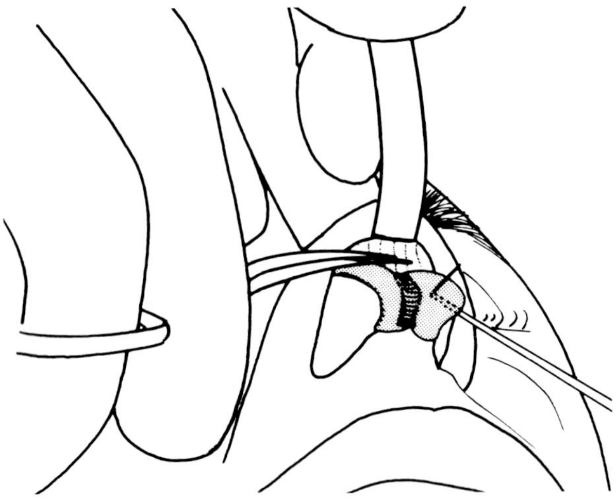

Figure 5-91A

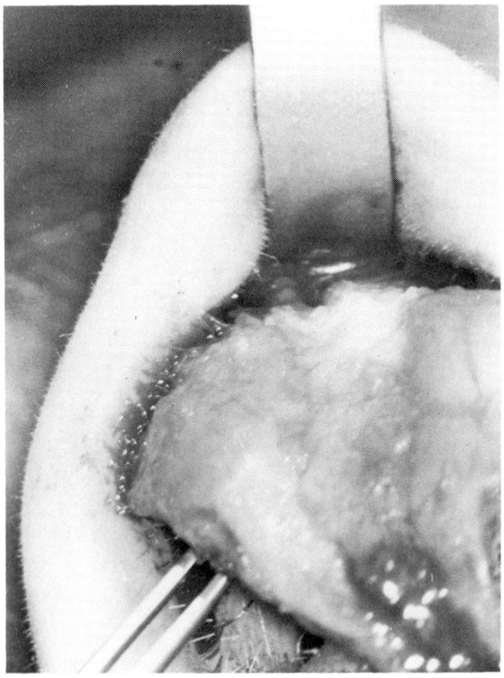

Figure 5-91B

The dissection of the soft tissue is later facilitated with a right-angled hook. The Park or Aufricht retractor is used to protect the cut edge superiorly by rolling the tip skin beneath the retractor. Note the intercrural sling between the medial crura as shown in Figure 5-91A and B.

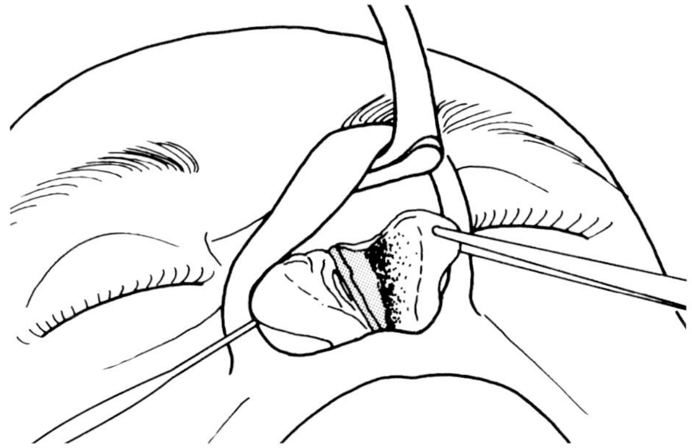

Figure 5-92A

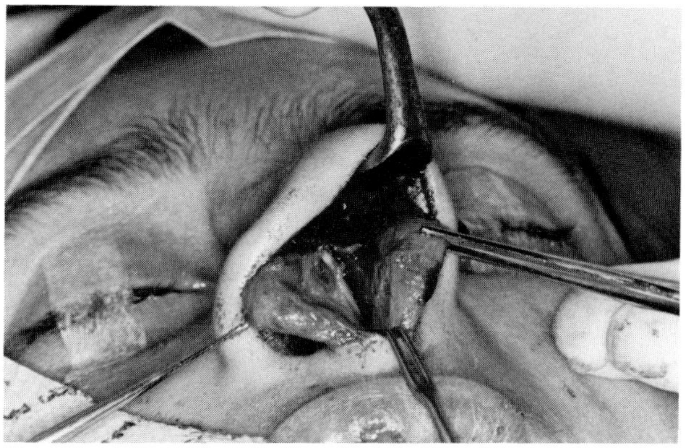

Figure 5-92B

The crural sling (interdomal) is cut, thus exposing the septal angle and providing an unparalleled view of the upper laterals and rhinion (Figure 5-92A and B).

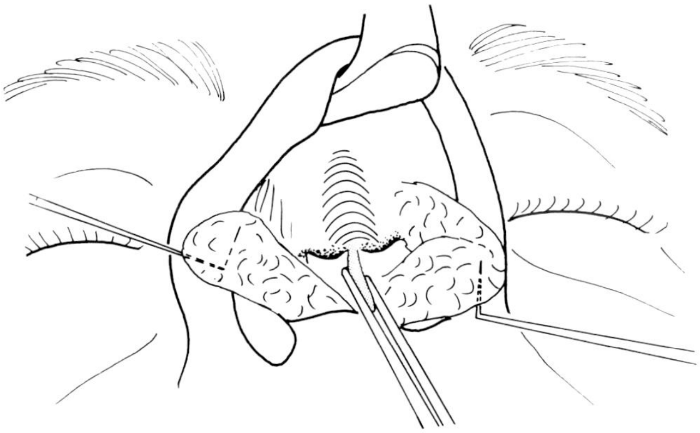

Figure 5-93A

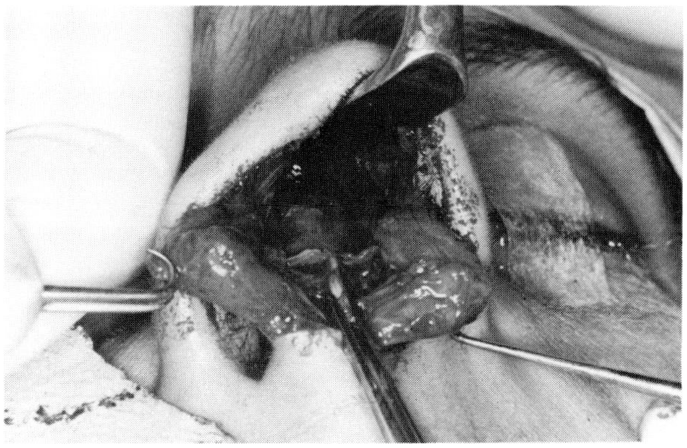

Figure 5-93B

In Figure 93A and B the septum is held between the pickups.

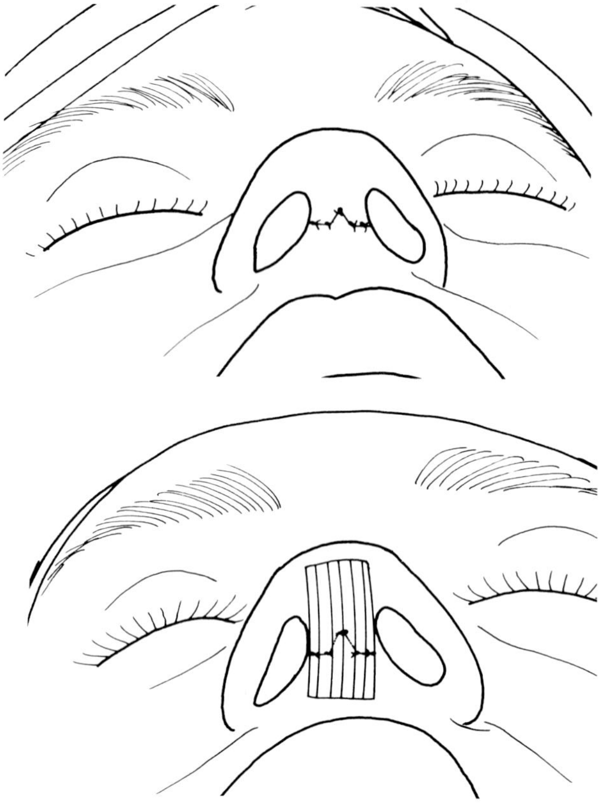

Figure 5-94A

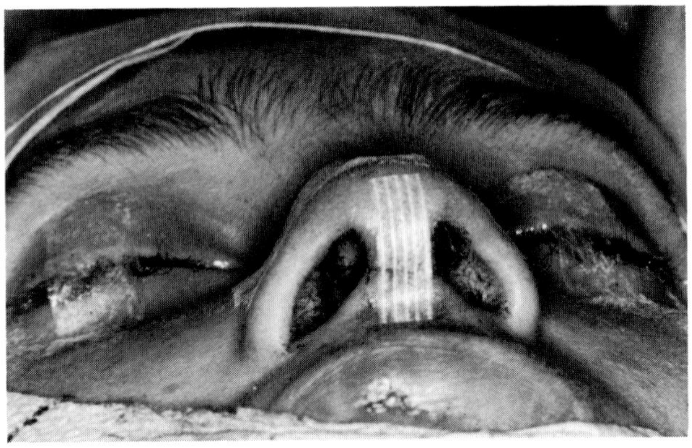

Figure 5-94B

After the surgery of the septum, tip, supratip, and bony framework, the wound is meticulously closed with 5-0 plain under direct vision. This wound is then reinforced with a Steristrip (Figure 5-94A and B).

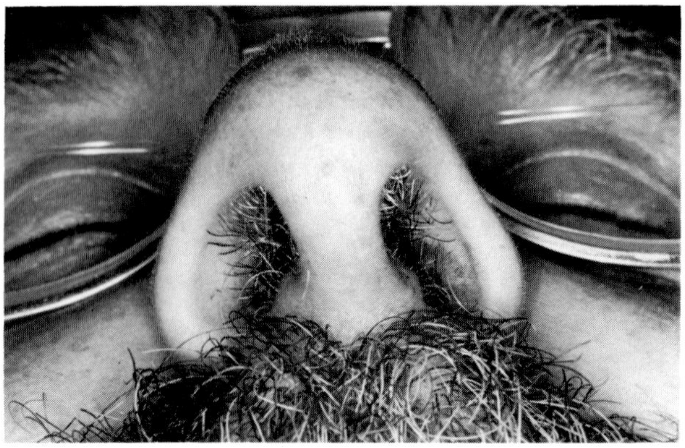

Figure 5-95

Figure 5-95 shows a 1-year postoperative scar following an open rhinoplasty and successful repair of two septal perforations from two previous surgeries by two different surgeons.

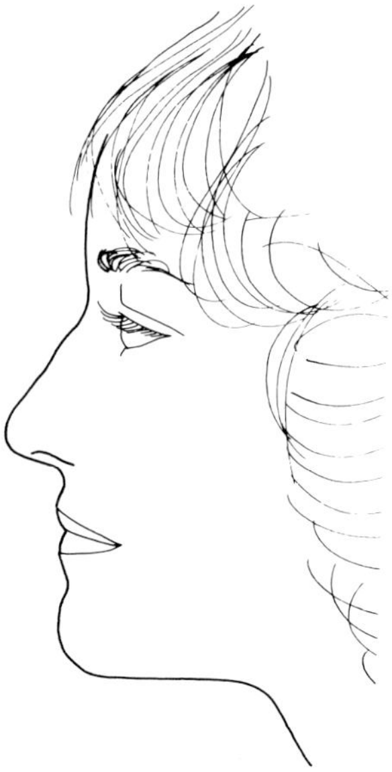

Figure 5-96A

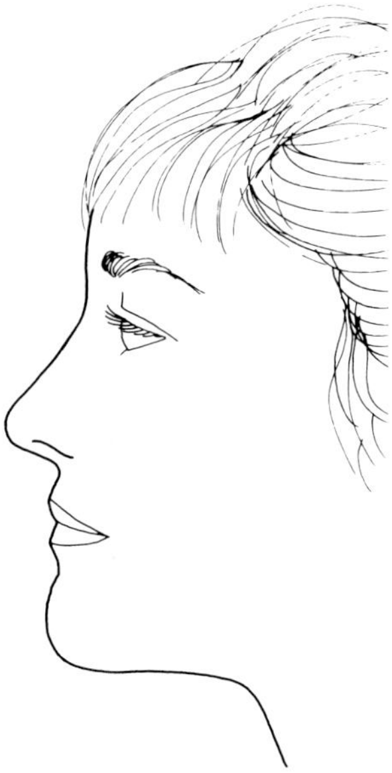

Figure 5-96B

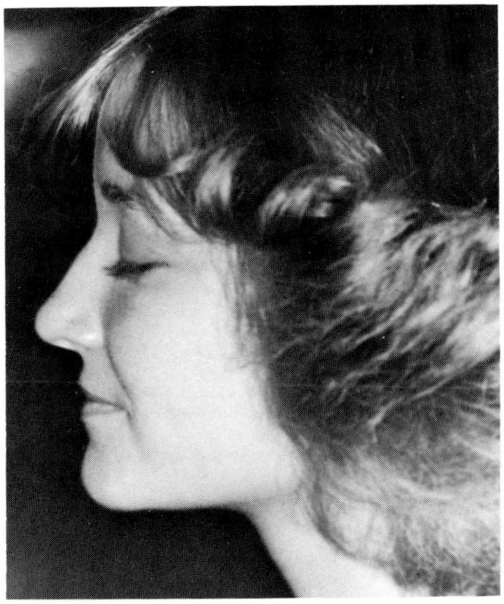

Figure 5-96C

Columellar Technique

There will be changes in the columella after tip surgery that involve rotation and or change in projection. Often these changes are desirable as in a slight dependent tip with poor lateral columellar show. With superior rotation of the tip the columellar show will improve as will the nasolabial angle (Figure 5-96A–D).

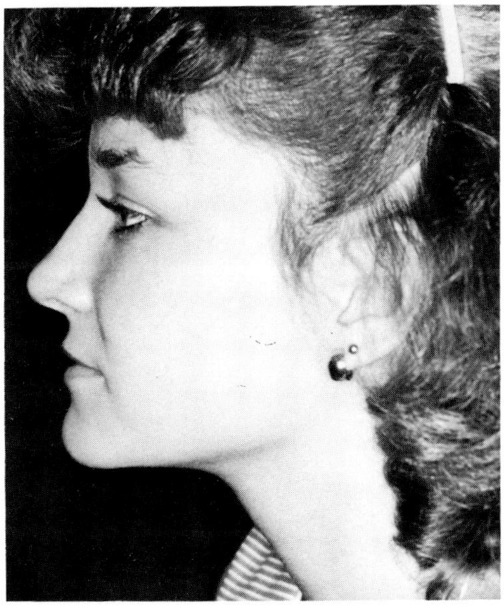

Figure 5-96D

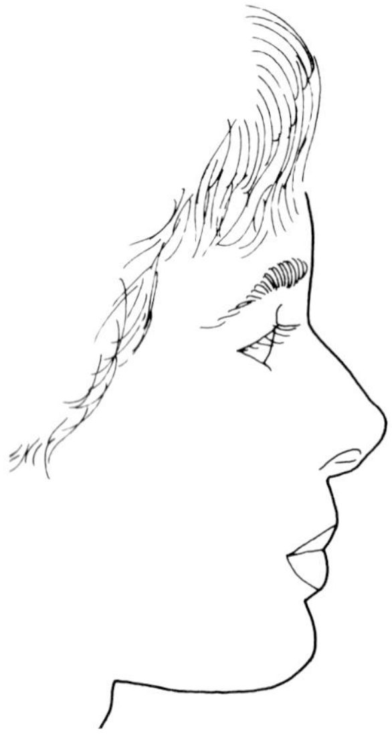

Figure 5-97A

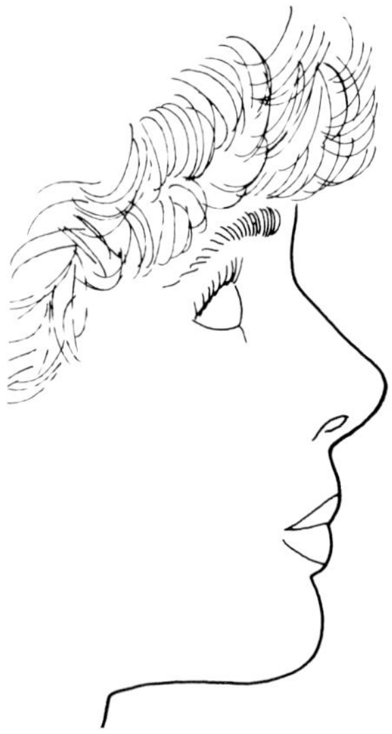

Figure 5-97B

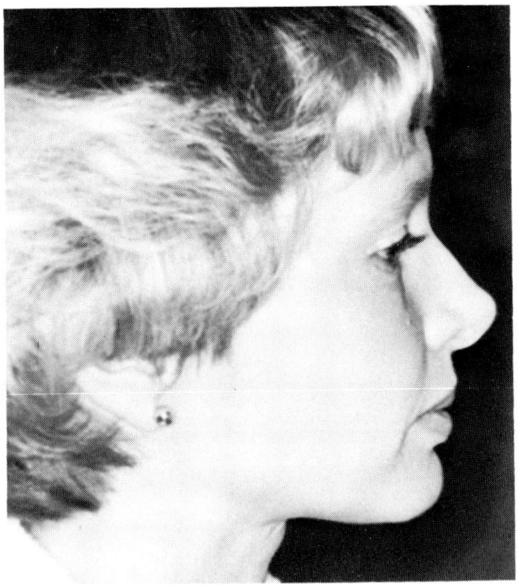

Figure 5-97C

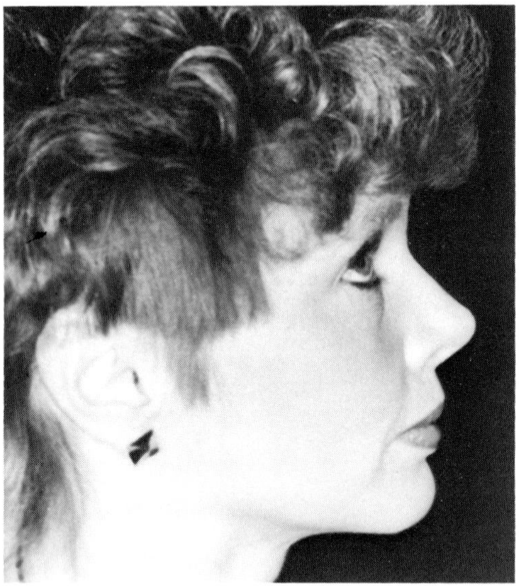

Figure 5-97D

If the changes with tip rotation result in excessive columellar show and/or open a nasolabial angle too widely, the etiology must be determined and corrected. The etiologies are the same as for a hanging columella: a caudally projecting septum, an excessive membranous columella, or commonly an unusually wide medial crura or any combination of the above. Figures 5-97A–D are examples of a columella with an abnormal columellar defining point secondary to too wide a medial crus. This is corrected by direct excision of both cartilage and vestibular skin of the medial cura through an extended marginal incision. The postoperative photograph is at 18 months (Figure 5-97D).

A retracted columella is difficult to correct. The use of a strut and/or battens plus plumping material is a generally effective manner of repair. Superior rotation is also helpful if the nose can take some shortening. Figures 5-78D–5-82 show an example of combining a wide strut of cartilage sutured between the medial crura, superior rotation, and plumping beneath the feet of the medial crura; Figures 5-81 and 5-82 were photographed preoperatively and 1 year postoperatively, respectively.

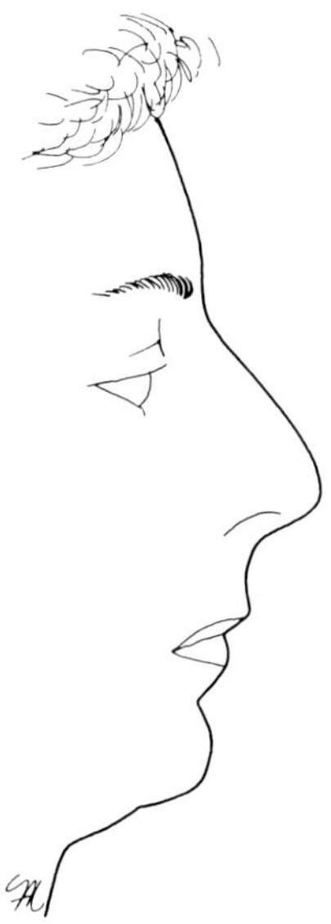

Figure 5-98A

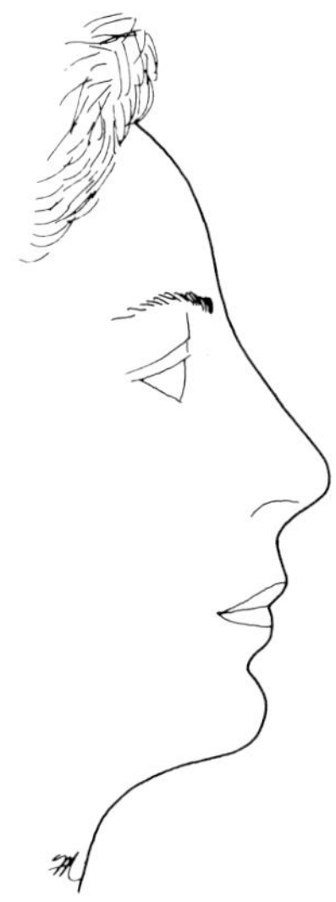

Figure 5-98B

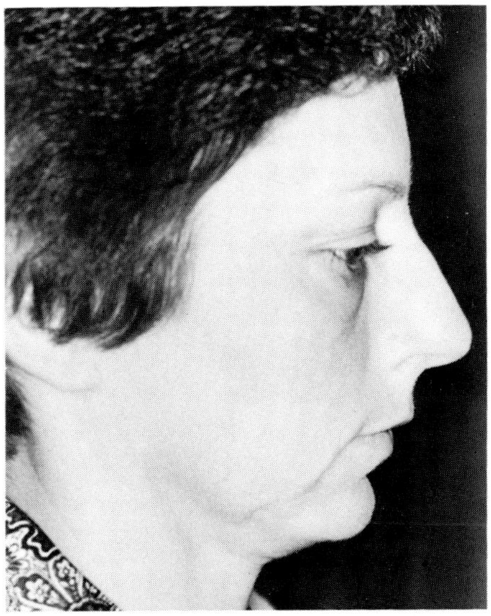

Figure 5-98C

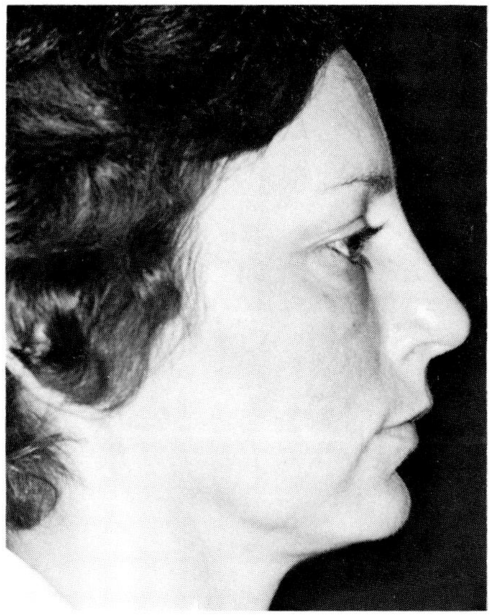

Figure 5-98D

The nasolabial angle may be distorted by an excessively anterior projection of the anterior nasal spine. This is determined by visualization and palpation. If it projects to too great a degree, it may be shortened by resecting a portion of it. Excess resection will result in an undesirable retraction. In Figure 5-98A–D the resection is accurately accomplished with a 2-mm chisel or a small pair of Takahashi Forceps. Note also the apparent strength given to the chin by the overall nasal reduction and in particular by the change in the vertical plane of the upper lip; see Figure 5-84A–C for base view. The postoperative photograph is at 18 months (Figure 5-98D).

The wide or clefted columella from base view can be consistently repaired by removing the soft tissue from between the medial crura. The soft-tissue removal must be down to the perichondrium on the medial aspect of the medial crura. This can be accomplished through existing incisions. A transfixion incision can be everted with a wide skin hook and the soft tissue removed retrograde with scissors and pickups. If an extended marginal incision has been used, the soft-tissue removal can be accomplished through that incision. It is easiest if an open rhinoplasty transcolumellar incision has been used.

After removal of the soft tissues, the medial crura must be approximated. The suturing must be accurate in both the anteroposterior plane and the inferosuperior plane, or there will be subsequent tip asymmetry. A Keith needle is useful for this alignment of the cartilages. This has the disadvantage of placing the knot internasally, which may occasionally become infected. An absorbable suture is used. They may also be approximated by using a small curved needle and burying the knot between the medial crura. Technically this is difficult to do unless the exposure is through an open rhinoplasty. This procedure should be done wih an absorbable suture [polyglactin (Vicryl)] as the columella will widen slightly in the postoperative period for a more natural appearance. In some patients there will be a slight increase in tip projection secondary to the approximation of the medial crura.

In Figure 5-99 the dashed Keith needle is not properly aligned, and because it is a straight needle the error is easily identified. The solid needle is correctly aligned. If the improperly aligned suture were tied, the asymmetry could be identified at the table. If a curved needle is used, it is much more difficult to make the suture placement correctly.

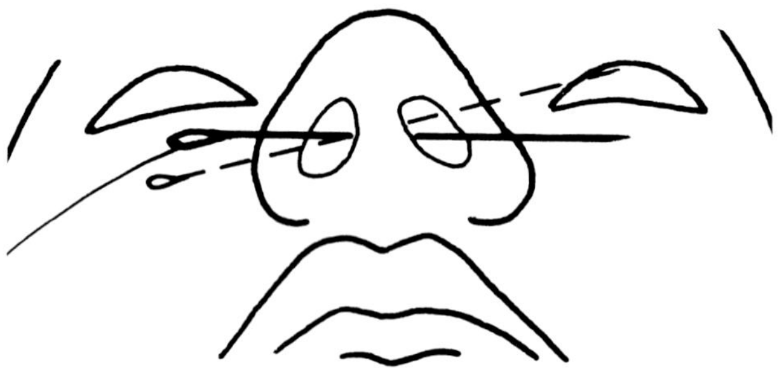

Figure 5-99

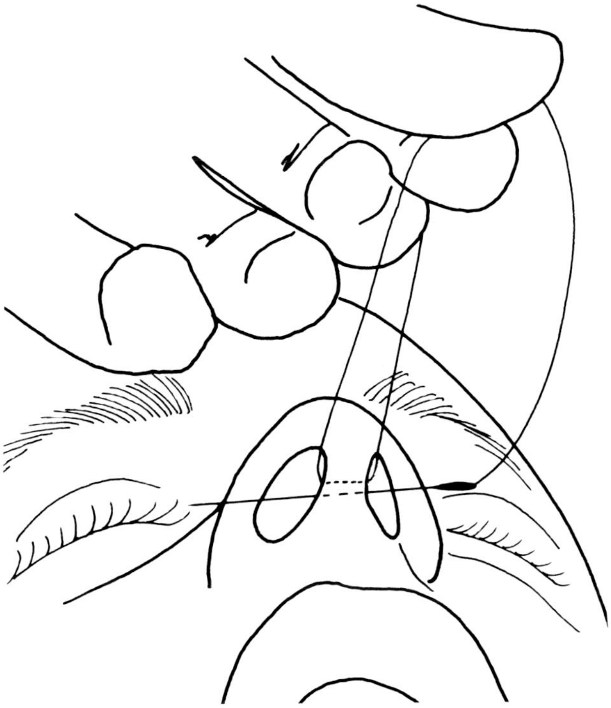

Figure 5-100A

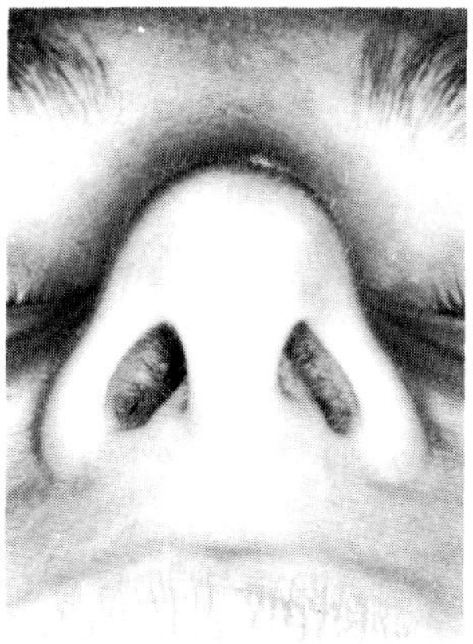

Figure 5-100B

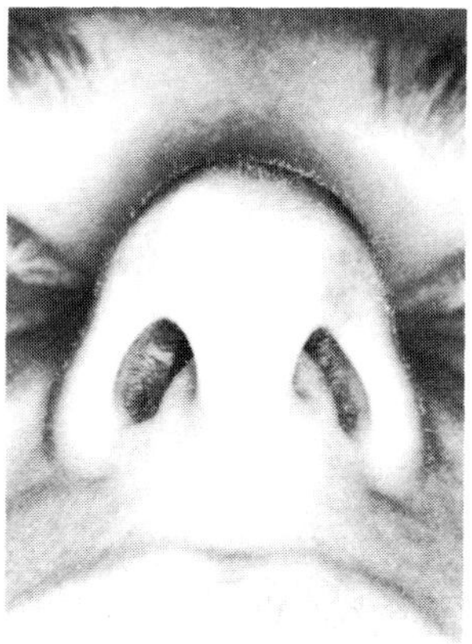

Figure 5-100C

Figure 5-100A shows a properly placed suture just before tying. These may be multiple if necessary. Figures 5-100B and 5-100C are preoperative and 1 year postoperative, respectively, of a clefted columella and tip repaired as just described.

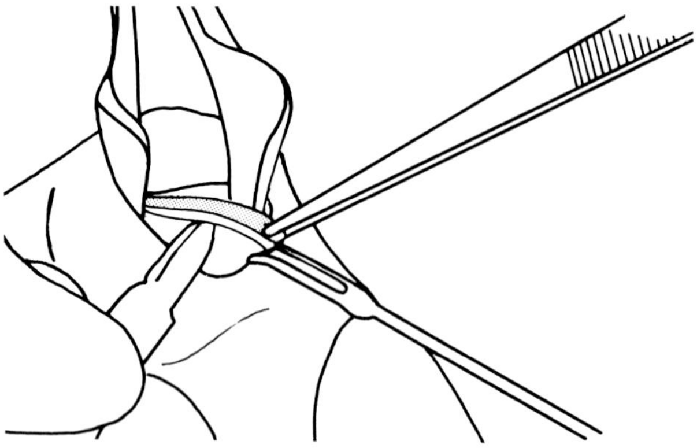

Figure 5-101A

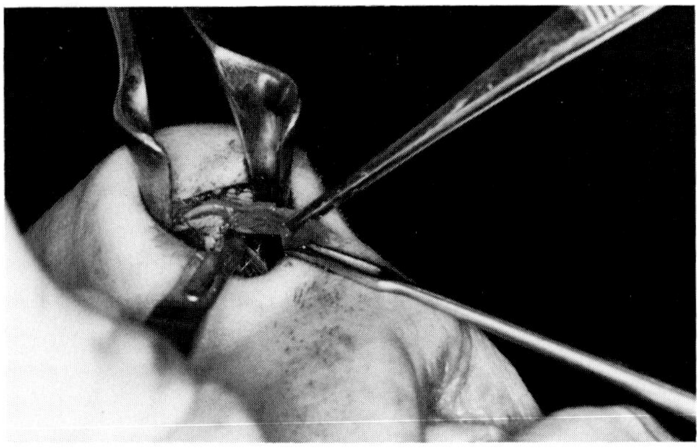

Figure 5-101B

CAUDAL SEPTUM

Surgery of the caudal septum may shorten the nose, facilitate rotation of the nose, change the nasolabial angle, and affect or eliminate the columellar defining point. This surgery must be precise and is best done in increments. Generally an attached portion of mucous membrane should also be excised. Because of the contraction of mucous membrane this should be approximately one-half the width of the resected cartilage. The caudal end of the quadrangular cartilage is not straight, so the excision should be curvilinear in nature. The columellar defining point may be moved superiorly or occasionally inferiorly as indicated with this excision, if the medial crura are not over developed. In Figure 5-101 the columella is displaced and the selected caudal end of the septum and attached mucous membrane is resected.

A major contribution to these poor results has been excessive resection of the anterior septal angle and straight line excision of the caudal septum. The dotted lines in Figures 5-102 and 5-103 represent the caudal septum as found at revision surgery. (Preoperative photographs could not be obtained).

Figure 5-102 shows the result of removing an excessive amount of anterior septal angle.

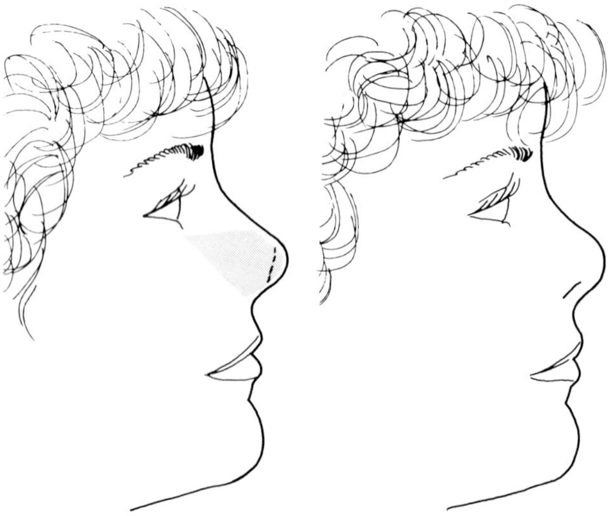

Figure 5-102

Figure 5-103 shows the result of a straight-line excision of the caudal septum.

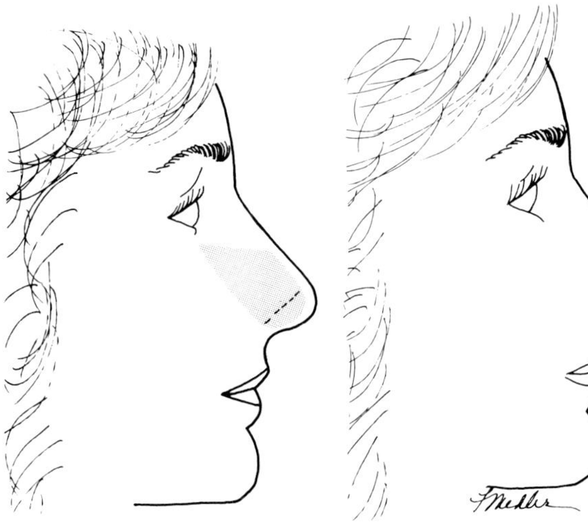

Figure 5-103

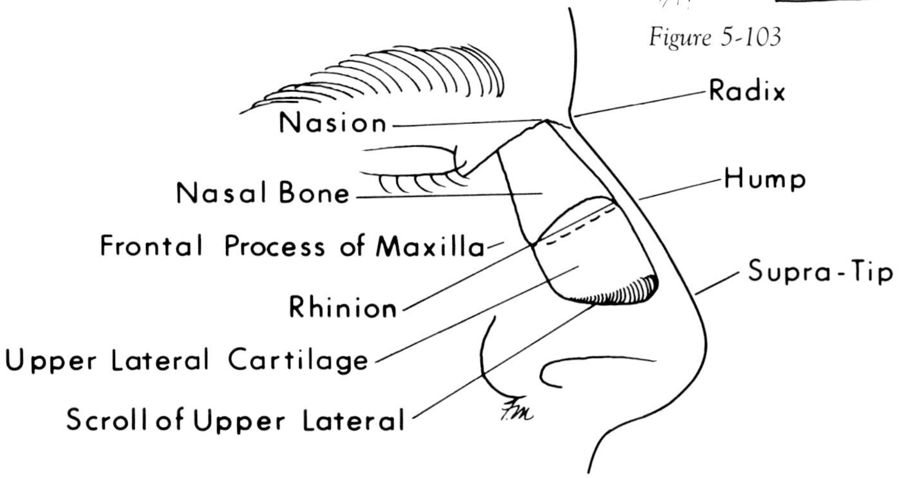

Figure 5-104

DORSUM

Surgery of the bony cartilaginous dorsum is difficult because much of the operator's information is obtained by palpation. Visualization of the structures involved is restricted by the skin and soft tissues. The open rhinoplasty has greatly increased the visibility and is an excellent teaching technique for both the operator and observers. Another problem is the great variation in the thickness of the frontal process of the maxilla, the nasal bones, and the nasal process of the frontal bone. Previous fractures greatly effect the lateral osteotomies, as does the thickness of the bone at the radix (see Figure 5-104).

The technique presented here relies on keeping as much periosteum intact as possible, as this provides stability and predictability. Remember also that the bones involved have periosteum on both sides. Surgery of the cartilaginous dorsum is presented in a manner that depends on direct visualization for accuracy. If this visualization is not present, further undermining should be performed until the cartilages are visible. It is important to remember that thickness of the skin and subcutaneous tissue varies greatly from one individual to another. The skin is thinner overlying the rhinion in all patients, and this must be allowed for at the time of the surgery.

The basic goals of dorsum surgery are to augment, reduce, and straighten the dorsum and to narrow the dorsum and lateral walls. There are specific terms that pertain to anatomy of the dorsum. Anatomically, the *nasion* is the junction of the nasal frontal sutures with the internasal suture; clinically, this is the *radix*. Anatomically, the *rhinion* is the fibrous union of the paired upper laterals with the paired nasal bones; clinically, this is the hump. Anatomically, the *frontal maxillary process* is the portion of the maxilla that articulates with the nasal bones laterally; clinically, it is fractured during the lateral osteotomy. Anatomically, the paired *upper lateral cartilages* meet in the midline with the quadrangular cartilage and form a single unit. The caudal edge of the upper laterals generally have an upward-turning scroll, which is greatest medially and tapers out laterally. Clinically the cartilaginous dorsum and its overlying soft tissue are responsible for the supratip area.

TECHNIQUE

The exposure of the bony cartilaginous dorsum is obtained through the incisions used for the exposure of the septum and the tip—either an intercartilaginous incision or cartilage splitting incision, which is joined with a partial or complete transfixion incision, or the external rhinoplasty incision (see Figures 5-68A and B, 5-69A and B, 5-85A and B, and 5-86A and B).

In Figures 5-105 and 5-106 the rhinoplasty scissors are introduced through the intercartilaginous incision. The Park retractor helps by placing tension on the soft tissues, thereby facilitating the exposure of the perichondrium of the upper laterals.

These scissors dissect when spread apart as a result of the taper of the lateral border of blades. This feature helps to maintain the plane of dissection at the relatively avascular perichondrial level. The scapel can be used for this exposure, but it is easier to stay in the proper plane with scissors.

After elevating the soft tissue off of the upper lateral cartilages up to the rhinion, the decision is made to either continue in this plane and leave the periosteum attached to the nasal bones or to attempt to elevate it off of the nasal bones.

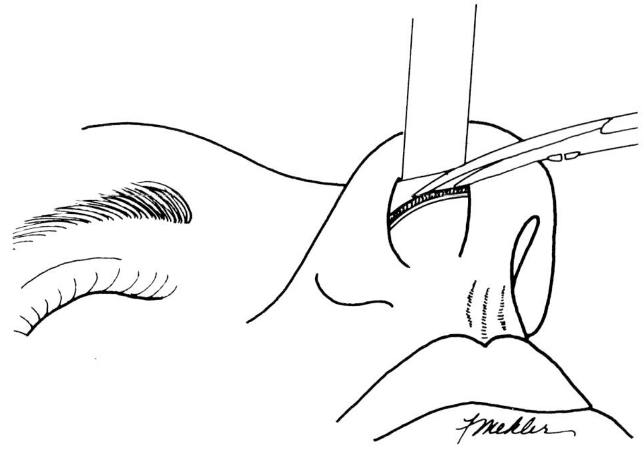

Figure 5-105

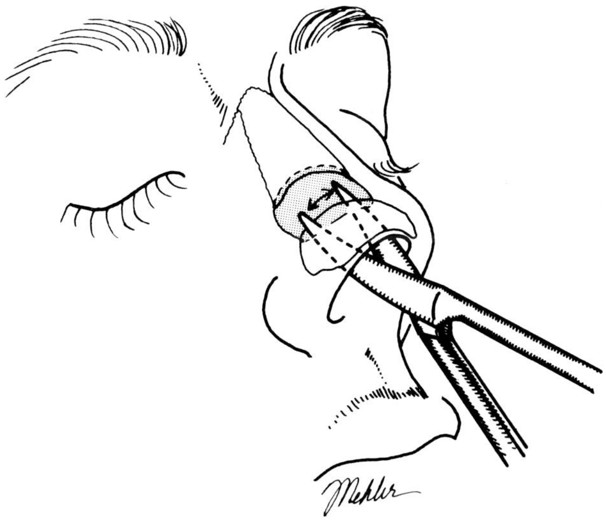

Figure 5-106

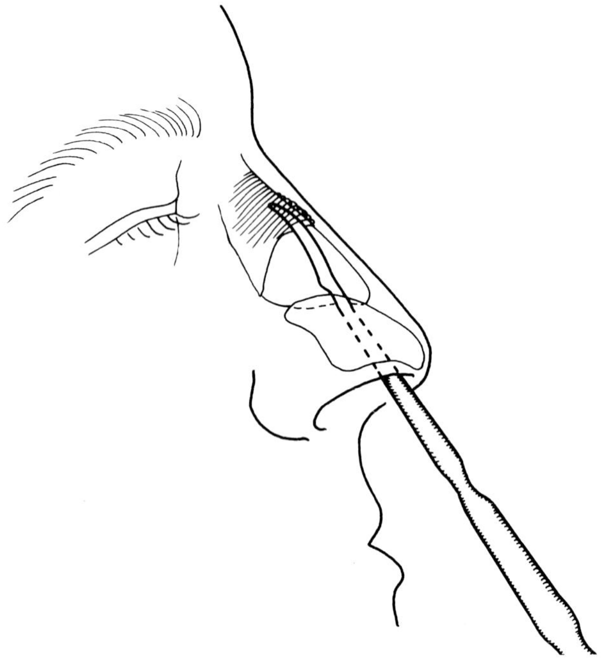

Figure 5-107

As shown in Figure 5-107, the Joseph periosteal elevator is used to elevate the periosteum over just that portion of the bony dorsum to be removed.

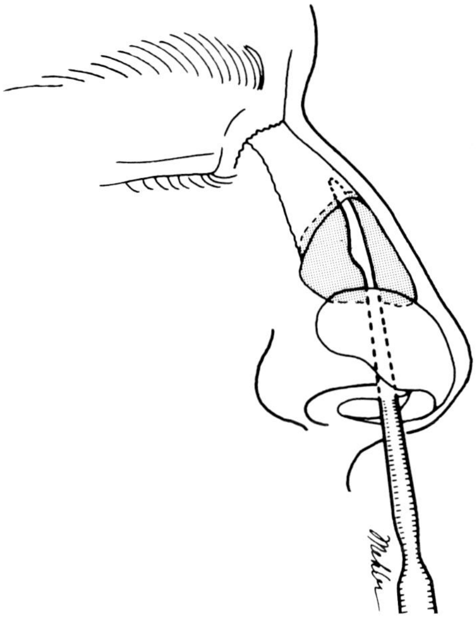

Figure 5-108A

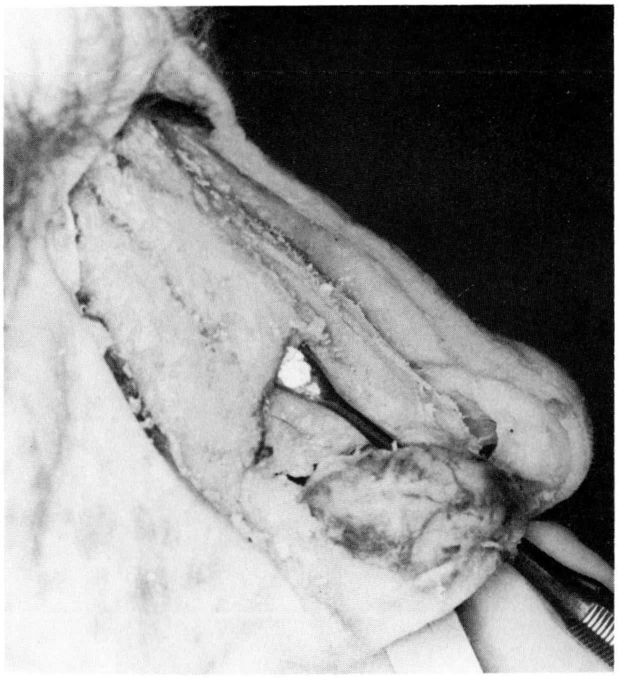

Figure 5-108B

The Joseph periosteal elevator shown in Figure 5-108A is in the wrong plane. The upper lateral cartilage is held to the nasal bone by a dense fibrous tissue, and this connection must not be interrupted, or the upper lateral cartilage may be avulsed from the nasal bone. If this avulsion occurs, a depression will develop in the postoperative nose, giving the overall impression of a crooked result. Figure 5-108B shows the modified Woodson improperly placed just beneath the nasal bone on top of the upper lateral cartilage.

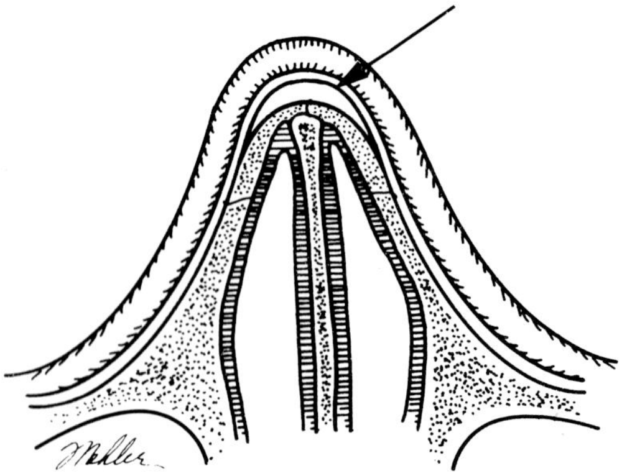

Figure 5-109

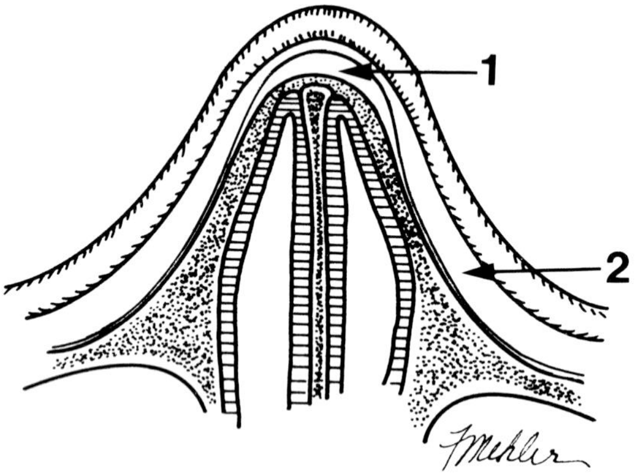

Figure 5-110

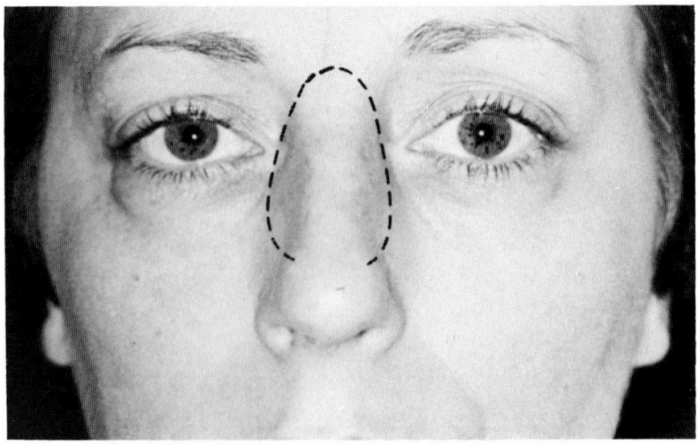

Figure 5-111

Figure 5-109 demonstrates the "ideal" periosteal pocket preparation for subsequent bony work with a rasp or osteotome. The periosteum left attached to the nasal bones provides a stabilizing force for the nasal bones following lateral osteotomy. The arrow points to the elevated periosteum.

For soft-tissue redraping to occur following reduction of nasal size or upward rotation of the tip, the skin and subcutaneous tissue must be elevated lateral to the periosteum. The Shea vein scissors are well suited to this elevation in a spread and cut manner. The greater the redraping, the wider the undermining necessary, and the more the postoperative ecchymosis. In cases where no rotation of the tip or reduction in the length of the nose is necessary, minimal to no soft-tissue elevation is necessary. The extreme example is the creation of a soft-tissue pocket for dorsal graft placement where the elevation is just large enough to accept the graft.

Figure 5-110 shows the creation of a subperiosteal pocket for the bony dorsal work and a supraperiosteal (or extraperiosteal) soft-tissue pocket for skin redraping. Arrow 1 is within the subperiosteal pocket. Arrow 2 is within the supraperiosteal pocket resulting from the soft-tissue undermining.

If the soft-tissue undermining is inadequate, there is often a false sense of successful rotation and improved tip projection intraoperatively, but postoperatively a mild tip ptosis or downward rotation will develop (see Figure 5-64C).

Figure 5-111 exemplifies wide undermining necessary for a large reduction.

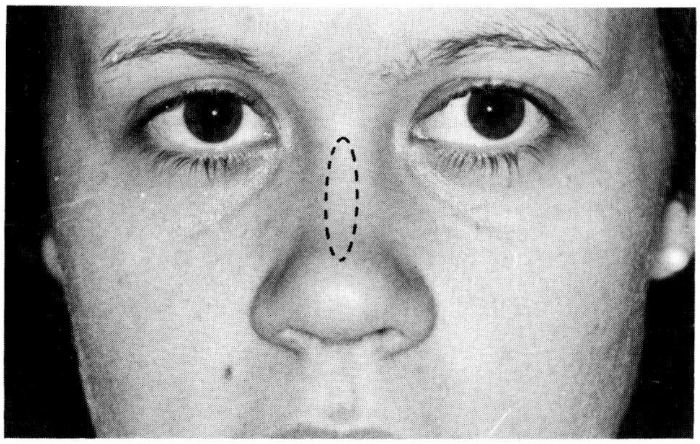

Figure 5-112

Figure 5-112 represents minimal undermining for a graft implant (see Figure 5-156D for patient's postoperative after-graft placement).

Dorsal reduction follows a specific sequence, which usually begins with small hump removal. If the amount of dorsum to be resected is small, the bony hump is first removed with a rasp. Next, the cartilaginous hump is resected with a broken-tipped No. 11 scalpel. When this is small, there will be very little or no open roof deformity created. The cartilaginous trimming is difficult and is aided by first removing the fibrous tissue between the upper laterals on top of the septal cartilage. This can be stripped out with a mosquito hemostat.

The Fomon rasp is well suited for this bony removal, as it minimizes the possibility of avulsing the upper lateral cartilage from the nasal bone (see Figure 5-113).

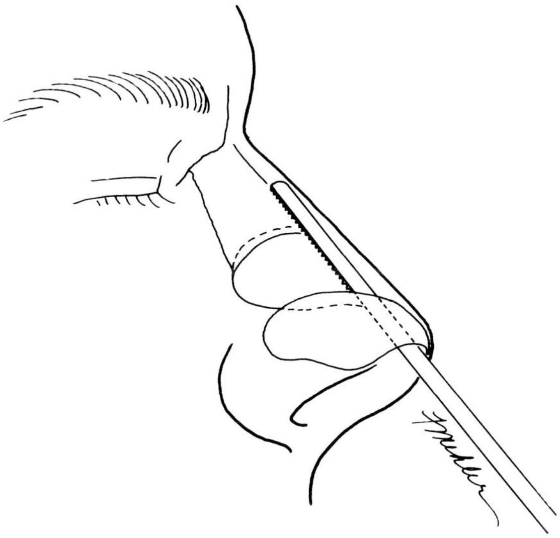

Figure 5-113

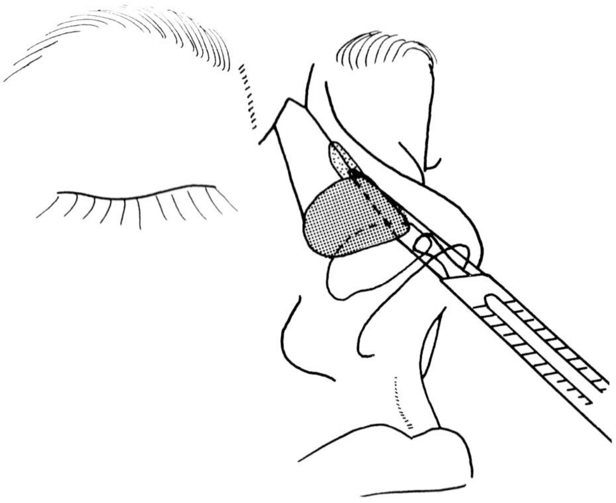

Figure 5-114

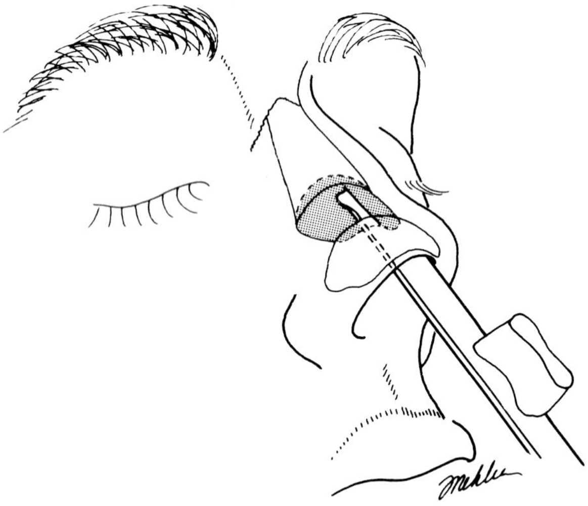

Figure 5-115

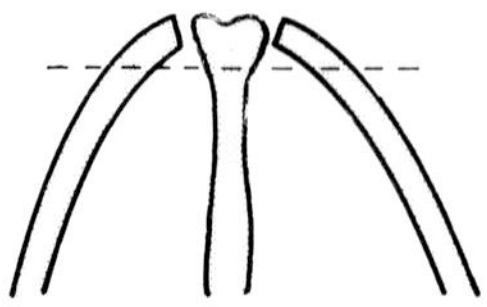

Figure 5-116

Following the removal of the bony hump, the cephalad portion of the upper lateral cartilage is often more exposed or seems to swell up. This is removed by sliver shaving with the belly of a No. 15 Bard-Parker or broken-tipped No. 11 blade (Figure 5-114). The Park or Aufricht retractor provides exposure and protects the soft tissue.

A medium-sized hump with a small cartilaginous component can be removed with a sharp Rubin osteotome. By using the osteotome it is easier to ensure that the cut is perpendicular to the septal plane. The cartilaginous cut is made with finger pressure under direct visualization up to the contact with the nasal bones. The osteotome is then set firmly into the nasal bones. Then the bony hump is removed by tapping the osteotome in series of two. The osteotome can have a tendency to cut the cartilage too deeply at the rhinion. This is best avoided by first making an incision with a No. 15 blade through the dorsal cartilaginous structures up to the nasal bones. Then the scalpel is removed and the Rubin osteotome is introduced.

The shaded area in Figure 5-115 represents the cartilaginous dorsum composed of the junction of the paired upper laterals and the septal cartilage. The dashed line in Figure 5-116 represents the level of the cut as seen from below.

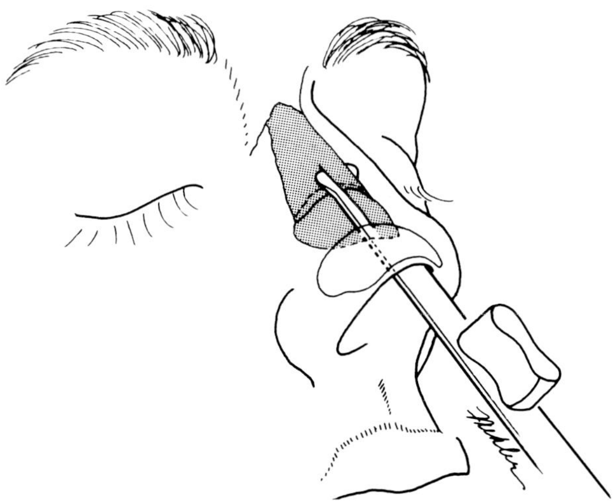

Figure 5-117A

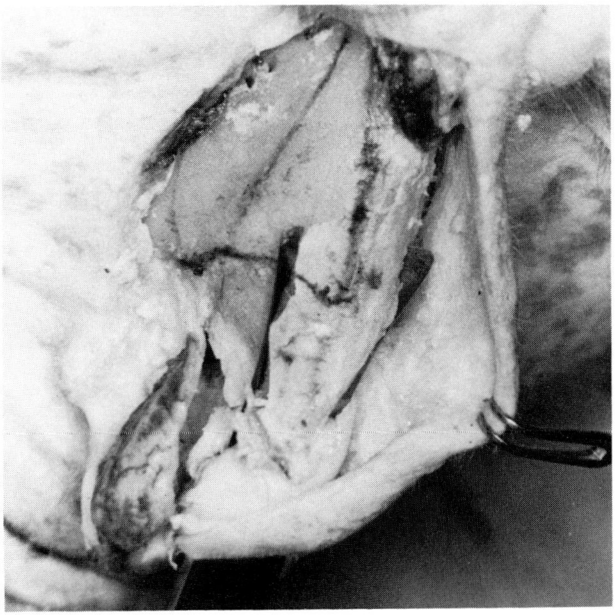

Figure 5-117B

The bony hump (Figure 5-117A and B) is then removed in continuity with the upper lateral cartilages. Caution is exercised at this time as the osteotome can very quickly cut too deeply with the first few taps of the mallet.

Figure 5-118 shows complete excision of cartilaginous and bony hump with a sharp osteotome. Depending on the contribution of the upper lateral cartilage to the hump, the caudal end of the upper laterals and their attachment to the quadrangular cartilage may not be excised. Note the rounded edges of the Rubin osteotome. This minimizes the possibility of inadvertently cutting the dermis of the skin overlying the nasal bones. If the dermis is scored, there is apt to be an indentation of the skin visable in the postoperative period. Guarded edges tend to require too large a soft-tissue pocket to accommodate them.

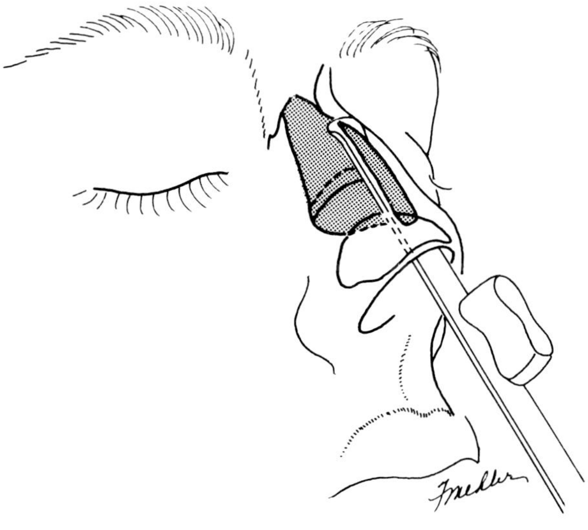

Figure 5-118

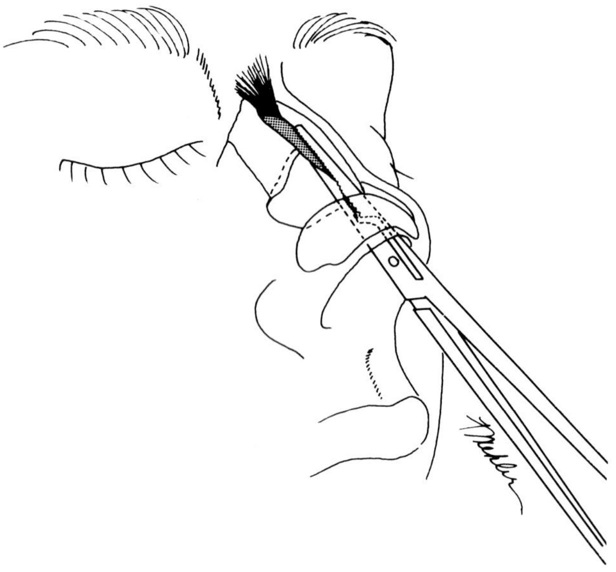

Figure 5-119

In Figure 5-119 the hump is often still attached superiorly by the procerus muscle. After the osteotome is removed, a small straight hemostat is introduced, which will grasp the hump firmly enough to allow the necessary traction to avulse the attachment of the procerus.

After removal of the hump, any irregularities are corrected at this time with a rasp. Particular reference is made to any portion of bone that will be later mobilized with lateral osteotomies.

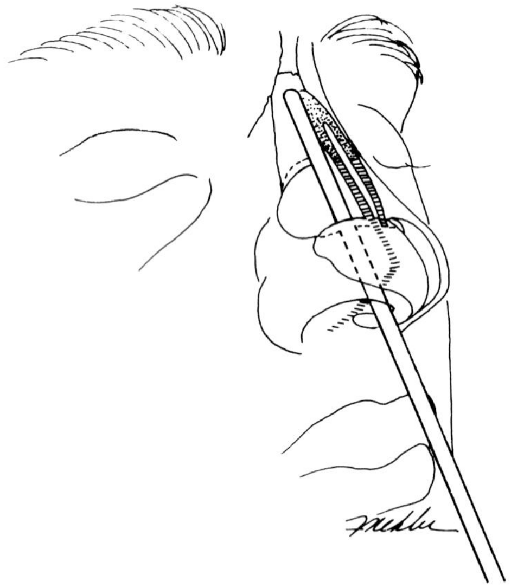

Figure 5-120

Figure 5-120 shows a Fomon rasp reducing a right nasal bone, which is higher than the left. This resulted from the Rubin osteotome not being perpendicular during the hump removal. If the rasping is not done prior to the lateral osteotomy, it cannot be done on any mobile pieces of bone because of the risk of avulsing the bone and subsequent collapse. Becker scissors may be used on mobile pieces if this occurs.

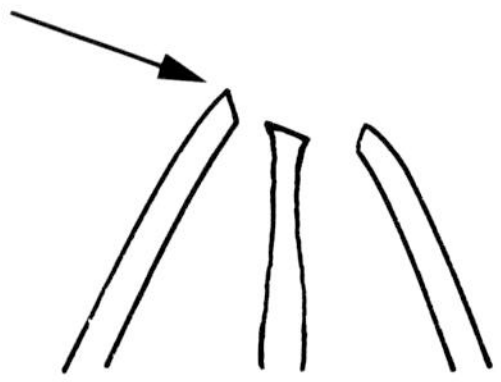

Figure 5-121

The arrow in Figure 5-121 points to the high spot to be rasped. Note the slightly high perpendicular plate also.

Figure 5-122 shows the rasp working on the left side.

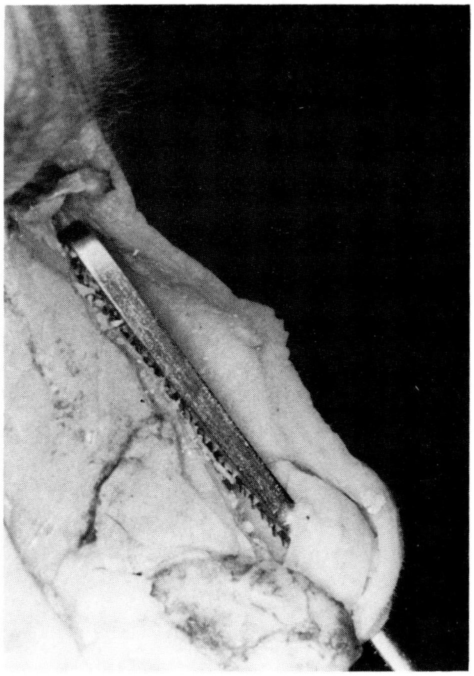

Figure 5-122

In removing a larger hump, it is best to first cut the upper laterals free from the septal cartilage in a submucosal plane (Figure 5-123). This then allows individual trimming of the cartilaginous hump. It is best to remove less than anticipated at first. The initial removal will allow the proper placement of an osteotome to remove the bony hump. Then after rasping and smoothing the bony work, further trimming of the cartilaginous components may be done. If the nasal bones are short, or if a large hump is removed, it is often best to save the final trimming of the upper lateral dorsal edge until the lateral osteotomies have been completed. Once the lateral osteotomies are performed and the upper laterals moved into their new position by infracturing, the amount to be resected may be significantly altered.

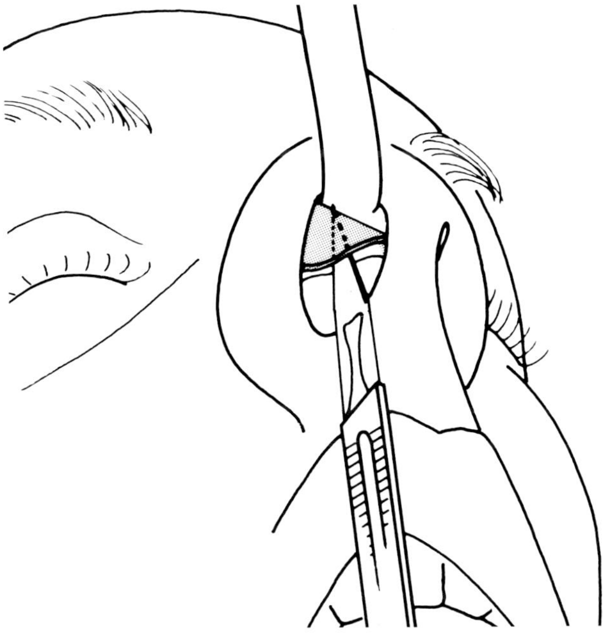

Figure 5-123

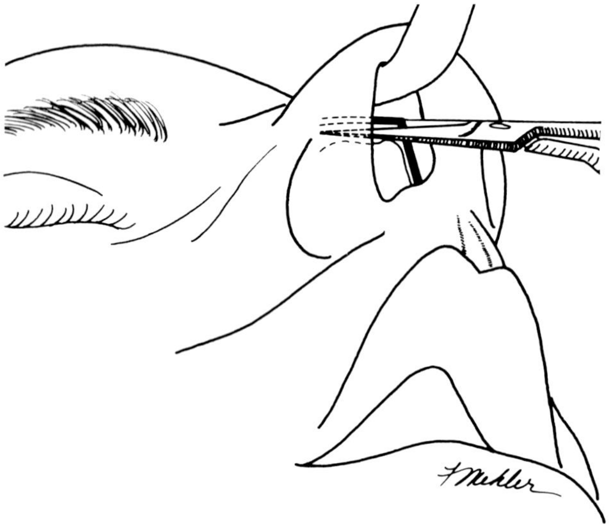

Figure 5-124

Fomon angled scissors are used to trim the dorsal edge of the septum (Figure 5-124). A scalpel can also be used to further trim or sliver shave the cut edges of the septum and the cut edge of the upper lateral cartilages.

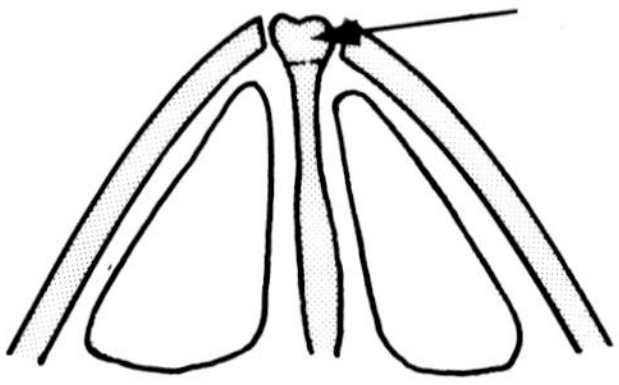

Figure 5-125

The arrow in Figure 5-125 points to the amount of septal cartilage to be resected.

After the upper laterals have been freed from the septal cartilage, they are ready for individual trimming. Trimming of the dorsal edge of the upper lateral cartilage with Fomon angled scissors is illustrated in Figure 5-126. A scalpel can be used for this also; however, the scissors offer a straight edge to sight along prior to cutting.

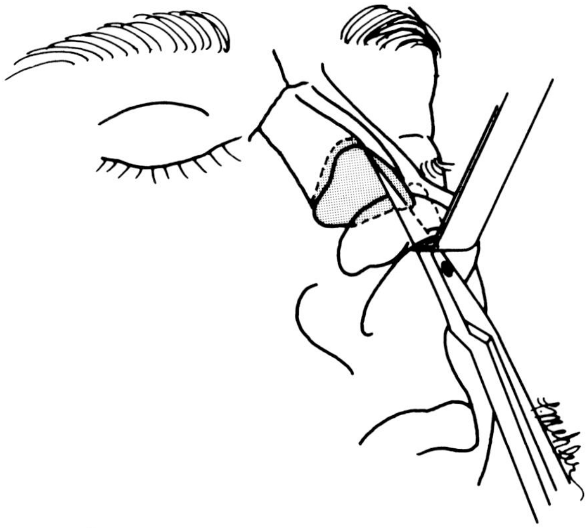

Figure 5-126

In Figure 5-127 the arrows point to the amount of upper lateral to resect to bring it flush with the septal cartilage, which has previously been trimmed (see Figure 5-124). If the scroll of the upper lateral is significant, this is the time to trim that also. If a large scroll is present, it can be the cause of postoperative supratip fullness. The upper laterals are shortened at this time also, if that is indicated.

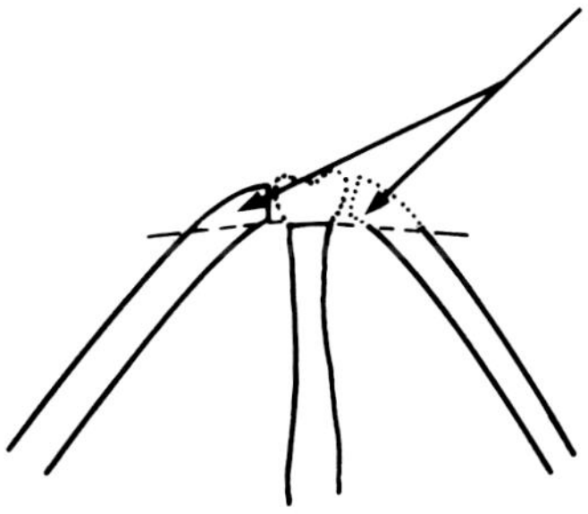

Figure 5-127

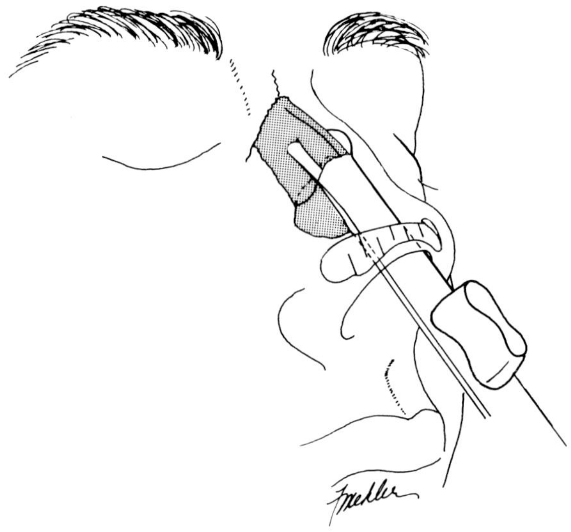

Figure 5-128

After the initial trimming of the septum and upper lateral cartilage, the osteotome is introduced and then the bony hump is removed (Figure 5-128).

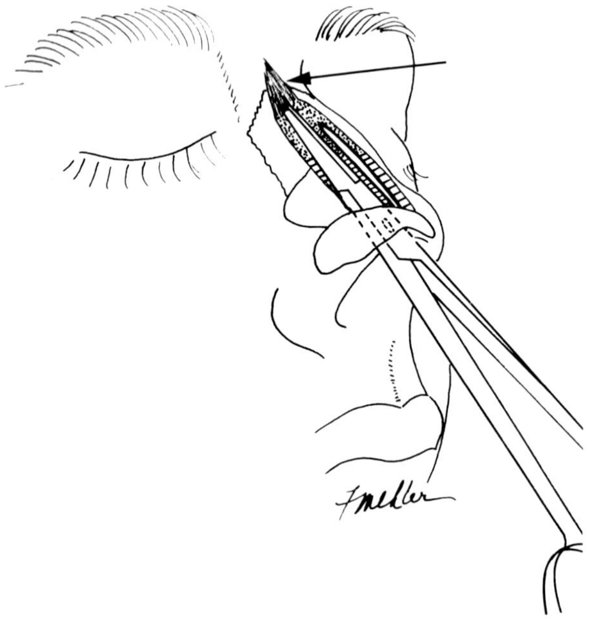

Figure 5-129

For reduction of the nasofrontal angle, the procerus muscle is removed by avulsing with a small hemostat. This must be done with care to avoid injury to the underlying dermis. Firm digital pressure for 5 minutes will markedly help to reduce the postoperative swelling. These patients must be watched closely postoperatively to ensure that they do not fill this area with fibrous tissue. If this starts, subcutaneous injections of steroids 2–3 times at weekly intervals will be helpful in preventing this recurrence of fibrous tissue. The arrow in Figure 5-129 points to the muscle fibers.

For bone removal, a push type of glabellar rasp will accomplish a surprising amount of reduction of the nasofrontal angle and is certainly the safest (see Figure 5-130).

Excellent results are possible with the use of a rotating burr through an open rhinoplasty approach. The long-shafted burrs must be available and sharp. The skin and soft tissue must be guarded to prevent them from being caught by the shaft of the burr.

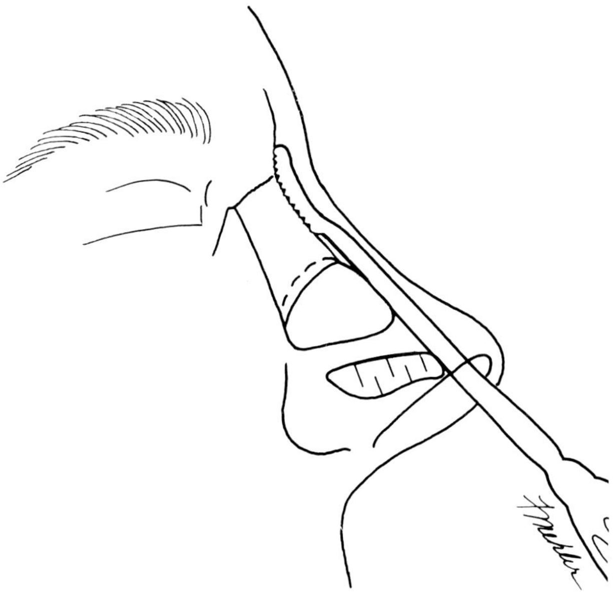

Figure 5-130

Lateral Osteotomies

The purpose of lateral osteotomy in dorsum surgery is to close an open-roof deformity created by hump removal, to narrow either all or a portion of the upper two-thirds of the nose, and to enhance straightening of a deviated bony pyramid. Further objectives are to create a stable controlled fracture of the frontal process of the maxilla and the nasal bones with their attached upper lateral cartilages and to have these symmetric and to avoid creating nasal obstruction.

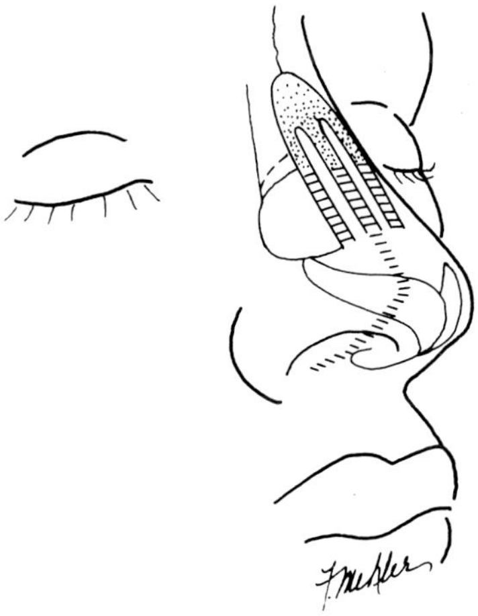

Figure 5-131A

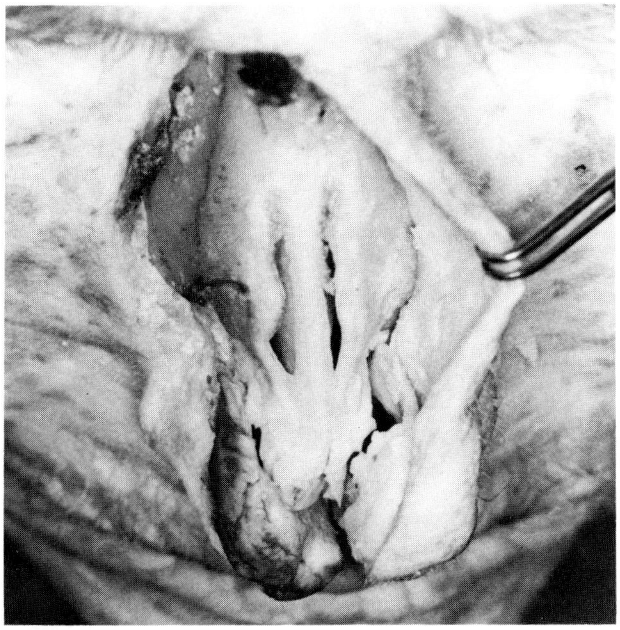

Figure 5-131B

The components of the open roof are the cut dorsal edge of the nasal bones, the cut dorsal edge of the upper lateral cartilages, the cut dorsal edge of the quadrangular cartilage, and the cut dorsal edge of the perpendicular plate (see Figure 5-131A and B).

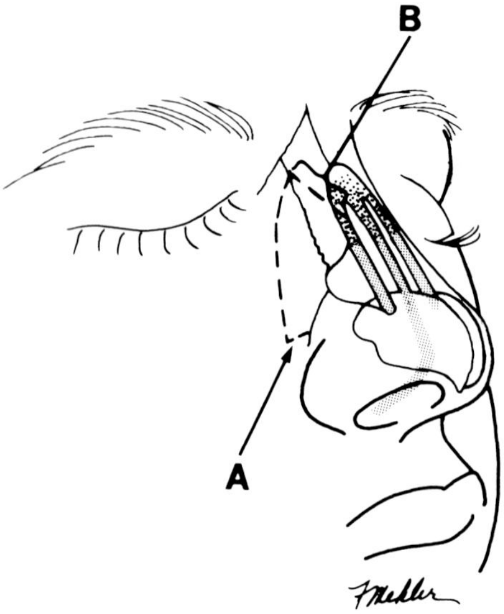

Figure 5-132

The dashed line in Figure 5-132 indicates the proposed line of the lateral osteotomy. The back cut at the very beginning preserves a buttress of bone that protects the airway at the level of the pyriform aperture. The long second cut curves gently toward the radix. The third and final line represents the back fracture. A medial osteotomy can replace the back fracture. The advantage of back fracturing is its greater stability due to the intact periosteum. The arrow labeled "A" points to the preserved buttress. The bracket labeled "B" indicates the area of intended back fracture.

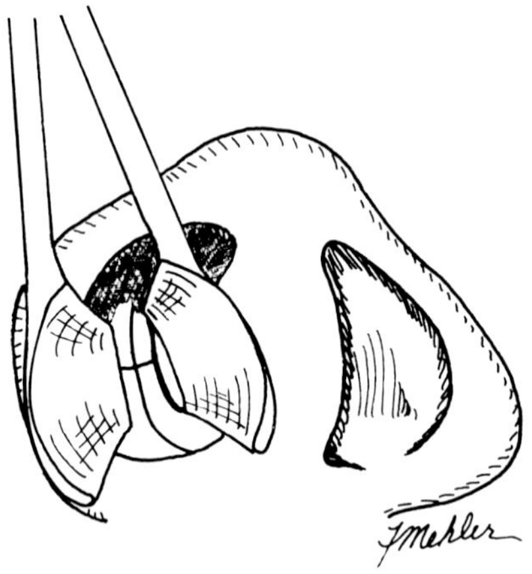

Figure 5-133

As shown in Figure 5-133, initially a small nasal speculum is used to help to expose and compress the vestibular skin against the pyrifrom aperture at the turbinate level. Then an incision, just long enough to allow passage of the guard of the osteotome, is made down to the bone of the pyriform aperture.

The osteotome is then placed firmly against and perpendicular to the edge of the pyriform aperture. This is at the approximate level of the anterior attachment of the inferior turbinate. The osteotome is then tapped by an assistant in series of twos. The osteotome placement is determined by the shape of the pyriform aperture and must initially be placed high enough to preserve the buttress, thus protecting the nasal airway.

As shown in Figure 5-134, this initial cut creates the buttress of bone and is nearly perpendicular to the next leg of the lateral osteotomy.

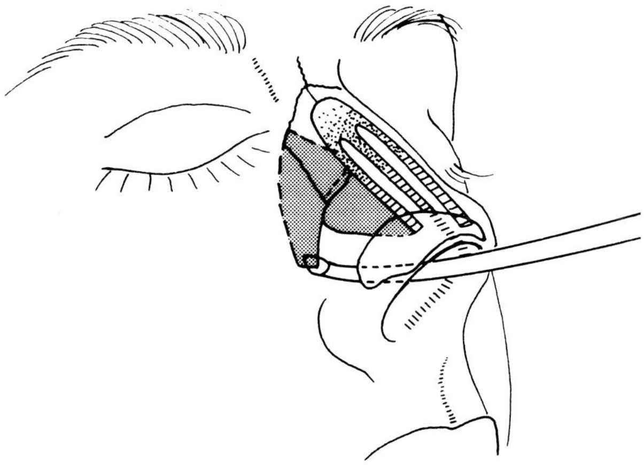

Figure 5-134

Figure 5-135 represents the pyriform aperture; the arrow points to the open roof.

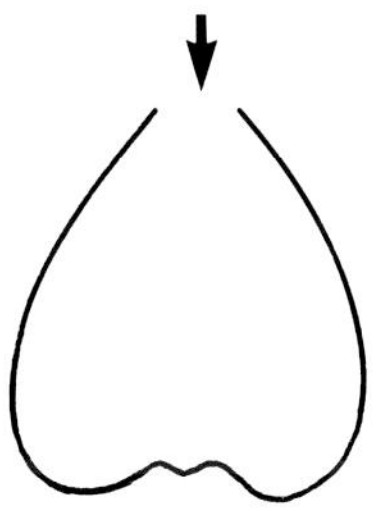

Figure 5-135

Figure 5-136 represents the same following a lateral osteotomy. The arrow points to the buttress referred to throughout the text.

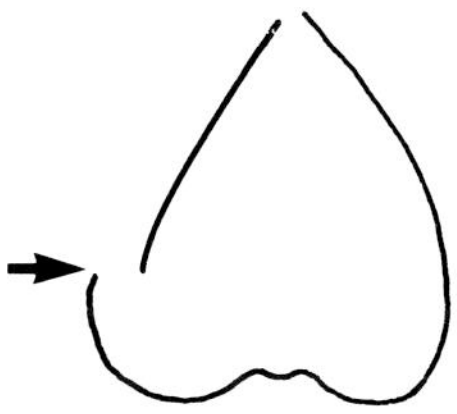

Figure 5-136

The osteotome is then rotated to start the long cephalad leg of the osteotomy. Continual palpation is the key to correctly guiding the osteotome. Slight lifting of the handle of the osteotome is also helpful in directing it to the desired place. It is also desirable to keep the cutting edge perpendicular to the bone being cut at the time. This requires several changes in the attitude of the osteotome during the osteotomy.

In Figure 5-137 note the gentle curve of this leg of the osteotomy. It will continue up to the approximate level of the infraorbital rim. The level is variable depending on the thickness of the bone and the desired level of back fracture. The nasal bone becomes much thicker toward the nasion, and it is important not to extend the osteotomy too high, certainly not to the frontal bone. The greatest potential problem would be the creation of a rocker, and secondary to this is the fact that anatomically this area is solid bone and no narrowing will occur.

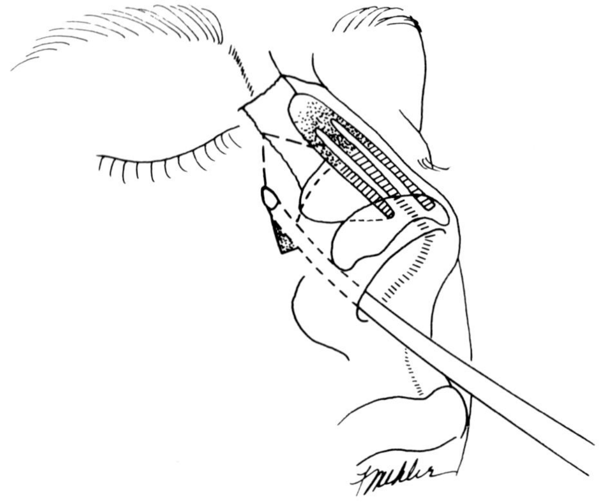

Figure 5-137

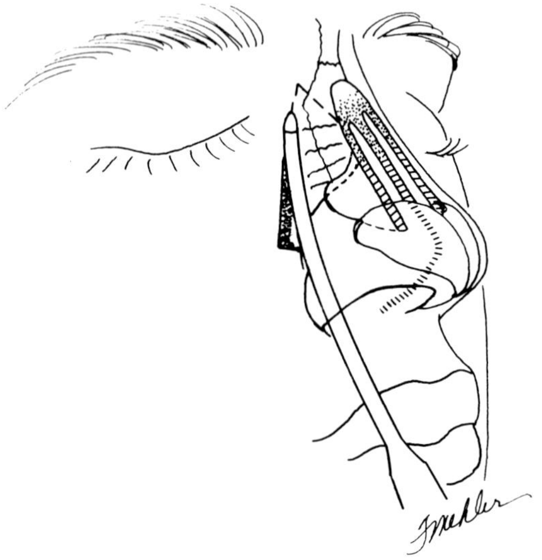

Figure 5-138

In Figure 5-138 note the small fractures radiating from the osteotomy line. These are desirable as they will allow more molding of the nasal bones. The thicker the osteotome, the more of these linear fractures and the greater the ultimate control of the osteotomy.

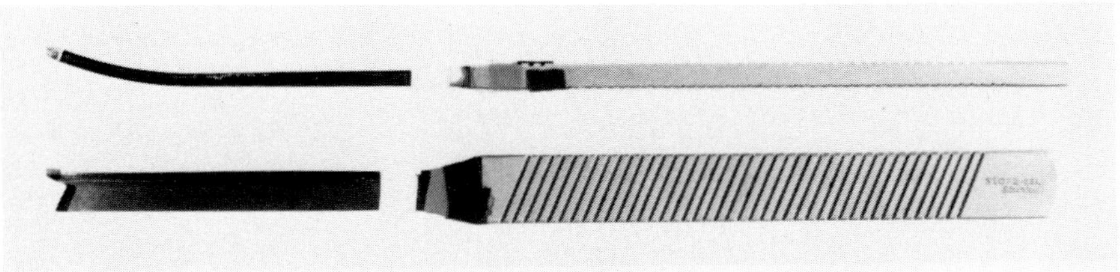

Figure 5-139

The curved Silver osteotome is excellent for this type of osteotomy. The guard is very large and drags in the soft tissue. This can be greatly reduced on a bench grinder as a modification (see modified Silver osteotome in Figure 5-139).

The next step is to create the back fracture. The osteotome is again redirected more medially, and an inward rotation of the handle is started. The fracture will occur along a natural stress line. This is often a greenstick fracture, which is desirable as it makes a very stable bony dorsum. However, it must not be incomplete and spring back out at the distal end of the nasal bone. This is readily determined by palpation. If this spring does occur, it is a simple matter to reintroduce the osteotome and go slightly further. Often the small Anderson-Neivert osteotome is useful for this maneuver. Digital pressure is also very useful at this time, but care should be taken not to overmobilize the segment.

Figure 5-140 represents the completed osteotomy, including the frontal process of the maxilla, the nasal bone, and its attached upper lateral cartilage.

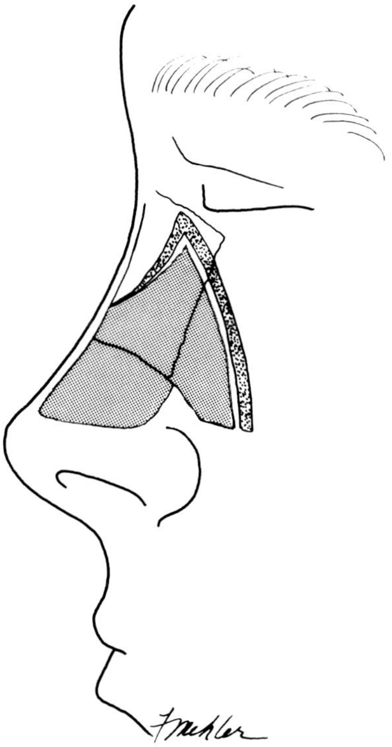

Figure 5-140

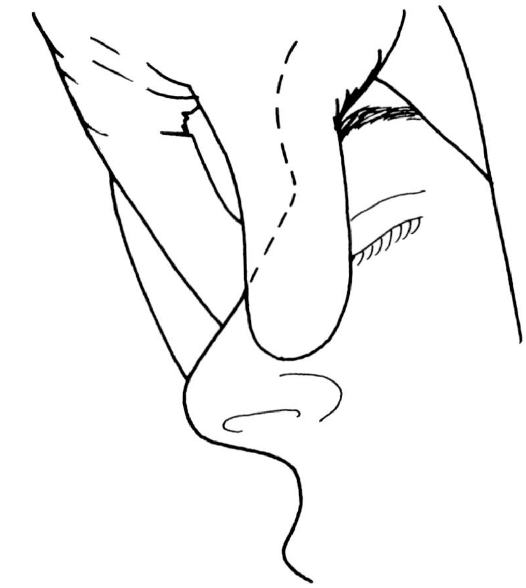

Figure 5-141

If the patient's right lateral osteotomy is done first, the right-handed operator's left thumb can be placed over the osteotomy site (Figure 5-141), allowing that operator to apply constant pressure while performing the left osteotomy. It also allows constant feedback, thus permitting continual adjustment of the left osteotomy, increasing the possibility of obtaining symmetric osteotomies. After completing the osteotomy, pressure should be applied on both sides. This reduces postoperative edema more than any other single thing (steroids, head elevation, cold packs, drain, etc.). After the application of pressure, the soft tissues can be gently milked or massaged. This will allow the careful palpation and visualization for final bony and cartilaginous trimming.

Failure to create back fracture, a potential problem, may represent a failure to have carried the osteotomy close enough to the midline. This can be corrected by reintroducing and completing the osteotomy. If the lateral osteotomy has been carried too high, it is best to use a Rubin nasofrontal osteotome or a percutaneous 2-mm osteotome to create the backfracture. If instead the lateral osteotomy is continued superiorly or more force is applied, the probability of rocker formation is high.

The Rubin nasofrontal osteotome is an excellent instrument to help create a back fracture in the desired place. It would be better to score the nasal bone prior to the lateral osteotomy with the Quisling osteotome. However, it can also be used "after the fact." Care must be exercised not to completely separate the nasal bone from its attachment above.

In Figure 5-142 the arrow points to the undesirable extension of a lateral osteotomy. The dashed line represents the desired back fracture line with the Rubin nasofrontal osteotome in place.

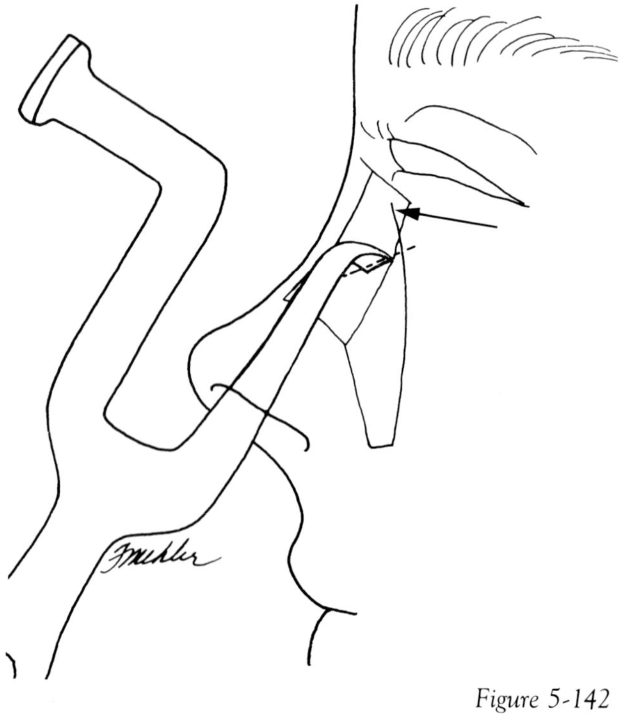

Figure 5-142

Bony irregularities of the solid unfractured radix can be safely and effectively removed with a good sharp rasp. Care must be taken to avoid inadvertently tearing the periosteum of the now mobile nasal bones. In Figure 5-143 the arrow points to an irregularity that could be well treated by rasping.

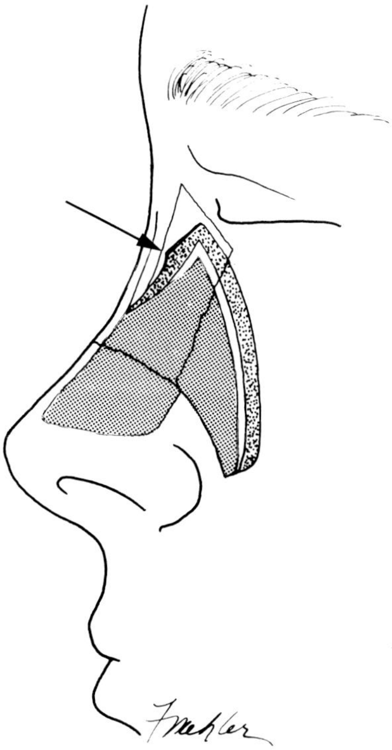

Figure 5-143

In asymmetric osteotomies, one side may fracture higher than the other, either from poor placement or because of an old fracture. A second lower osteotomy will correct or improve the symmetry. Figure 5-144 demonstrates the use of a second osteotomy to further fracture the frontal process of the maxilla.

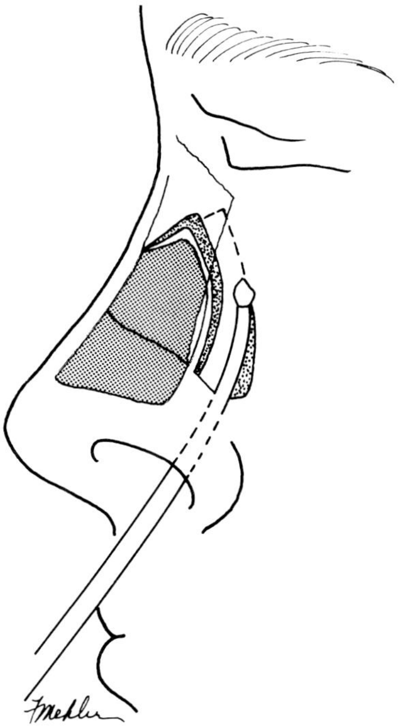

Figure 5-144

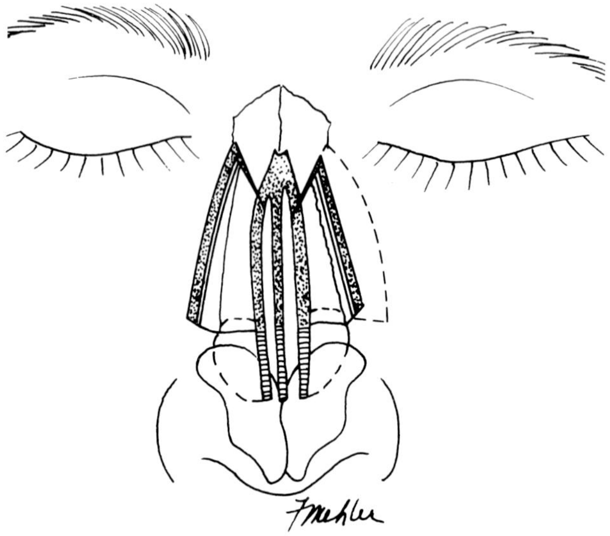

Figure 5-145

Figure 5-145 illustrates a frontal view of a unilateral double osteotomy. Generally the double osteotomy is done bilaterally. These are usually stable as a result of the dense periosteal support. The dashed line on the left in Figure 5-145 represents the proposed second osteotomy.

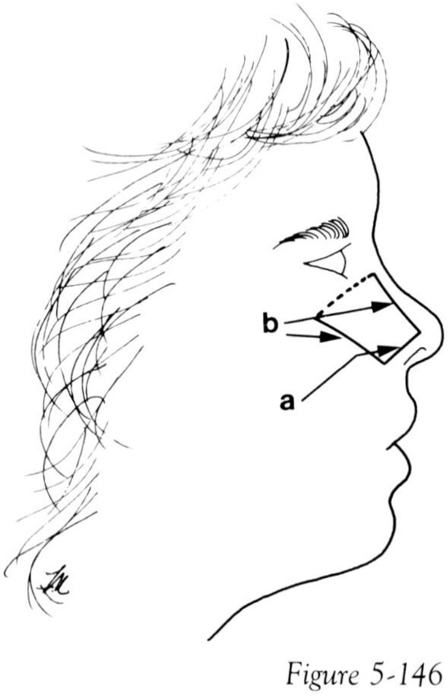

Figure 5-146

Implants

When augmenting the nasal dorsum with a graft (regardless of the choice of the material), the recipient pocket must be carefully prepared in the midline, and ideally just large enough to receive the graft. Large pieces of septum can be harvested in the following manner. Incision a in Figure 5-146 is made with the spade end of a Woodson No. 1, approximately 1 cm from the caudal border of the quadrangular cartilage. The superior and inferior cuts (arrow b) are made with Becker scissors to avoid fracturing of the perpendicular plate. The dashed line represents the last and most difficult cut. These are small fractures made with the tip of a long nasal speculum and or the spade end of the Cottle elevator. The graft material is then removed with broad forceps.

Figure 5-147 shows a graft removal in this manner. Note that the osseocartilaginous junction is intact. The dots are guides for cutting the graft into three segments, which will then be stacked.

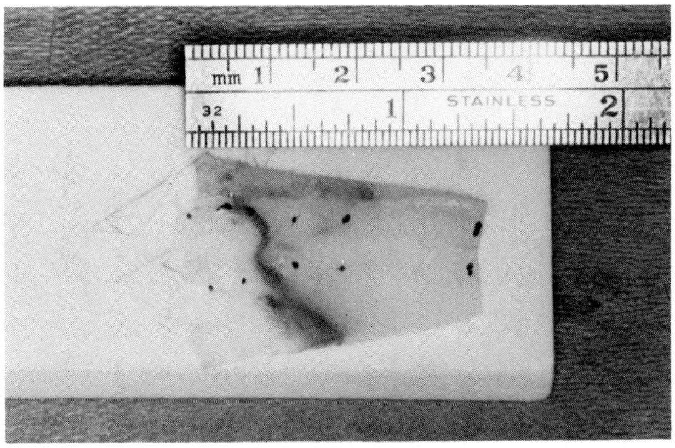

Figure 5-147

Figure 5-148 shows one of the three segments to be stacked. Note that with this graft source, bone will be placed over the patient's nasal bone, and cartilage will be placed over cartilage.

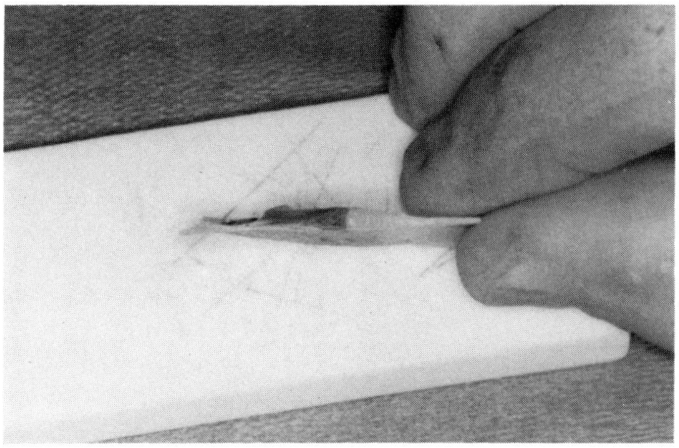
Figure 5-148

Figure 5-149 shows finished stacked graft covered with a single layer of Vicryl mesh just prior to placement. The use of Vicryl or polyamide mesh provides for a smooth graft without palpable steps in the postoperative result.

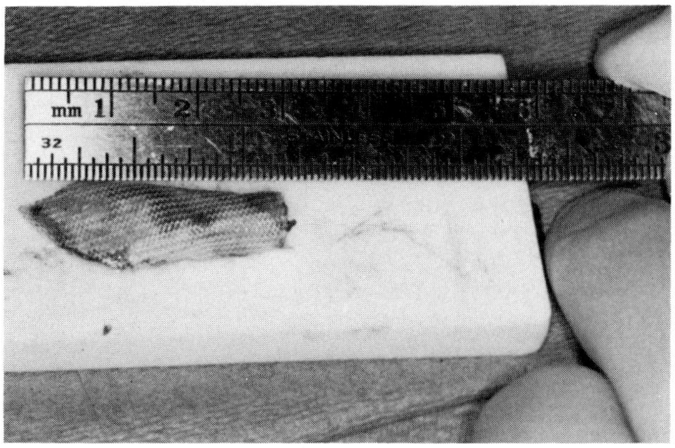

Figure 5-149

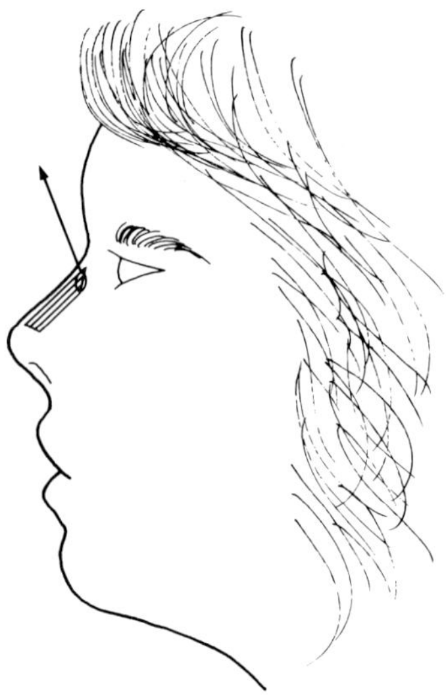

Figure 5-150

Any grafting material, whether autogenous or alloplastic, is soaked in an antibiotic solution prior to placement. The recipient site is prepared while the graft soaks. The incision for creation of the site ideally is as far removed from the site as possible. Next, the graft is placed into the pocket. Often several attempts are made before the pocket is large enough. If the pocket is too large, it is useful to place a suture through the proximal end of the graft with a Keith needle and pass it through the site percutaneously at the level of the nasofrontal angle. This is then used for traction and can be taped to the skin for stability at the end of the case. The chromic suture is then cut flush with the skin when the cast is removed (see Figure 5-150).

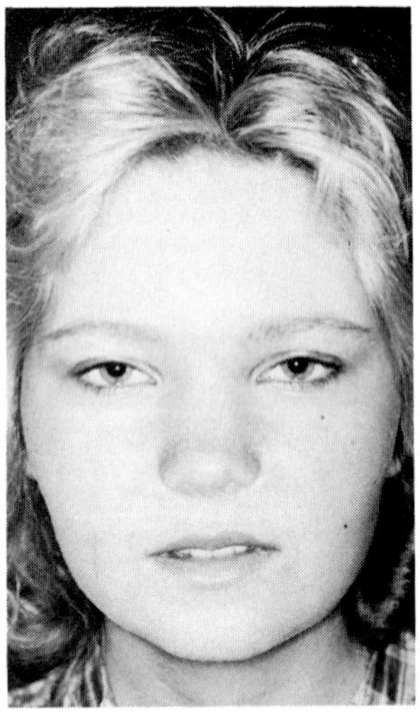

Figure 5-151A

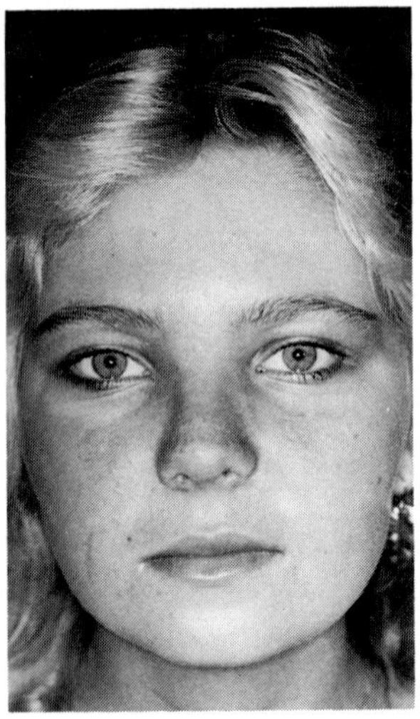

Figure 5-151B

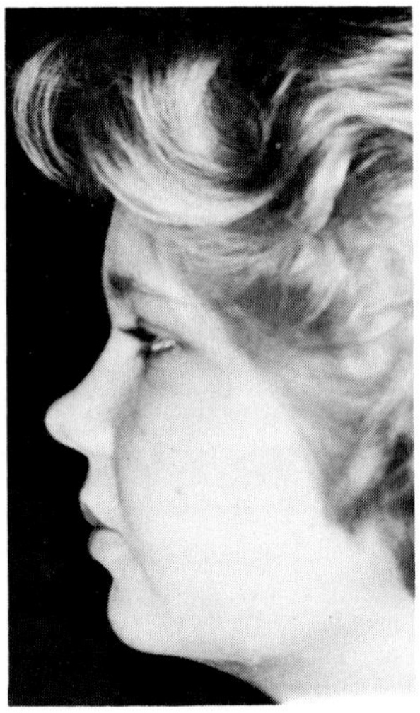

Figure 5-151C

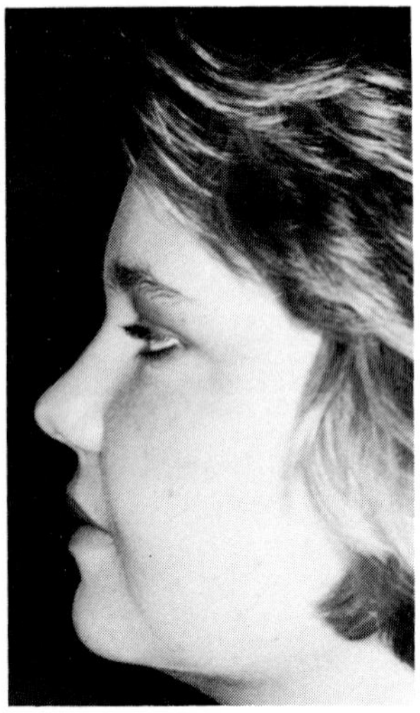

Figure 5-151D

Figure 5-151A–D shows this particular graft in place at 1 year postoperative (Figure 5-151B). Note the limited resorption with the use of the large pieces of graft. A Supramed graft would be placed in an identical manner. The only difference is the graft size, as autogenous material should be large enough to allow for slight resorption noted within the first postoperative year. The larger the graft pieces used, the less the resorption.

Figures 5-152–5-153 show a very wide quadrangular cartilage and abnormal upper lateral development at the level of the rhinion that was reduced by a wedge-shaped excision with a No. 64 Beaver blade. It included both upper lateral cartilage and quadrangular cartilage.

In Figure 5-152A the arrow points to the ellipse that was removed of both septal cartilage and upper lateral; Figure 5-152B is a cross section of the same.

Note the very wide rhinion in the preoperative photograph (Figure 5-153A). The postoperative photograph (Figure 5-153B) shows the narrowing achieved with the above-described resection and lateral osteotomies. Figures 5-96B and 5-96C are of this same patient's profile. Finally, the upper laterals vary greatly in the size of the scroll and overall length. The upper laterals should be well visualized and always symmetrical at the end of the procedure. Excision of the medial aspect of the scroll is often necessary to prevent a postoperative supratip fullness. In view of these variables, meticulous examination at the end of the procedure is essential to a symmetrical result.

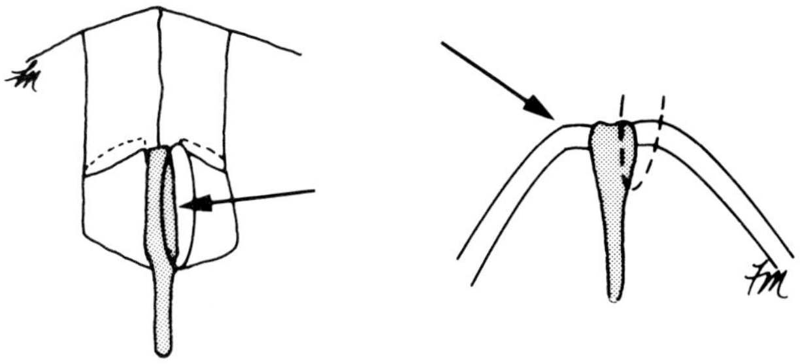

Figure 5-152

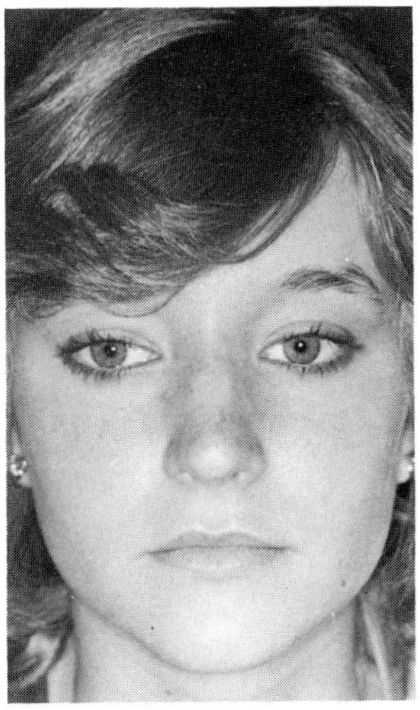

Figure 5-153A

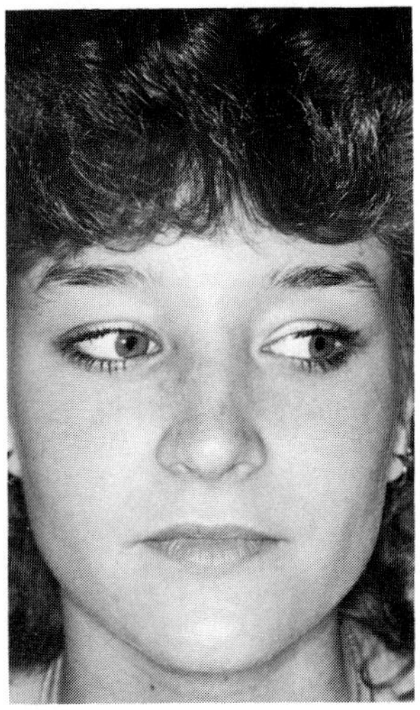

Figure 5-153B

ALAR RESECTION

When the alar lobules and/or nostrils are wide preoperatively or assume a relative increase in width secondary to reduction rhinoplasty, they need to be resected. Basically two changes are noted following alar resection. One is the size, shape, and orientation of the nostril (the internal opening). The second is the size, shape, and orientation of the alae (Figure 5-154). The dashed line represents the nostril and the solid line, the alae. The surgical resection can involve the alar lobule only, the alar lobule and the nostril, or the nostril only; each affects the other. Each resection is individually tailored. It can be just alae resection with no incision of the nostril or the reverse with just nostril resection and no alae incision. If the nostril border is incised, great care must be taken not to create a visible notching, giving a surgical appearance.

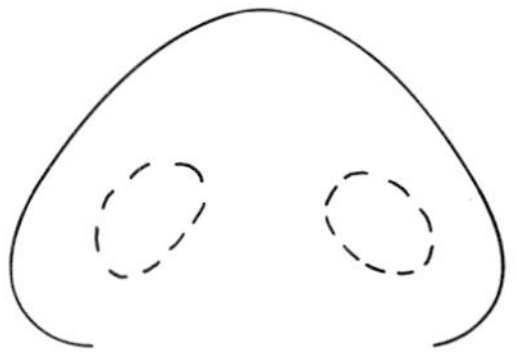

Figure 5-154

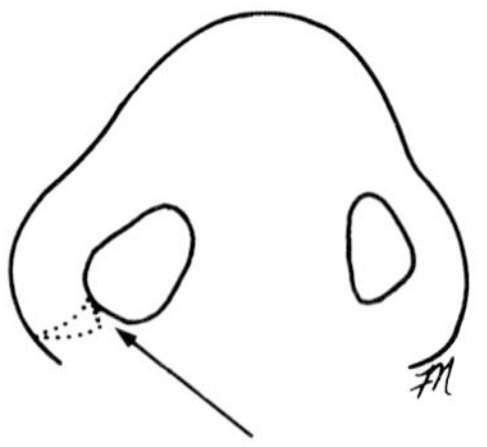

Figure 5-155

The creation of a medially based flap as advocated by Jack H. Sheen,[6] solves this problem. Figure 5-155 shows a proposed resection of a 4-mm nostril resection and a 2-mm alae resection. The arrow in Figure 5-155 points to the very important medial flap of nostril skin, which will provide a smooth border postoperatively. The use of a No. 11 blade is helpful for the inferior incision as it is made from the alae to the nostril approximately 1–2 mm above the alae facial groove. If the incision is made within the alae facial groove, accurate closure is much more difficult and the sebaceous nature of the facial skin makes the scar less desirable.

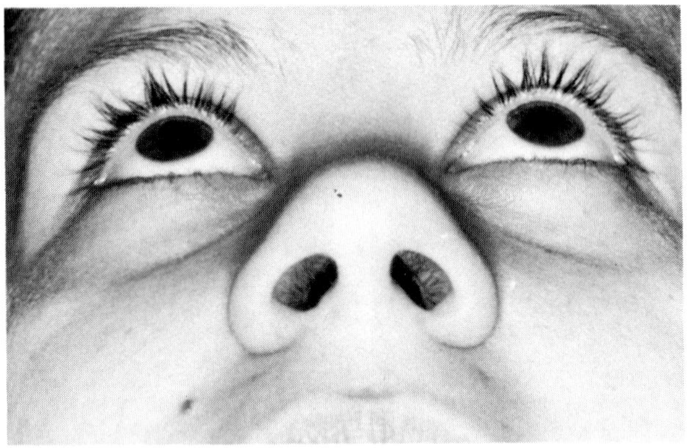

Figure 5-156A

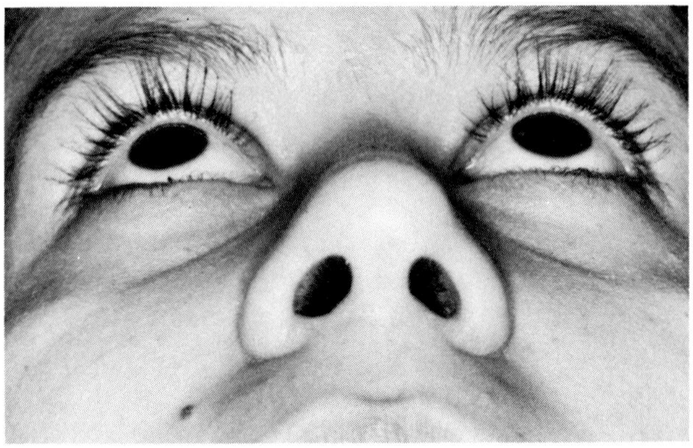

Figure 5-156B

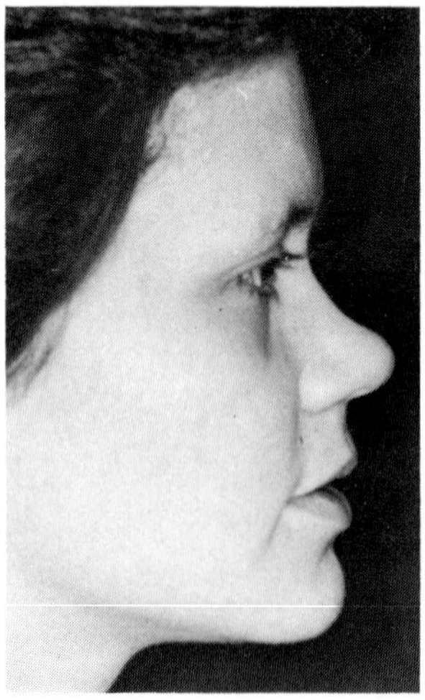

Figure 5-156C

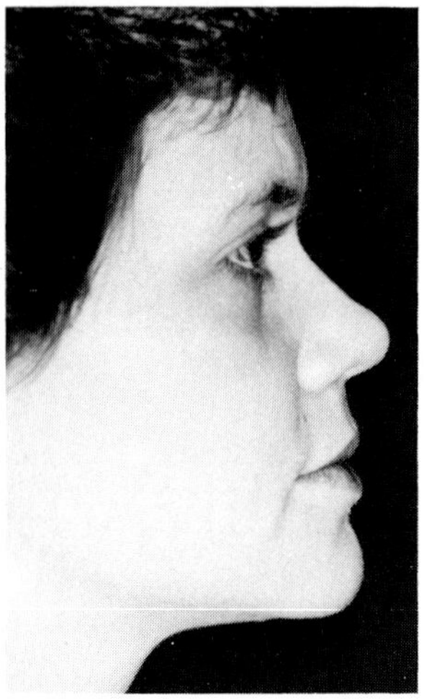

Figure 5-156D

If the first incision—the inferior one—is stopped just short of transecting the nostril border, the second incision can be made much more accurately. Generally this is made with a No. 15 blade from nostril border to alar border. One to two deep chromics are used for approximation and the silk skin sutures, which are removed in 3–5 days. In Figure 5-156A–D these photographs were intentionally taken at 3 months, so that the scar is still visible. Note the smooth nostril border with no evidence of notching. This represents a combination of nostril vestibular skin excision and alar excision with a medial base flap technique. Note the change in both the nostril and the alae. The excised segment measured 2 mm of vestibular and 4 mm of alae. Profile photographs (Figures 5-156C and 5-156D) also show a subtle but important change in the relationship of the alae to the columellar lip complex. This patient had a stacked cartilage bone graft of septal origin. The decrease in projection of the tip will continue for at least 3 more months secondary to using the full delivery technique for tip exposure and modification.

NASAL PACKING

If septal surgery or turbinate surgery has been performed, the patient is packed overnight. A standard finger cot is first lubricated with an ointment and then placed over a large nasal speculum and placed intranasally (Figure 5-157).

Then it is packed with petrolatum (Vaseline) gauze as in Figure 5-158. The use of a lubricated gauze greatly facilitates its removal the next day.

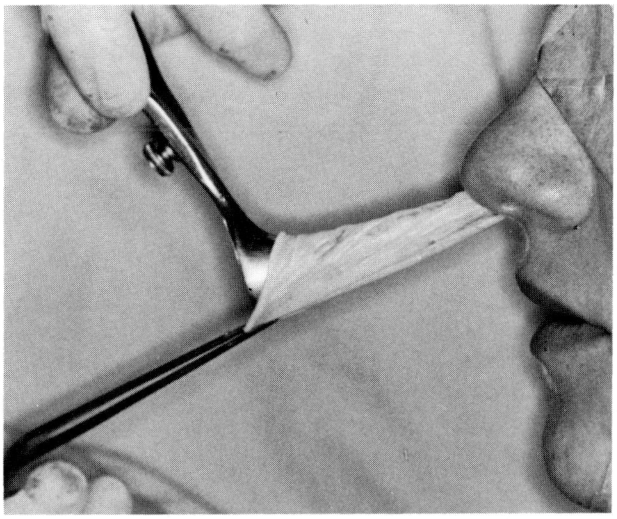

Figure 5-157

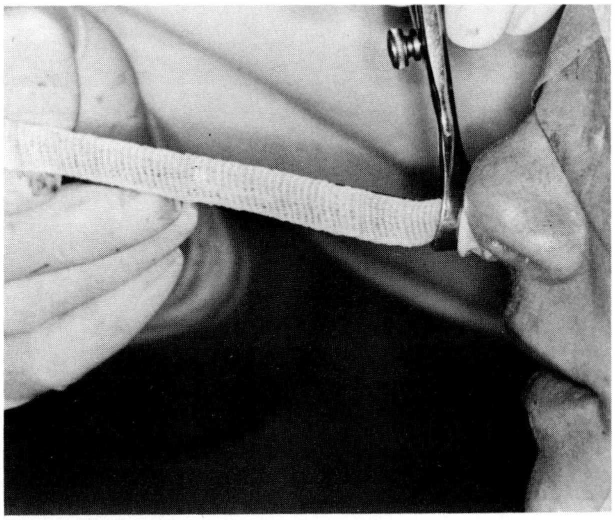

Figure 5-158

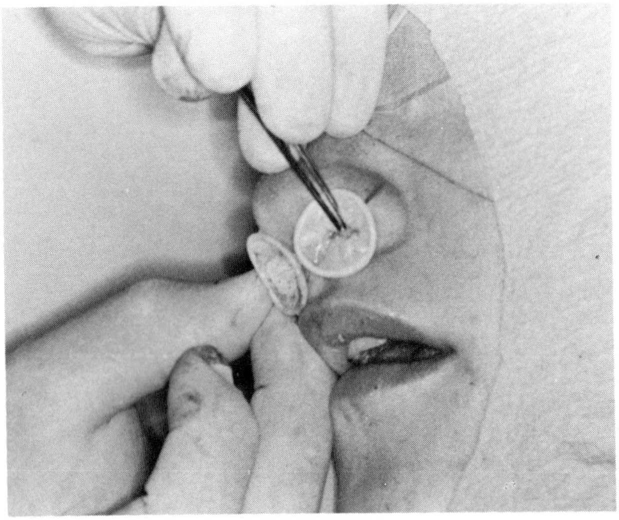

Figure 5-159

Next, the finger cots are sutured together with silk on a Keith needle to prevent any possible posterior displacement and aspiration (Figure 5-159). The following morning the suture is cut; the Vaseline gauze is removed first, and then the empty finger cot. This eliminates any discomfort associated with packing removal, and generally there is no bleeding following removal.

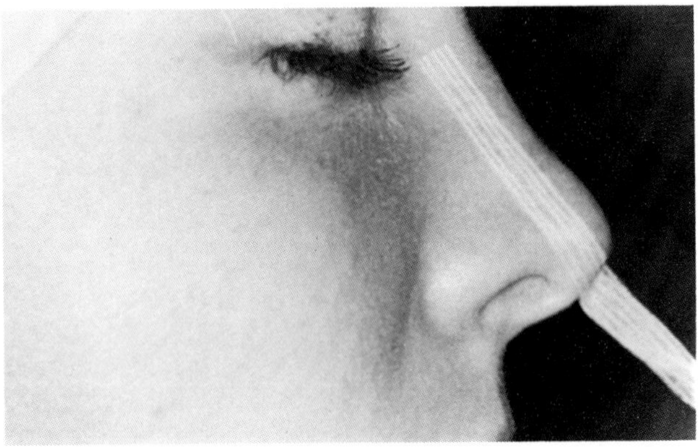

Figure 5-160

CASTING

The casting is important for reduction of edema as well as to allow final molding if the nose is intentionally overpacked. Skin gel by Hollster is first applied to the nose to allow good tape adhesion. Next, long $\frac{1}{4}$-inch-wide Steristrips are placed to help approximate the lower lateral cartilages (Figure 5-160).

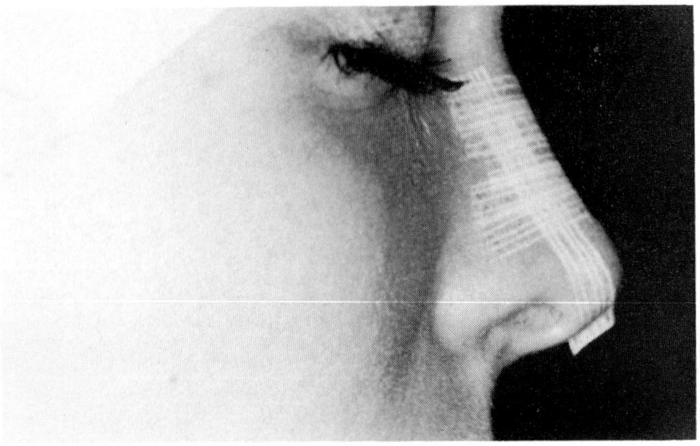

Figure 5-161

Then individual $\frac{1}{4}$-inch strips are applied (Figure 5-161).

Note that they do not extend past the lateral osteotomy site. Another layer of $\frac{1}{2}$-inch-Steristrips is then similarly applied. Next, standard adhesive tape is applied; the size corresponds to that of the plaster to be applied next (Figure 5-162).

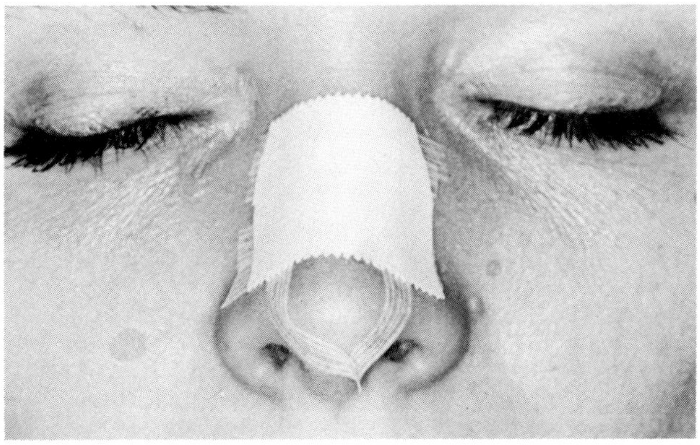

Figure 5-162

The final step is the application of a fast-drying plaster cast, which covers only the area between the lateral osteotomies (Figure 5-163). The cast is routinely removed in 4–7 days following surgery.

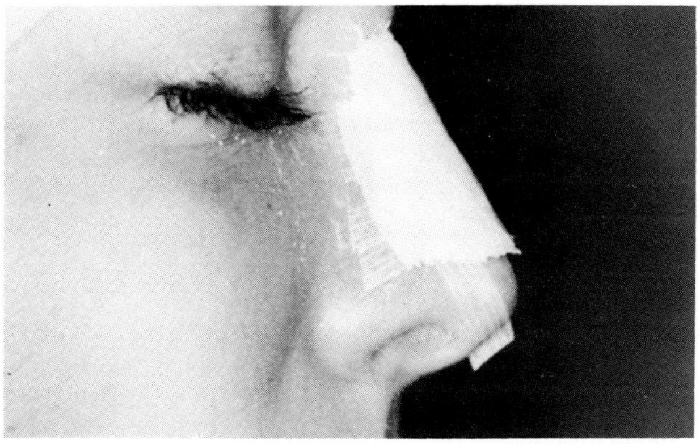

Figure 5-163

CHIN IMPLANTS

The two common approaches are intraoral placement with a buccal gingival incision or percutaneous with submental incision. The intraoral approach is presented as that is the author's preference, thus avoiding the submental scar. The submental approach is reserved for patients who need a concomitant submental lipectomy or have a very shallow labial sulcus. Alloplastic material is used; the major difference is whether it is preformed and thus symmetrical or is an implant that can be tailored in the operating room. The preformed gel-filled Heyer-Schulte chin prosthesis is used routinely on patients with symmetrical chins. The gel-fill provides a normal feeling chin postoperatively. The Beekhuis polyamide implant is used in the asymmetrical cases as it can be tailored to accommodate the patient's asymmetry. Any implant is first soaked in an antibiotic solution prior to placement.

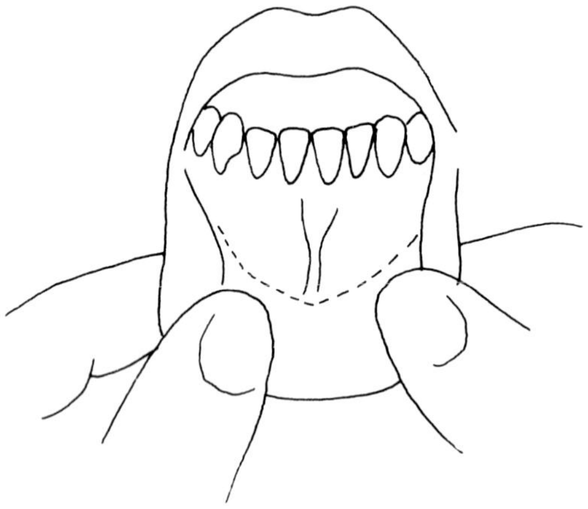

Figure 5-164

Initially the incision is made 3–4 mm on the buccal side of the buccal gingival groove (Figure 5-164), thus allowing easier subsequent closure with 4-0 chromic. Next, the dissection is carried down to the mentalis muscle, which is spread apart vertically in the midline. With all except the smallest implants it is necessary to transect at least a portion of this muscle to accommodate the implant. Then a Joseph periosteal elevator is used to elevate the periosteum, as in all implants the pocket is just large enough to accept the implant. Midline placement of the implant is key, and the frenulum of the lower lip serves as a useful reference point.

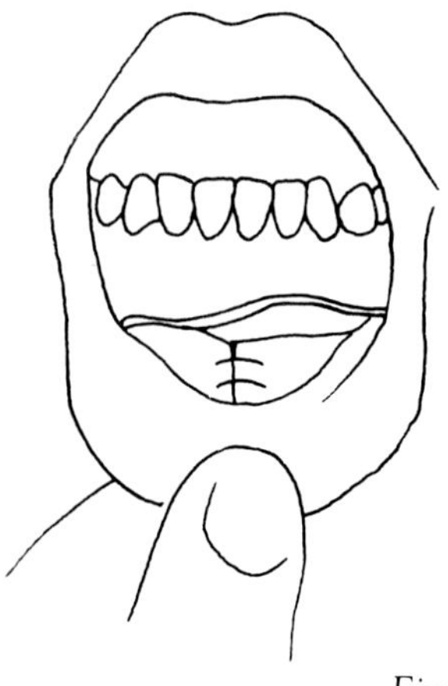

Figure 5-165

After placing the implant, meticulous closure of the mentalis muscle in one or preferably two layers in a vertical orientation is desirable (Figure 5-165). Then the mucosal incision is a watertight vertical mattress closure in the horizontal plane. A compression dressing is applied in a basket-weave pattern with Elastoplast. The reported bone erosion beneath the implant has not proved to be of clinical importance and appears to be self-limiting.

POSTOPERATIVE CARE

Antibiotics are not routinely given. If any implants are placed, or if the patient has a mustache or beard, a cephalosporin-class drug is given IV prior to any incisions, and then three additional oral doses are given at 6-hour intervals postoperatively. The nasal packings are routinely removed the following morning. The patients are given 60 mg of glucocorticoid triamcinolone (Aristocort) orally to help reduce intranasal edema. After packing removal they are discharged with instructions to use a nasal spray 4 times daily and also instructed to irrigate their noses with warm saline solution and a bulb syringe as needed for removal of secretions. They are advised to use the irrigation only if they feel it is beneficial. On their return 4–7 days postoperatively their casts are removed, splints are removed, and their noses are suctioned of secretions. The next visit is at 3 weeks, after which the patients return at 6 weeks postoperative for their first postoperative photographs.

DISCUSSION

ANESTHESIA

The purpose of local anesthesia infiltration is to obtain a field block for total anesthesia and the best possible hemostasis. If small amounts are injected slowly, there will be no significant distortion or distention of the tissues. It is the rapidity of an injection that causes pain; therefore, it is done slowly. A full 10 minutes should be allowed for the local to take effect in order to provide the best hemostasis. It is a good time to write orders, prep the patient, and scrub. The better the anesthetic technique, the less preoperative and intraoperative medications needed. Patients in general respond much better to less drugs as they are able to maintain their awareness and sense of control. Also, they feel much better in the immediate postoperative period. General anesthesia is necessary for some patients; patients with very poor self-control, revision cases, or patients who have had complications during previous surgery; and cases where the surgery time is expected to exceed 2 hours (i.e., rhinoplasty-otoplasty combination). The final truth is that general anesthesia is often easier on the surgeon, and this also must be taken into consideration.

TECHNIQUE

Regarding turbinate surgery, turbinate reduction is an extremely useful adjunct to septorhinoplasty. The increase in useful airway is essential to a functional result. The majority of rhinoplasty surgery narrows the airway, and this must be compensated for at the initial surgery. The greatest advantages of submucous resection are negligible postoperative bleeding and the simultaneous reduction of both components of the turbinate—the bone by direct removal and the functioning mucosa through surgical trauma, the elevation, and subsequent fibrous healing. Also, if the reduction has been excessive, the mucosa retains the ability to compensate through hypertrophy. The chief disadvantage is that initially it is a time-consuming and frustrating surgical experience. Thin instruments will greatly increase the available space for manipulation and are essential.

Surgery for correction of septal and caudal septal disorders is progressive, and at its completion the columella may still be deviated. If this is the case, the medial crura may be fractured or twisted, in which case they must be exposed, repaired, and sutured together. In addition, the soft tissues at the base of the columella and anterior to the anterior nasal spine may need to be dissected in order for them to redrape in the now straight plane. Finally, the anterior nasal spine itself may not be in the midline. This can be checked by aligning it to the space between the maxillary central incisors. If the anterior nasal spine is fractured, it may be placed back in the midline. Finally, in a severely distorted cartilaginous septum it is commonly necessary to elevate both mucoperichondral flaps in order to correct the septal cartilage.

Concerning nasal tip surgery, the tip segment of rhinoplasty is frequently stated to be the most difficult procedure. However, the tip will appear to be the causative factor in an unsatisfactory result when the error is actually in the initial analysis. The use of a chin implant will reduce the amount of reduction that a large or projecting tip needs. The use of a dorsal graft will often be a much better choice than reducing a tip. Augmentation of the premaxilla or plumping of the anterior nasal spine area will increase tip projection more naturally than will transecting the medial crura and suturing them together. Poor surgery of the upper laterals (supratip) or late fibrosis in the supratip area is another example of the tip appearing at fault when it is in reality an anatomically close-by error.

The tip techniques presented are safe and predictable but are still difficult and require meticulous surgery. Many other tip surgical techniques have not been presented here, and the reader is referred to the literature for these. Several techniques have been avoided because of their unpredictability. Tip grafts have not been presented because of the author's personal lack of long-term experience with this technique. Finally, if it appears that the tip needs a major change, one must reanalyze the face as a whole and be prepared to compromise.

There are two major schools of thought concerning the periosteum of the nasal bones. Proponents for elevation state that this provides an extra layer for redraping and covering of any minor postoperative irregularities of the nasal dorsum. Proponents for leaving the periosteum state that the periosteum is so tightly adherent to the bones that it cannot be elevated without shredding it. Also, the periosteum provides for more stable osteotomies. Ideally, if the periosteum were elevated (or shredded) only over the bone to be removed, then all possible periosteal support would remain, and the maximum soft tissue would be available for redraping. The elevation is begun just cephalically to the lower border of the nasal bones, with care taken not to elevate between the upper laterals and the nasal bone. The periosteum is very tightly adherent to the midline and must be sharply cut there in order to create a subperiosteal tunnel.

Regarding hump removal in dorsum surgery, any rasping should be accomplished prior to the lateral osteotomies. If not, the mobile segments of bone are not safe to rasp after the fact. Becker scissors can be used for trimming of thin bone irregularities after lateral osteotomy. A dull osteotome should not be used and must be guarded against as it will not run true. Saws for hump removal were not discussed in this chapter because the surgeon needs a good deal of experience to know just how much greater the loss of height will be due to the saw kerf. Greater deepening of the nasal frontal angle with the use of large gouges or by fracturing larger segments of bone is approached with great caution because of the unpredictable results secondary to the variation in the thickness of bone in the radix. This is a solid area anatomically and will not reduce through infracture.

Regarding augmentation of the dorsum, ideally this would place bone over bone and cartilage, with its flexibility, over cartilage. There are two commonly available sources of material for augmentation: autogenous and alloplastic material. All autogenous sources from a second site have the common disadvantages of added scar, time, and dressings. In addition, each has its special restrictions. For instance, the use of ear cartilage in augmentation is limited as cartilaginous material is limited in quantity and subject to warpage. Rib is also subject to warpage. Also, with use of the iliac crest, the patient is vulnerable to postoperative pain. All bone grafts generally require wiring in place creating a stiff lower two-thirds of the nose, which is susceptible to fracture. The septum appears to be the material of choice, if it is available in sufficient quantity. It has both bone and cartilage, is readily available without a second donor site, and adds no significant time to the procedure.

All alloplastic materials have the advantages of being free of warpage, easily shaped, and available in unlimited amounts. Moreover, no added surgery is needed to harvest the material. The disadvantage has been surgically induced infection, rejection of some materials, and in one, a poor color choice. Supramed mesh has an exceptional track record with follow-up now at 12 years.

In a recent conversation with this author, G. Jan Beekhuis, M.D., who now has 12-year follow-up using Supramed mesh, stated that there has been no true immune rejection of polyamide mesh. There has been surgically induced infection with rejection. This has been nearly eliminated by presoaking the implant in an antibiotic solution just prior to placement. He also stated that there has been some late reduction in the size of the implant as it is replaced by scar tissue many years following its implantation. If septum is available in significant quantity, quality, and strength, it is the graft of choice because it is autogenous and allows bone over bone and cartilage over cartilage. If this source is not available, Supramed mesh is used.

A final word on dorsum surgery: anatomically, this is difficult at best because of the many variables, all of which are important. The thickness and texture of the skin and subcutaneous tissue within the same patient, which is thinner at the rhinion, and the marked variation between individuals that must always be taken into consideration—the clinical radix with its variations in size and strength of the nasal process of the frontal bone, as well as the variations in the thickness of the most cephalad portion of the nasal bones, and the variable width of the underlying perpendicular plate. This anatomy does not allow narrowing by infracture without very extensive and unpredictable bone removal. The choice is sculpturing with rasps and burrs, which is far safer and predictable. The next great variation is in the nature of the frontal process of the maxilla and the attached nasal bones. Previous fractures will often become apparent during the lateral osteotomy. The concept of intact periosteum over the line of back fracture provides the necessary stability and is the main contraindication to the use of a separate medial osteotomy. With hump removal and a curved lateral osteotomy, a significant degree of medial osteotomy has been accomplished. In closing an open roof, if the perpendicular plate and or the dorsum of the septum is deviated or thick, this must be recognized and corrected.

REFERENCES

1. Beekhuis, G.J.: Saddle Nose Deformity—Etiology, Prevention, and Treatment; Augmentation Rhinoplasty with Polyamide. *Laryngoscope,* 84:2–42, 1974.
2. Goodman, W.S. and Charbonneau, P.A.: External Approach to Rhinoplasty. *Laryngoscope,* 84: 2195–2201, 1974.

3. Lipsett, E.M.: A New Approach to Surgery of the Lower Cartilaginous Vault. A.M.A. *Arch. Otol.*, 70:42–47, 1959.
4. Patterson, C.N. and Powell, D.G.: Facial Analysis in Patient Evaluation for Physiologic and Cosmetic Surgery. *Laryngoscope,* 84:1004–1019, 1974.
5. Rees, T.D.: Aesthetic Plastic Surgery, Vol. I. W.B. Saunders Co., Philadelphia, 1980.
6. Sheen, J.H.: Aesthetic Rhinoplasty. C.V. Mosby Co., St. Louis, 1978.
7. Smith, T.W.: Osteotomy and Infarction in Rhinoplasty. *Arch. Otolaryngol.*, 100:266–268, 1974.
8. Webster, R.C.: Advances in Surgery of the Tip: Intact Rim Cartilage Techniques and the Tip-Columella-Lip Esthetic Complex. *Otol. Clin. North Am.*, 8(3):615–644, 1975.
9. Wright, W.K. and Kridel, R.W.H.: External Septorhinoplasty—A Tool For Teaching and For Improved Results. *Laryngoscope,* 91:945–951, 1981.
10. Wright, W.K.: Surgery of the Bony and Cartilaginous Dorsum. *Otol. Clin. North Am.*, 575–598, 1975.

6
Hair Replacement and Scalp Reduction

John A. McCurdy, Jr.
Bruce B. Chrisman

GENERAL CONSIDERATIONS

Recession of the frontal and temporal hairline begins in almost all males during adolescence. Although progressive diffuse thinning of the hair continues at a slow rate with increasing age, a significant percentage of the male population experiences accelerated hair loss at age 20–40—a condition known as *male pattern baldness* (MPB) (see Figure 6-1). This process is termed MPB because hair loss occurs in distinct patterns and shows predictable progression as demonstrated in the classification by Norwood.[9]

Although some men have used baldness to enhance their image and further their social or business endeavors, for most, adjustment to hair loss is emotionally painful as evidenced by sales of devices for hair replacement, as well as aggressive merchandising of products that promise to preserve hair or stimulate its growth. Hair replacement surgery provides another option in dealing with baldness. Recent refinements in technique have significantly improved the results and extended the application of such surgery to men with more extensive degrees of baldness.

MALE PATTERN BALDNESS

Male pattern baldness is characterized by diffuse thinning of scalp hair in the frontal, upper temporal area, and vertex. This thinning tends to become confluent with increasing age. Such progres-

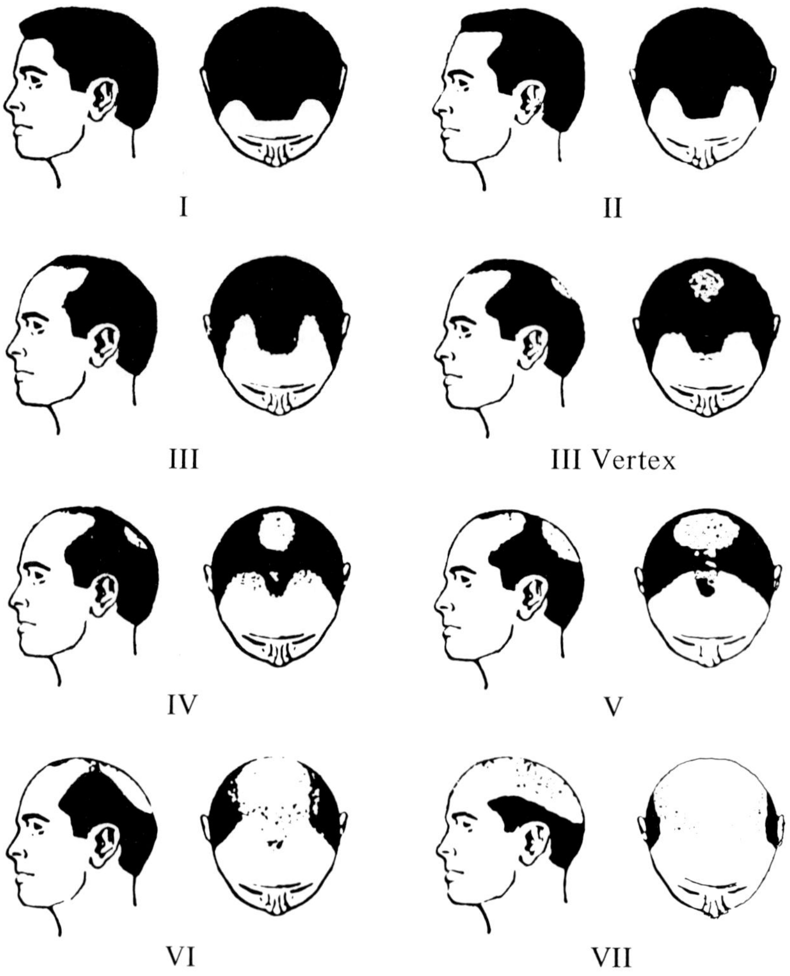

Figure 6-1

sive alopecia, the rate and extent of which show individual variation, is related to interaction of three etiologic factors: genetics, androgens, and age.

Histopathologic evaluation of MPB shows that the number of hair follicles in affected scalps is not diminished but that their size is reduced. As alopecia progresses, the shed telogen (resting) hairs exhibit shafts of reduced diameter consistent with a progressive miniaturization of genetically susceptible hair follicles in response to the effects of dihydrotestosterone. With each cycle the percentage of "miniaturized" follicles in the affected scalp increases, and the density of hair in these areas diminishes. The hairs also tend to be shorter since the anagen (growing) phase is shortened. In the final analysis, therefore, MPB is not caused by a loss of hair follicles but rather by a time-dependent, hormonally mediated and genetically determined miniaturization of follicles associated with a diminution in the anagen or growing phase of each affected follicle.

The principles of surgical hair replacement in MPB are based on two observations related to this progress:

1. Hair loss occurs in a predictable pattern, allowing reliable, although not precise, estimation of hair-bearing areas that will remain unaffected by the process.
2. A phenomenon termed *donor dominance* may occur, where hair follicles transplanted into an area of alopecia maintain the growth characteristics of their donor regions.

CLASSIFICATION OF HAIR REPLACEMENT SURGERY

Punch Grafts

Transplantation of punch grafts of hair-bearing scalp obtained from fringe areas in the parietooccipital region is currently the most popular method of surgical hair replacement. These punch grafts, usually 3.5–4.5 mm in diameter, contain about 8–15 follicles and are placed in the surgically created recipient sites in the area of alopecia. In most patients 4–10 sessions at 3-week to 3-month intervals are necessary to achieve an optimum result. One disadvantage of punch grafting relates to the hair cycle. Shortly following transplantation, the hair in each plug is shed as follicles enter the telogen phase as a result of the "shock" of transplantation. This telogen phase lasts for 10–12 weeks, after which time hair growth (anagen phase) begins at the rate of approximately 1 cm per month. A lapse of 12–15 months is required before transplanted hair reaches sufficient length to produce full cosmetic benefit, although significant improvement may be noted as early as 8 or 9 months after starting transplantation.

Punch grafting cannot produce hair of entirely normal density over the whole scalp, and in order to provide the illusion of increased density, professional hair styling is beneficial.

Strip Grafts

Transplantation of strips of hair-bearing scalp would seem to offer a method of enhancing hair density in the frontal area. Although championed by some, most surgeons have found that strips produce a low yield of viable hair and have abandoned this method. In addition, placement of strips so that hair grows at the proper angle is often difficult.

Scalp Flaps

Recently, considerable interest has been generated in hair replacement using hair-bearing flaps. Such flaps have long been used for correction of traumatic alopecia, but it was not until the report by Juri[8] that the value of flaps for treatment of MPB was convincingly demonstrated.

A major advantage of flap surgery is that, in contrast to punch grafting, bald scalp is replaced with hair of normal density. A second advantage relates to the fact that follicles in the flap seldom enter a telogen phase following transposition and thus "instant hair" is produced.

A theoretical disadvantage of scalp flaps is that hair growth in the frontal hairline is in a posterior direction rather than in the natural anterior direction. Flap transposition involves a major surgical procedure and the consequences of possible complications are more significant and difficult to rectify than those associated with punch grafting. These controversies are discussed in more detail later in this chapter.

Scalp Reduction

A valuable addition to the armamentarium of the hair transplant surgeon, scalp reduction involves excision of segments of bald scalp, undermining of the scalp in a plane deep to the galea, and advancement of the residual scalp toward the midline with primary closure. This technique accomplishes two objectives. First, hair from the fringe area is advanced toward areas of alopecia, and the area of bald scalp requiring resurfacing with either punch grafts or flaps is reduced. The second objective is of more significance as it is estimated that each square centimeter of excised scalp saves as many as nine punch grafts. In an average case, the area of alopecia excised during the primary scalp reduction averages 40–45 cm^2, and serial, staged reduction procedures allow subsequent excision of even greater areas of bald scalp. Scalp reduction is a valuable adjunct to hair replacement using punch grafts, strip grafts, or flaps and in some cases may enhance the cosmetic result of hairpieces.

Tunnel Grafts

Tunnel grafts are adjuncts to hair replacement and are used in conjunction with hairpieces. Attachment of hairpieces to the scalp by use of adhesive tape, metal clips, Teflon-coated sutures, and the like is often fraught with problems, and tunnel grafts provide a secure and convenient method of fixation.

The tunnel graft consists of an epithelium-lined subcutaneous tract that is constructed by elevating a small strip of scalp and lining its undersurface with a graft of postauricular skin which is rolled into a cylindrical configuration around a small rubber tube. Following healing, a hairpiece can be securely attached to the subcutaneous tube without penetration of the scalp itself by sutures, clips, or other means. In most cases the prosthesis is fastened to two such tunnels. In some patients, accumulative daily stresses of hairpiece attachment may damage the tunnels, requiring repair or surgical construction of additional tunnels.

SELECTION OF PATIENTS FOR HAIR REPLACEMENT SURGERY

The extent of hair loss and density of remaining hair is of prime importance in selecting candidates for hair replacement surgery. Although the success of scalp reduction techniques has increased the acceptable recipient site : donor site ratio, the surgeon must ensure that sufficient donor hair is available to satisfy the desires of the patient.

Each surgeon has personal preferences concerning the ideal hair color, texture, and skin coloring which is most suitable for hair replacement surgery. Age per se is not a factor in the success of hair replacement surgery. Suggestions that older men risk a lower "take ratio" because of decreased scalp blood supply have been disproved. Young men, however, should be approached with caution, particularly those in whom hair loss has recently begun. Such candidates may be more impulsive in their desires for hair replacement. They tend to be more impatient in waiting for the results of surgery and thus may discontinue staged procedures before completion. The surgeon must also be cautious in determining the available donor site, as the final extent of hair loss is more unpredictable in younger patients. Family history may provide a rough guide in this regard and should be carefully elicited.

ANATOMY

THE SCALP

As shown in Figure 6-2; the scalp is composed of five soft-tissue layers easily remembered by the following single-letter acronyms: S, skin; C, connective tissue; A, aponeurosis (galea); L, loose areolar tissue; and P, pericranium. Three of these layers,

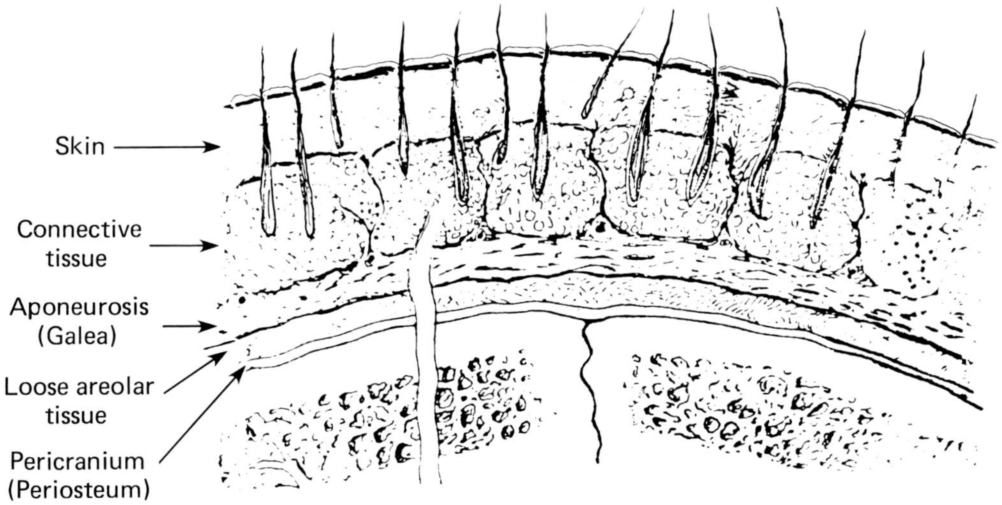

Figure 6-2

the connective tissue, loose areolar tissue, and the aponeurosis, are important in hair replacement surgery.

The subcutaneous connective tissue layer contains the blood and nerve supply of the scalp, an important consideration in gauging the depth of anesthetic injections. Hair follicles are also located within this layer. In scalp flap and scalp reduction procedures, the proper plane of dissection is in the loose areolar tissue (subgaleal).

The galea must be closed following scalp reduction procedures and when approximating the donor site of a scalp flap in order to prevent widening of the scar and relieve tension on the overlying skin. Some surgeons advocate placement of multiple relaxing incisions in the galea to facilitate closure of these wounds.

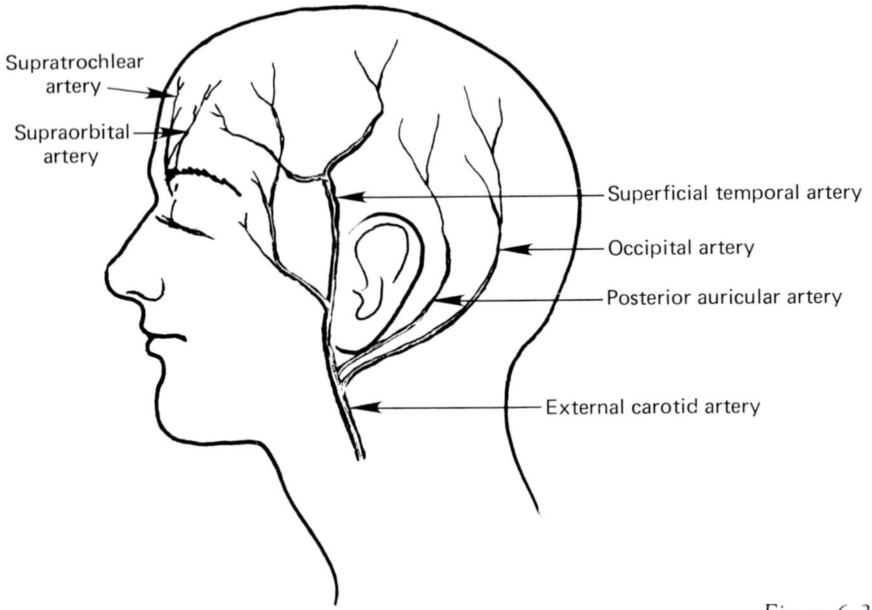

Figure 6-3

The pattern of blood supply within the scalp is illustrated in Figure 6-3. The profuse blood supply of the scalp originates mainly from branches of the external carotid artery. The frontal branch of the superficial temporal artery supplies blood to the anterior aspect of the scalp, and the posterior branch of the superficial temporal artery supplies blood to the central scalp. The posterior scalp and vertex are supplied blood by occipital and posterior auricular arteries.

Branches of the internal carotid artery anastomose with those of the external carotid, also contributing to the scalp blood supply in the frontal region; these branches are the supratrochlear and supraorbital arteries. The venous drainage of the scalp generally corresponds with the arterial supply, ultimately draining into the common facial, external jugular, and internal jugular (via supraorbital, supratrochlear) veins.

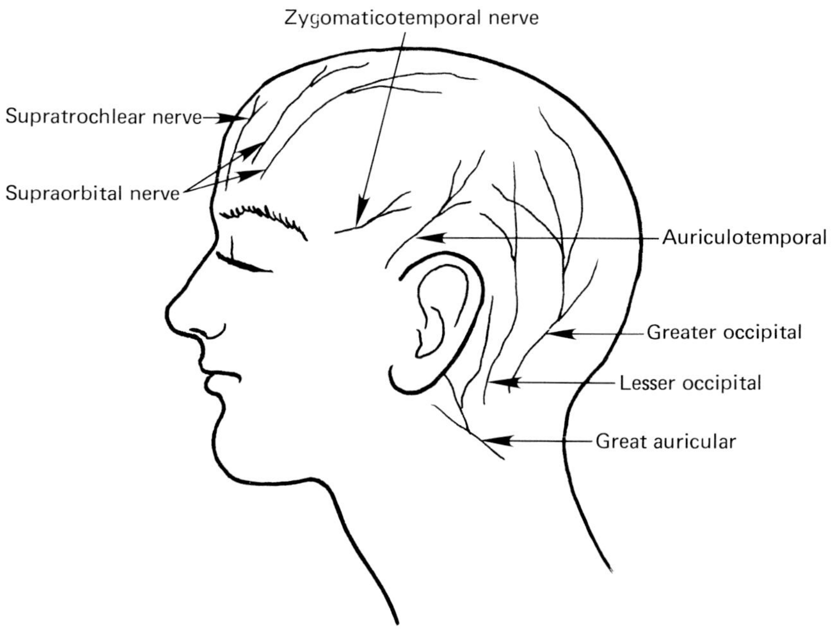

Figure 6-4

Figure 6-4 shows innervation of the scalp. Branches of four nerves supply sensory innervation to that portion of the scalp anterior to the auricle: supraorbital, supratrochlear, zygomaticotemporal, and auriculotemporal. Branches of four nerves supply sensory innervation to that portion of the scalp posterior to the auricle: great auricular, lesser occipital, greater occipital, and third occipital.

TECHNIQUE

PUNCH GRAFTING

In general, the hairline should be curvilinear in configuration, forming a somewhat open U shape. The dotted lines in Figure 6-5A and B show the anticipated regression of the temporal hairline. Establishment of the frontal hairline must allow for this hair loss (Figure 6-5B) and not extend laterally to fill in the temporal area (Figure 6-5A).

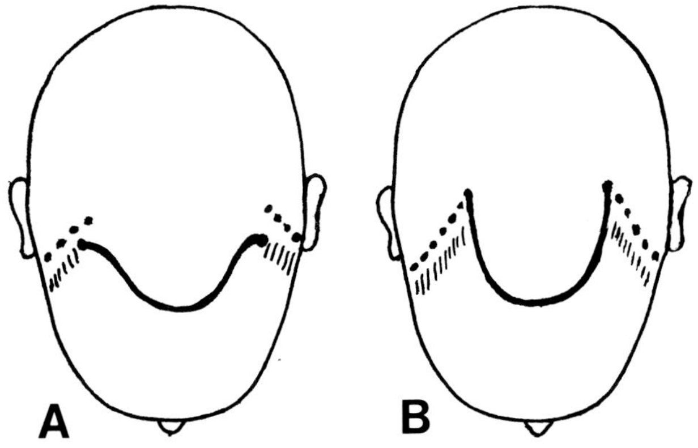

Figure 6-5

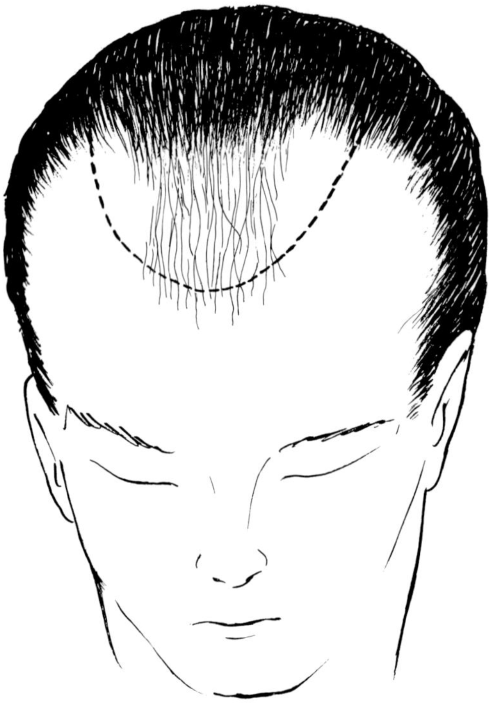

Figure 6-6

The hairline (see dotted line in Figure 6-6) should be placed posterior to any fine hairs that may persist in the frontal area. These hairs provide an illusion of natural recession and camouflage the abrupt look of densely planted plugs.

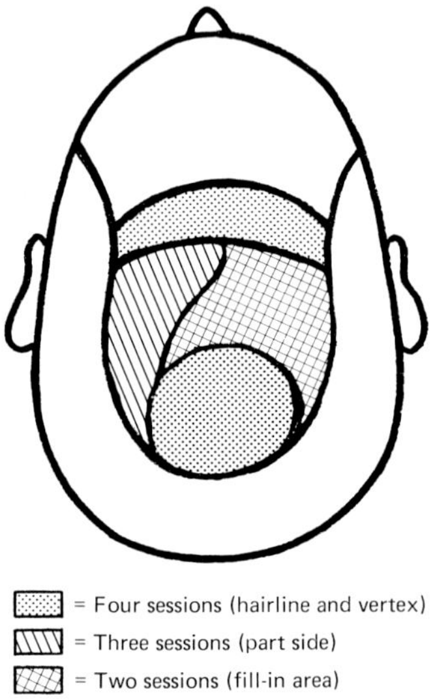

Figure 6-7

One factor to be considered when planning the frontal hairline is the donor site : recipient site ratio, that is, the number of plugs needed versus those available. As seen in Figure 6-7, the largest number of grafts will be required along the frontal hairline and in the vertex area. Each of these areas will probably require at least 200 plugs, and both areas will require a minimum of four grafting sessions to achieve maximum density. Other areas generally require at least two sessions to avoid an excessive appearance of "tufting."

The method of harvesting the donor site is important in the ultimate yield of punch grafts. If the strip method is used, approximately 35–45 4.0-mm plugs can be harvested from each row extending from ear to ear across the occiput. Figure 6-8A shows the strip method using 18 plugs. Use 2.0–3.00 mm of space between the horizontal rows.

If the block method is used, each square inch of donor scalp will yield 25–30 4.0-mm plugs. Figure 6-8B shows the block method using 25 plugs. It is important to plan use of the donor area so that hair of essentially similar quality, thickness and color will be used for the critical frontal rows. If the right lateral occiput was used for rows 1, 3, and 5 at the first session, then the equivalent area of the left occiput should be used when later filling in these rows.

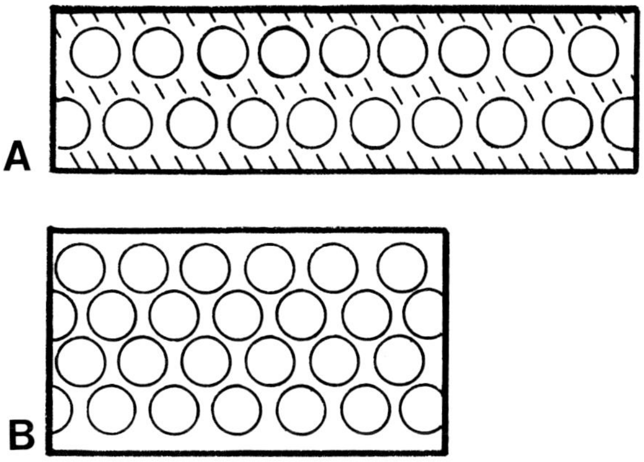

Figure 6-8

As shown in Figure 6-9, the face is divided into aesthetic units of equal size by horizontal lines drawn through the columellar base (C) and glabella (B). Rules of facial proportion and balance dictate that the hairline (A) should never be placed closer to the glabella (B) than the distance from the columellar base (C) to the chin (D). Often the hairline is placed higher.

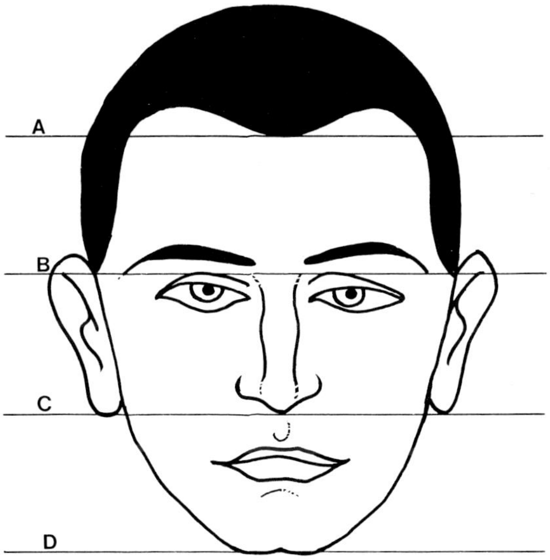

Figure 6-9

If scalp reduction (central shaded area in Figure 6-10) is to be part of the hair replacement program, the effect of such procedures on the frontal hairline must be taken into consideration. A useful rule of thumb is that the rearward limbs of the U-shaped hairline will each be pulled approximately 1 cm (distance between a [wider hairline] and a′ [planned reduction] in Figure 6-10) toward the midline each time an elliptical midline reduction procedure is performed. Figure 6-10A shows a standard hairline without scalp reduction and Figure 6-10B shows an altered hairline.

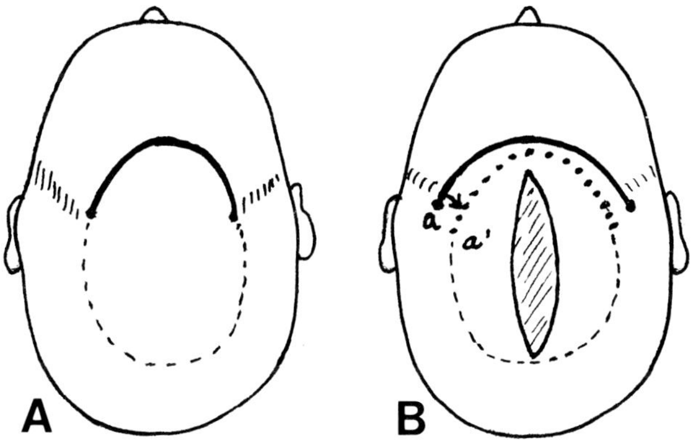

Figure 6-10

Punch grafting is performed under local anesthesia as an office procedure [0.25% bupivacaine (Marcaine) and/or 1% lidocaine (Xylocaine) with epinephrine (Adrenalin) 1 : 100,000]. Better hemostasis is usually obtained if fresh epinephrine (1 : 1000 vial) is used to prepare the local anesthetic immediately prior to infiltration. Adjunctive sedation is preferred by some physicians. Spraying the scalp with ethyl chloride or producing localized wheals of anesthetic using a Dermo-Jet® (Robbins Inst. Co.) prior to injection may minimize the pain of anesthetic infiltration.

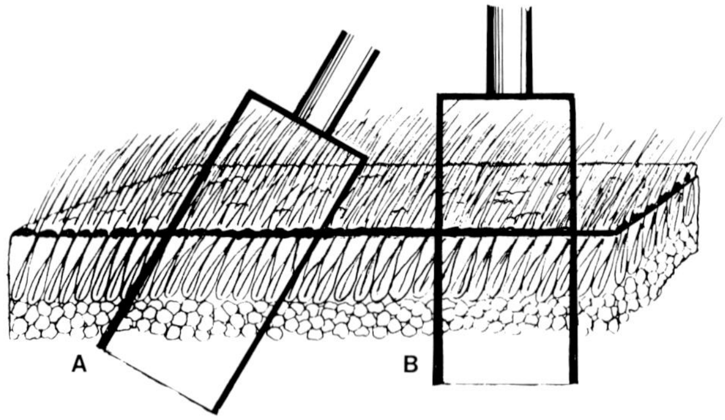

Figure 6-11

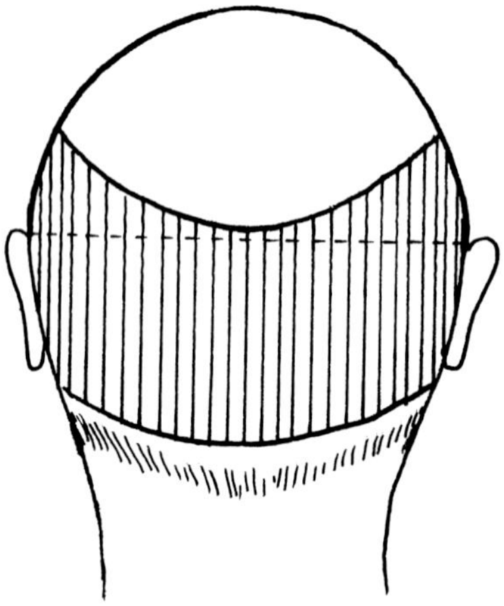

Figure 6-12

The proposed frontal hairline is marked. This should be done with extreme care according to the principles stated regarding selection of hairline in the Discussion section later in this chapter. The recipient sites are marked with methylene blue or other dye using a dull punch or Q-tip or other implement (wax pencil, eyebrow pencil). Recipient holes of at least rows 1, 2, and 3 should be separated by a distance just smaller than the plug size selected in order to allow overlapping of grafts placed in subsequent sessions. Such overlapping enhances density in the frontal hairline and aids in reducing a "tufted" appearance (see Figure 6-14, later).

Before donor plugs are cut, hair in the donor areas is trimmed to a length of 2 mm in order to allow determination of the direction of hair growth (Figure 6-11). Plugs are then cut, ensuring that the direction of the punch is parallel to the orientation of hair follicles in the donor area. Figure 6-11 shows the correct (A) and incorrect (B) direction of the punch. Visual inspection of each fifth plug harvested will alert the surgeon to subtle variations in follicle direction.

The maximum extent of eventual recession in the rear midline of the parietooccipital fringe can be estimated by a horizontal line at the level of the superior aspect of the ears (Figure 6-12). In order to avoid future alopecic loss of hair in donor plugs, plugs should be harvested in the area below this line.

The plugs are removed by grasping gently with forceps, lifting them from the donor sites, and cutting them loose with small-angled hair transplant scissors well below the follicle level. Following their removal, the donor plugs are immersed in a petri dish of saline. The best plugs should be reserved for use in the central frontal hairline region. Plugs exhibiting a more wispy hair growth and density should be reserved for use near the area of temporal recession.

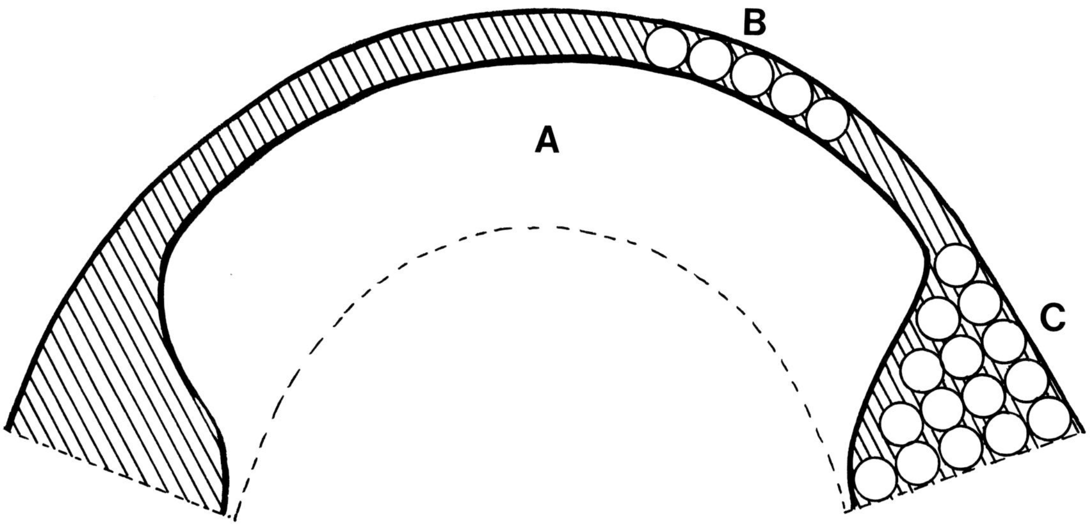

Figure 6-13

As shown in Figure 6-13, the densest plugs generally should go in rows 2–6 (A). More delicate plugs should be placed in the first row of the frontal hairline (B) and especially near the temporal recessions (C) in order to provide a slightly thinning look that produces a more natural appearance.

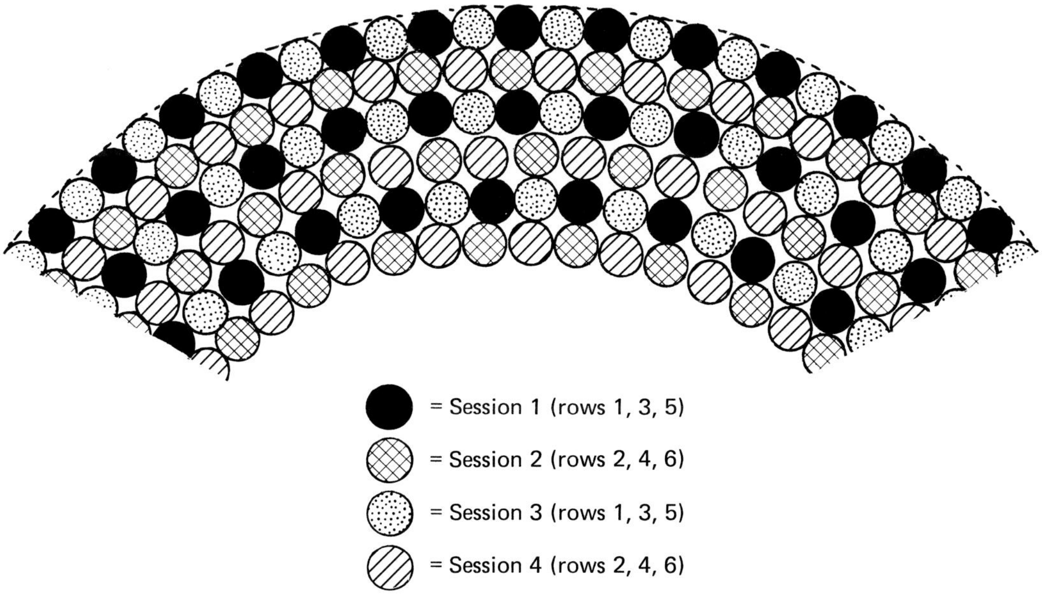

Figure 6-14

Figure 6-14 shows placement of plugs in each individual session; at least four sessions are recommended for sufficiently dense coverage.

Following boring of the recipient sites (done after donor plugs are cut and prepared), bleeding is controlled with pressure or injection of the anesthetic or saline containing 1 : 100,000 epinephrine. Boring is done at a natural, forward hair angle.

After sorting of donor plugs, the punch grafts are placed in recipient holes, with care being taken to ensure that the orientation of hair follicles is consistent with the natural orientation of hair in each recipient site area. (Opinion varies as to whether or not donor site holes should be sutured.)

Following completion of the procedure, a Telfa pad is placed over the donor plugs and a bulky compression dressing applied. The dressing is removed on the first postoperative day and the plugs inspected to ensure that each lies flush with the recipient scalp. Plugs that appear slightly elevated should be gently pressed back into place.

The patient's head must be elevated on two or three pillows for the first 24 hours postoperatively, and vigorous activity should be avoided during the first week. The patient should be instructed that if bleeding occurs, it can almost always be controlled by applying pressure for 10–15 minutes. Gentle rinsing of the hair under a low-pressure shower is allowed on the fourth postoperative day. Normal shampooing may resume in 5–7 days. The patient should be reminded that a crust forms over each donor plug and usually remains for 2–3 weeks.

Finesse

Punches should be maintained in razor-sharp condition. Transplant surgeons should learn proper techniques for sharpening their own punches. Donor plugs should always be graded when transplanting the frontal lines. The less dense and wispy plugs and also those with only moderate growth potential should be separated. Better hemostasis is generally obtained if fresh epinephrine 1 : 1000 is mixed with plain Marcaine or lidocaine in order to achieve an epinephrine concentration of 1 : 100,000. A record of the donor area used for each session should be kept, noting where the punch grafts were placed. This will ensure that grafts from comparable areas are used in each given recipient area for subsequent fill in sessions.

Following trimming of the donor site, it is helpful to strip it of residual hair spicules by pressing the area with sections of 1-inch paper tape, held between the thumbs. The donor area should be ballooned generously with saline solution to increase its rigidity. This facilitates harvesting plugs that are truly cylindrical, with maximal hair follicles. Every fifth to tenth plug should be carefully examined to ensure that they are being cut precisely parallel to the hair shafts. Wetting the hair adjacent to the donor area facilitates its control while harvesting punch grafts. Pressure will control most bleeding in the donor site. If this does not suffice, however, the site should be immediately injected with a small amount of anesthetic-epinephrine solution in order to constrict the bleeding vessel. If bleeding persists, the hole can be filled with powdered thrombin or Surgicel or sutured.

The recipient hole should be cut as deeply as possible and should always be cut at a slight angle corresponding to the angulation of remnant residual hairs in the area. It is probably best to use a fairly standard angulation, perhaps 20–25°, so that later transplants will not cut into previously planted follicles. Most plugs over the crown will be oriented slightly forward and/or away from the midline. Recipient sites in the vertex are cut in radial fashion corresponding to the usual growth or whorl.

As the recipient scalp is generally 20 percent thinner than donor scalp, it is often necessary to trim plugs in order to allow proper seating and thus lessen cobblestoning. Plugs should be trimmed under bright illumination. With handling of the plug top with fine forceps, fat should be carefully trimmed, approaching the hair matrices by about 1 mm. Less experienced surgeons should err on the side of very conservative fat removal. The plugs should be trimmed while immersed in saline.

If a properly trimmed plug is not well seated, it should be removed and the recipient hole inspected for presence of a blood clot or infolded hair.

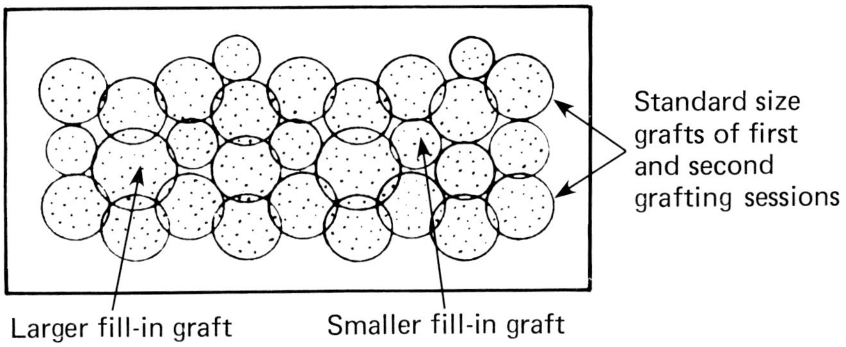

Figure 6-15

For fill-in grafts, the frontal hairline and midvertex require careful attention in order to achieve maximum hair density. In these areas it is generally best to wait 3–4 months between the second and third and third and fourth procedures. This allows adequate time for hair growth in transplanted punch grafts, thus allowing the surgeon to determine what size spaces remain to perhaps be filled in by grafts of varying size (fill-in grafts). Note that the grafts shown in Figure 6-15 overlap.

It is difficult to cut satisfactory plugs smaller than 3.5 mm. If smaller-sized fill-in grafts are needed, it is preferable to trim larger plugs in order to fit recipient holes in the 2.0–3.0-mm range.

For improvement of the transplanted hairline, in patients having considerable problems with color match or surface irregularity following completion of punch grafting, the following procedures may be considered:

1. Use of 5-fluorouracil cream can be applied over the entire forehead, blending it well into the scalp. This agent will eradicate early actinic keratoses and, following resolution of erythema, the sun-damaged skin will blend more satisfactorily with the grafted plugs.
2. Persistent elevations of individuals grafts can be treated by light desiccation with a fine epilation needle, carefully working around each individual hair to flatten the raised tissue without damaging hair shafts.

Complications

Syncopal episodes. Syncope usually occurs as a vagal response to the pain of anesthetic injections or cutting plugs in poorly anesthetized areas. Occasionally the sight of blood may precipitate syncope. Blood and needles should be kept out of the patient's sight. Reassurance of the patient combined with lowering of the head and elevation of the lower extremities generally produces resolution of a syncopal spell. Treatment with atropine or other medications is rarely indicated.

Infection. Infection is estimated to occur in approximately 1 in 500 patients following punch grafting. Such infection is usually superficial, often presenting as pustules or localized erythema. (New hair growth is another cause of pustules.) Small pustules may be treated by incision and drainage, with culture and sensitivity as indicated. Systemic antibiotics are rarely indicated in such infections. Some surgeons, however, routinely institute short courses of prophylactic antibiotics.

Scarring. Scarring in the donor area may occur as a consequence of removal of an excessive number of plugs from a small area or necrosis secondary to overly tight suture placement. Occasionally scarring may result from infection. The most common type of scarring in the recipient area is the phenomenon of "cobblestoning." Cobblestoning occurs when there is disparity in the height of the plug relative to the level of the surrounding scalp. This most commonly results when persistent bleeding following plug placement causes partial extrusion of the graft. Cobblestoning may also result from inadequate trimming of fat from the inferior surface of grafts. Rarely, cobblestoning may result from recipient holes that have not been bored to a sufficient depth. Blood clots in recipient holes may cause similar problems and should be removed by forceps. All plugs should be examined to ensure that no hairs are trapped beneath them. Such entrapped hairs may be a factor causing "popping up" of plugs. Inspection of the grafts on the first postoperative day allows manipulation of any elevated grafts. Occasionally, use of surgical tape is beneficial in helping maintain proper graft level.

Several methods have been advocated to correct cobblestoning. Slight elevation of plugs is most often due to the edema of the inflammatory response and generally clears spontaneously in 6–12 months. Persistent elevation may be treated by dermabrasion or shave excision. Another method is light desiccation of the elevated areas. Hypertrophic scarring or keloid formation is rare following punch grafting. Intralesional steroid injection is the treatment of choice.

Foreign body reaction. Foreign-body reaction most commonly occurs secondary to hair shaft entrapment beneath plugs or in sutured donored site holes. Treatment consists of incision and drainage and/or excision.

Aneurysm or arteriovenous malformation. This rare complication is estimated to have an incidence of 1 in 5000 cases. Clinically a purple or red, gradually enlarging nodule appears in the donor area, becoming fluctuant and occasionally reaching 1–2 cm in diameter. Occasionally a bruit is audible on auscultation, and a palpable thrill may be present. In early stages a figure of eight sutures may be placed to strangulate a developing lesion. More mature lesions are best treated by excision after the nodule becomes nonpulsatile.

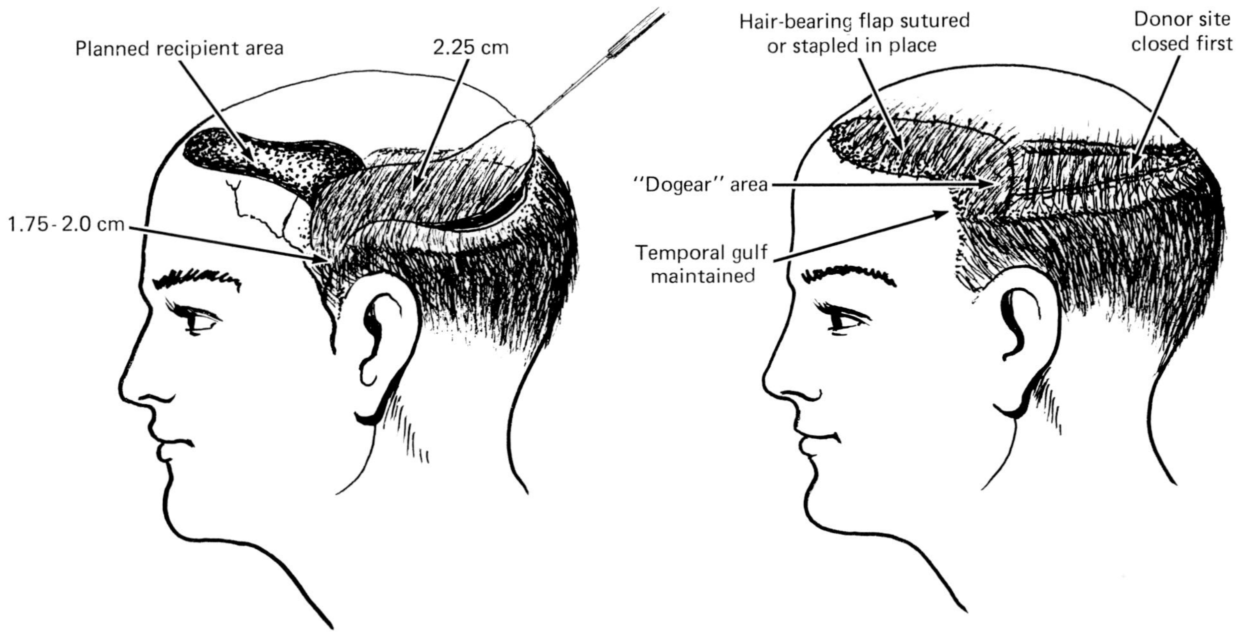

Figure 6-16

SCALP FLAPS

Design of short flaps (temporoparietal) is shown in Figure 6-16. The base of the flap is oriented vertically and centered over the posterior branch of the superficial temporal artery approximately 3 cm above and just anterior to the superior attachment of the auricle. The flap base is 1.75–2.0 cm wide.

The flap arches superiorly over the auricle then extends posteriorly and somewhat inferiorly below the temporoparietal fringe, maintaining a maximum width of 2.25 cm and tapering to a point at its end to facilitate donor site closure. The first flap (part side of scalp) is fashioned to extend 1–2 cm past the midline. This length is estimated by measuring the distance from the pivot point of the flap to the midpoint of the frontal hairline and adding 3 cm. The total flap length thus averages 12–14 cm and the length : width ratio, approximate 5–6 : 1. An appropriate amount of bald hairline is incised and the flap transposed to cover one-half of the frontal hairline. Final transposition of the flap is facilitated by first closing the donor site. This "opens" the recipient area so that less scalp is excised there. It is thus best not to cut away the proposed recipient site until the donor area has been closed.

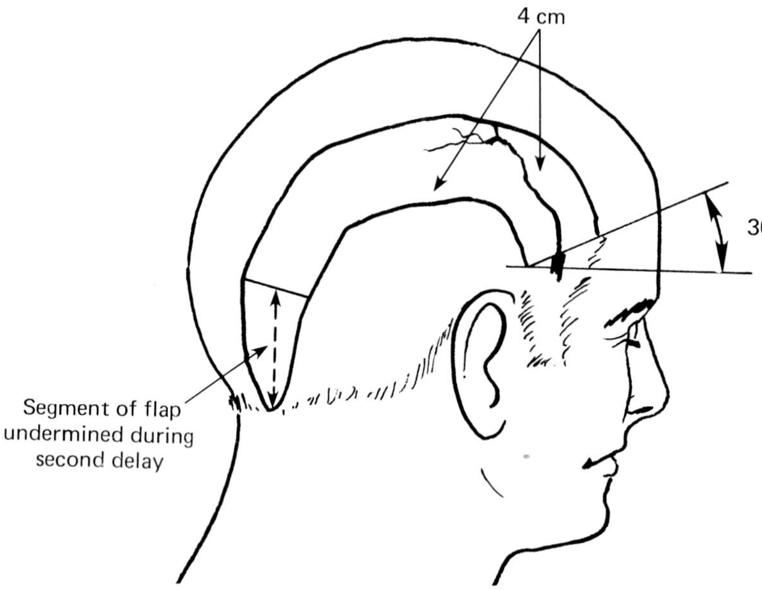

Figure 6-17A

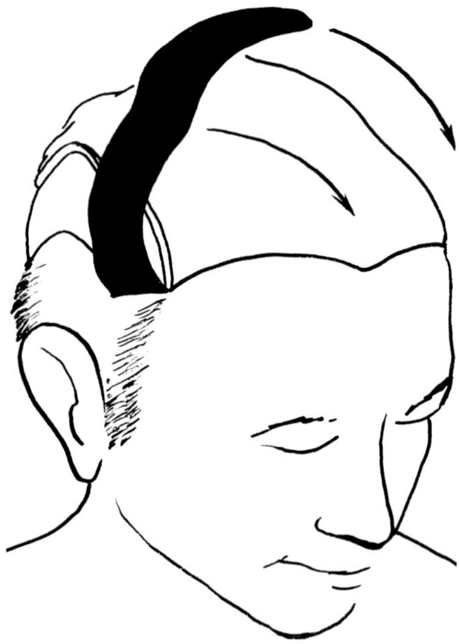

Figure 6-17B

Design of the Juri flap is illustrated in Figure 6-17A. The base of the flap is centered over the posterior branch of the superficial temporal artery at a point 3–4 cm above and just anterior to the attachment of the auricle. Some surgeons recommend use of a Doppler flow meter to assist in location of the artery. The flap base subtends an angle of 30–45° with the horizontal in order to enhance rotation and minimize "dog-ear" formation at the pivot point. The flap base is 4 cm in width, and the flap maintains this width as it arches superiorly over the auricle and then extends posteriorly and inferiorly in the parietal scalp, tapering near its end to facilitate donor site closure (Figure 6-17B). It does not cross the midline.

Flap length is determined by measuring the distance from the flap pivot point to the opposite frontal temporal junction and arbitrarily adding 3–4 cm to compensate for loss of length at the "dog-ear" and so on. The usual flap is 23–28 cm in length.

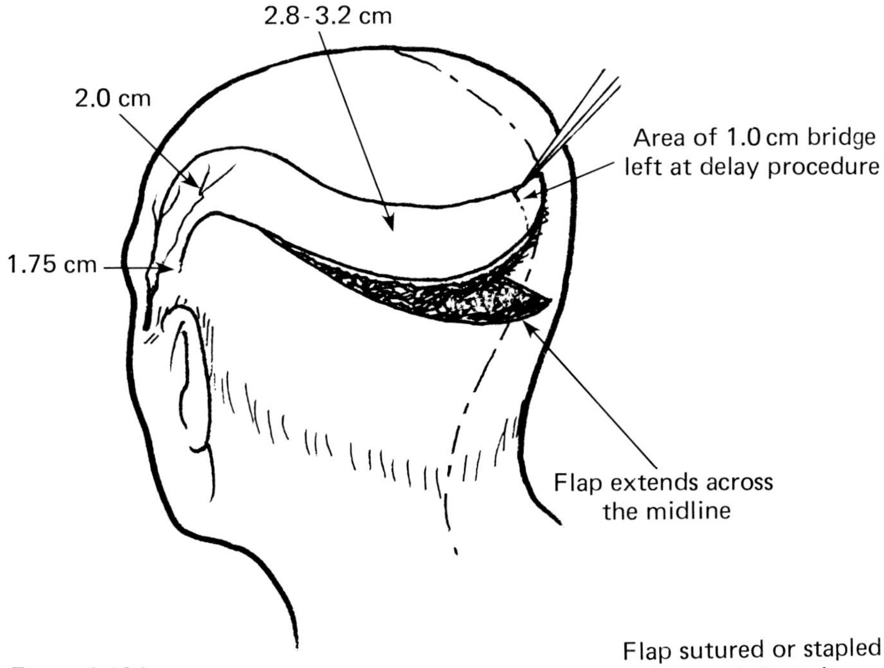

Figure 6-18A

Design of the temporoparietooccipital flap (similar to that of the temporoparietal flap) is shown in Figure 6-18A. The flap base (1.75 cm) is centered over the pulsation of the posterior branch of the superficial temporal artery and is oriented vertically and becomes 2.0 cm in width in the proximal third of the flap. The flap arches superiorly over the auricle and then curves in a posteroinferior direction toward the occipital region, maintaining a width of 2.8–3.2 cm. Flaps maintaining a width of 3 cm or more may extend past the occipital midline in order to gain sufficient length to cover at least three-fourths of the distance of the frontal hairline (and sometimes to reconstruct the entire frontal hairline) (Figure 6-18B). The flap is tapered near its end to facilitate closure of the donor site.

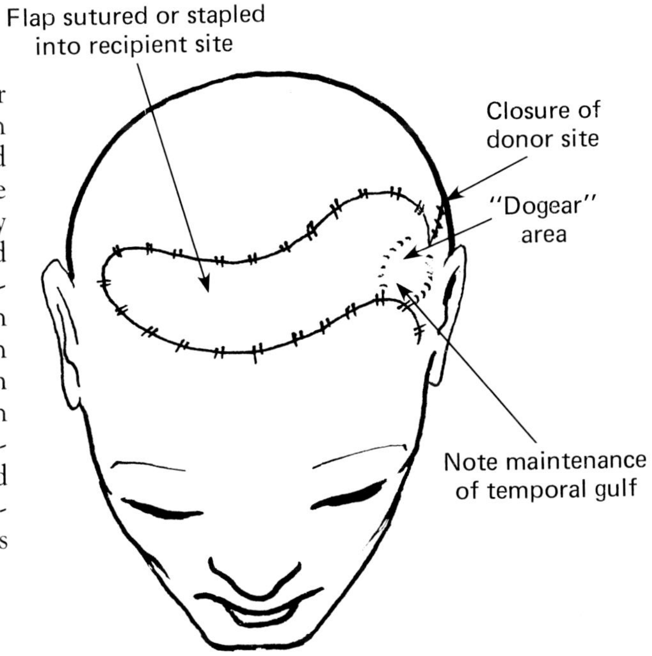

Figure 6-18B

Local anesthesia (0.5% Marcaine or 1% Xylocaine with epinephrine 1 : 100,000) with sedation is used for the temporoparietal flap and for delays of the Juri flap. The Juri flap is usually transposed under general anesthesia in a hospital operating room, although some surgeons perform this procedure under local anesthesia. The patient's head is usually elevated 20–30°. Hair is not cut; rather, it is controlled with moisture, braiding, and hair clips.

The Juri flap (Figure 6-17A) is delayed to enhance its viability. Two delays 7 days apart are recommended. At the first delay, incisions are made (parallel to the hair follicles and extending through the galea) along most of the superior and inferior margins of the flap and then closed with running sutures of 4-0 nylon. The second delay consists of elevating the tail of the flap (distal 5–6 cm) deep to the galea and resuturing it in its bed with 4-0 nylon. The flap is transposed 7–10 days later (see Figure 6-17B).

The temporoparietooccipital (TPO) flap is delayed 7–10 days prior to transposition. The flap (Figure 6-18A) is incised (parallel to the follicles) through the galea, maintaining an intact 1.0-cm bridge at the distal end of the flap. The flap is not elevated from its bed, and the incisions are closed with a running suture of 4-0 nylon or with surgical staples.

Elevation and transposition of the Juri flap, the temporoparietal flap, and the TPO flap are similar. Beginning at the tail of the flap, elevation proceeds in a plane deep to the galea. Hemostasis is secured with electrocautery and ligatures (electrocautery is not employed on the flap itself to minimize the danger of retrograde thrombosis).

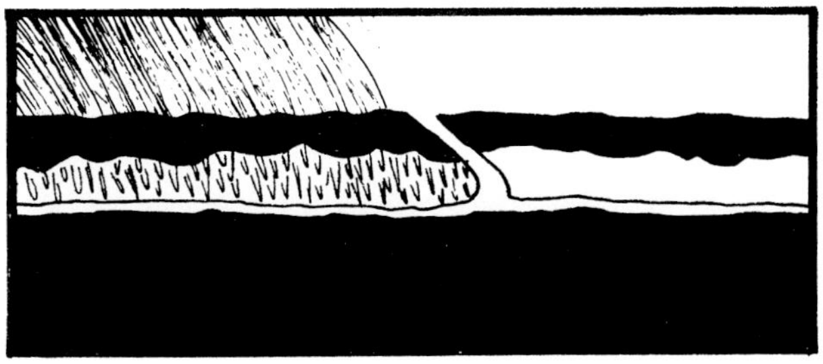

Figure 6-19

In Figure 6-19 the frontal hairline incision in the forehead is shown beveled inferiorly to correspond to the beveled superior incision of the flap (encouraging growth of hair through the scar), and the scalp posterior to the frontal incision is elevated for a distance corresponding to the flap width.

The donor site is undermined in a plane deep to the galea to allow closure without tension. The extent of undermining varies as a function of flap width and scalp elasticity. Closure of the Juri flap donor site often requires undermining into the posterior neck, over the posterior surface of the auricle and superiorly as far as possible over the central skull. Gaining closure from inferiorly is advisable in order to avoid "spreading" the bald scalp. Relaxing incisions in the galea are sometimes employed. Closure without tension is of utmost importance in preventing traction alopecia and scarring in the donor site as well as to minimize widening of the scar. The galea is approximated with interrupted sutures of 0 Vicryl and the skin closed with surgical staples.

Tension often occurs in the anterior portion of the donor site, and posteroinferior rotation and transposition of recipient site scalp into the area (Figure 6-20) is often helpful in achieving satisfactory closure.

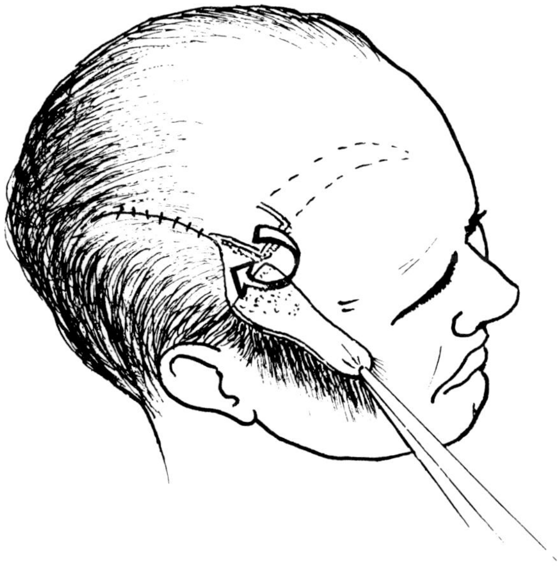

Figure 6-20

The flap is rotated into the recipient site and the necessary amount of bald scalp excised. As noted above, scalp near the anterior portion of the flap is often employed in donor site closure; thus excision of this area should be deferred until its possible need is ascertained. Scalp excision is planned so that the flap is under no tension in the recipient bed. Closure of the hairline proceeds from lateral to medial (5-0 nylon) in order to minimize "dog-ear" formation. Undermining the forehead 2–3 cm assists in distribution of the dog ear. The posterior incision is closed with surgical staples. Drains (penrose or suction type) are routinely employed beneath the flap. They are removed on the second postoperative day. All incisions are covered with antibiotic ointment and a bulky dressing applied. Pressure on the flap (dog ear) must be avoided so that circulation is not compromised. Hairline sutures are removed in 5 days and staples at 10–14 days. The flap may be advanced posteriorly ("stretched") 6–8 weeks following transposition. This is accomplished by incising its posterior margin, elevating the flap and posterior scalp, advancing these tissues with excision of an appropriate amount of bald scalp, and closing with sutures. Excision of galea beneath the flap may enhance its "stretchability."

Figure 6-21 shows the short flap outline.

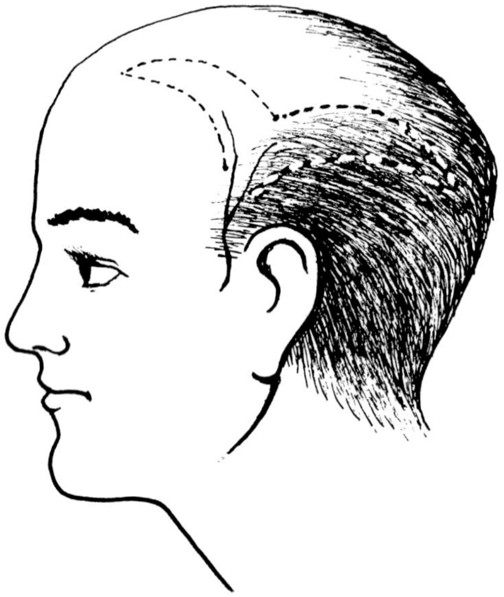

Figure 6-21

Finesse

Use of "advancement" suturing to mildly stretch the flap from lateral to medial across the frontal hairline helps to minimize the dog ear. For proper design of flap base, the base of the Juri flap should subtend an angle of 30–45° with the horizontal (Figure 6-17A) in order to enhance rotation and minimize dog-ear formation. Design of the temporoparietal and longer TPO flap so that the base is vertically oriented (centered over the posterior branch of the superficial temporal artery) minimizes the dog ear, as does the narrow width (2.0 cm) of the flap pedicle (Figures 6-16 and 6-18A and B). Undermining of the lateral aspect of the frontal region 2–3 cm is often of value in minimizing dog-ear formation.

For closure of the donor site, wide undermining of the donor area is essential in order to achieve adequate closure of the donor site. Approximation of the scalp tissue with towel clips assists in obtaining secure galeal closure. Galeal relaxing incisions (discussed later in this chapter) may assist in closure of the donor wound.

A through and through relaxing incision in the scalp 2.5–3.5 cm above the flap donor site may also be of benefit in closure. This relaxing incision is approximated in one layer following completion of donor site closure.

A rotation flap from the lateral aspect of the recipient site is often useful in achieving closure of the anterior aspect of the donor site near the flap pedicle.

For maintenance, blunting of the temporal gulf is more common with the Juri flap than with temporoparietal or TPO flaps because its base is wider and less flexible. Design of the temporoparietal and TPO flaps with the base oriented vertically facilitates preservation of the gulf (Figures 6-16 and 6-18 A and B). If the gulf is blunted, the flap can be advanced posteriorly in that area 4–8 weeks after transposition.

To minimize blood loss, the flap should be elevated in sections, securing hemostasis in one section prior to proceeding to the next section. Use of neurosurgical clips is also helpful in minimizing blood loss.

Complications

Complications of scalp flap surgery are similar to those encountered in other flap procedures in the head and neck area; these include bleeding, hematoma, flap necrosis, donor site necrosis, scar formation (at hairline or donor site), infection, ingrown hairs and cyst in the hairline, dog-ear formation, telogen effluvium (temporary "resting-phase") hair loss at flap or donor site, unnatural hairline (blunting of the temporal gulf), and hypesthesia of the scalp.

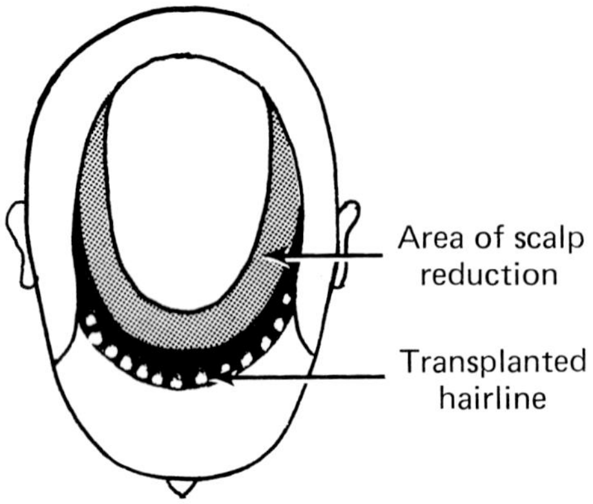

Figure 6-22

SCALP REDUCTION

A U-shaped pattern behind the frontal hairline may be useful for reduction of alopecia in the anterior portion of the scalp (Figure 6-22). (A reversed U shape can reduce the posterior scalp also.)

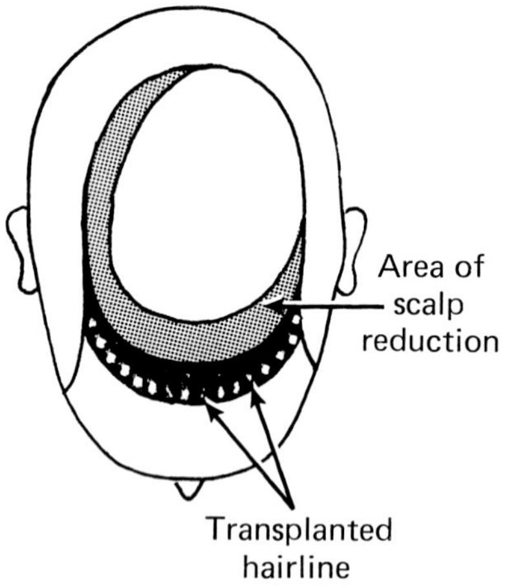

Figure 6-23

A J or C pattern originating behind the hairline and extending posteriorly along the lateral fringe on the part or nonpart sides may be used for reducing alopecia in the anterior and lateral scalp (Figure 6-23).

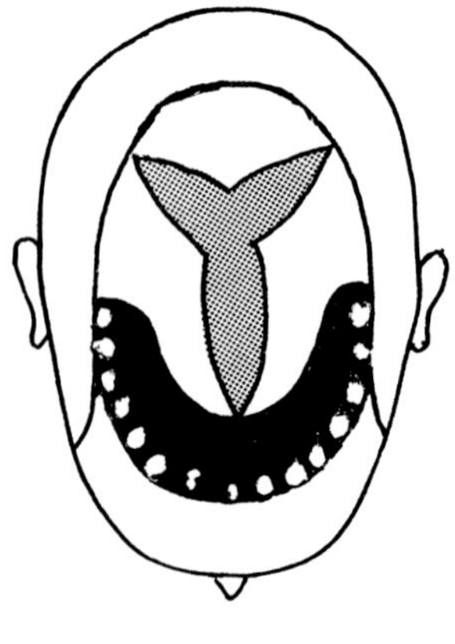

Figure 6-24

A Y-shaped ("Mercedes") (Figure 6-24) or T-shaped pattern (Figure 6-25) originating in the central scalp and extending into the vertex is useful for reduction of alopecia in the midcrown and vertex.

Figure 6-25 shows the T-shaped pattern for reduction in the midcrown and vertex.

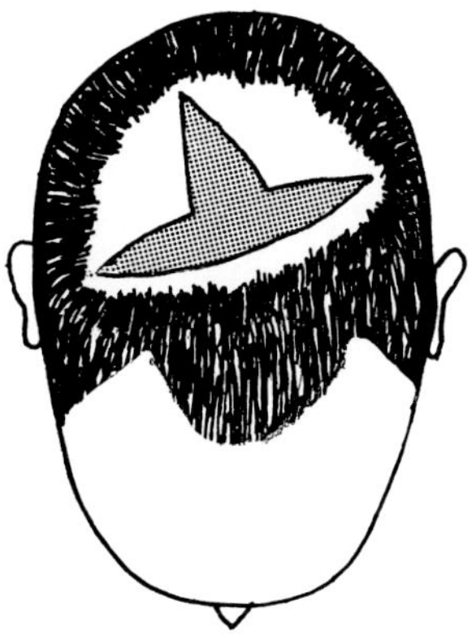

Figure 6-25

A longitudinal midline ellipse originating just posterior to the frontal hairline and extending into the vertex is a widely used pattern; an M-plasty is often incorporated into the posterior aspect of the ellipse in order to increase scalp excision without extending the length of the ellipse itself (Figure 6-26).

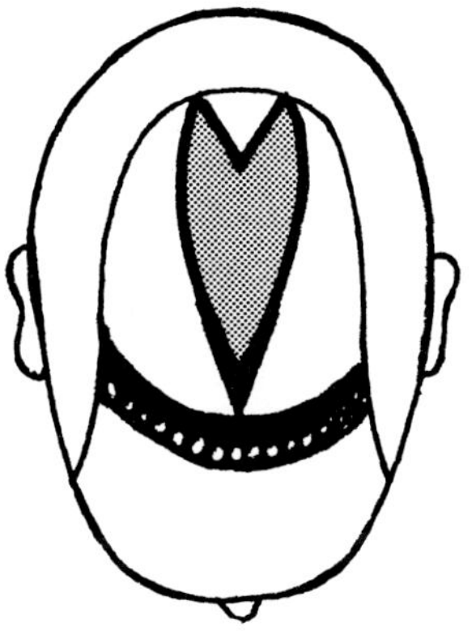

Figure 6-26

A paramedian crescent-shaped or "S" pattern originating just posterior to the frontal hairline, extending along the lateral fringe into the vertex, is useful for removing large amounts of alopecia in the crown and vertex (Figure 6-27).

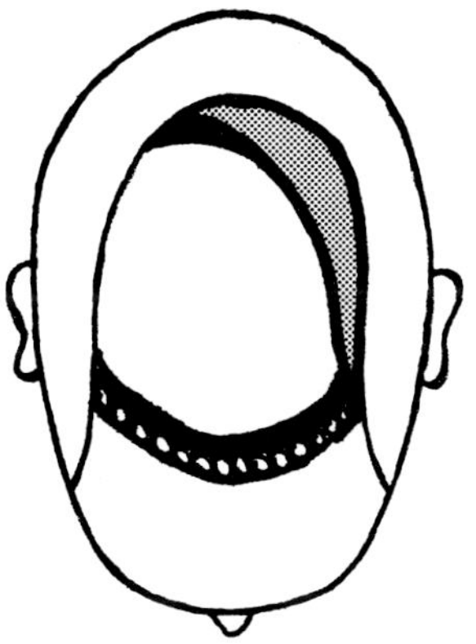

Figure 6-27

Scalp reduction is most commonly performed with the use of local anesthesia (0.25% Marcaine or 1% lidocaine with epinephrine 1 : 100,000) with or without sedation. Regional block is performed and the incision itself infiltrated with anesthetic solution in order to reduce bleeding. General anesthesia may be utilized if the patient desires. The operative site, however, should be infiltrated with anesthetic solution containing epinephrine in order to minimize blood loss.

The patient may be placed in a semisitting position in order to facilitate access to the operative site. Some surgeons recommend the supine or prone position in order to reduce the incidence of syncope.

In the surgical procedure, the proposed incision is made on one side of the pattern only, using the scalpel or electrocautery blade and extending through the galea. The scalp is undermined in the subgaleal plane as far as possible on both sides of the incision. Commonly, undermining extends to the upper ear attachments laterally and to the attachment of occipitalis muscle in the superior nuchal ridge posteriorly. Regardless of the pattern used, the frontal hairline and forehead area is not undermined in order to minimize elevation of the hairline.

Undermining can often be performed with blunt finger dissection over the central scalp, but dissection with scissors or a periosteal elevator is generally necessary over the vertex and posterior scalp. Care must be taken to avoid injury to the perforating vessels in the posterior scalp region as well as over the mastoid process and to avoid perforating the galea-muscle layer or periosteum. Following completion of undermining, redundant scalp is excised, with care taken to limit the amount of skin that can be removed without producing excessive tension at closure.

The galea is approximated with sutures of 2-0 Vicryl to reduce skin tension and the skin edges approximated with 4-0 nylon or surgical staples. Regular, not "wide," staples should be used in order to avoid bending. A bulky compression dressing is applied and removed on the first postoperative day. Sutures or staples are removed on postoperative day 10–14.

Finesse

Secure closure of the galea is essential in order to avoid wound separation or scar widening. This closure can be achieved with either permanent or absorbable sutures; 0 or 2-0 Vicryl is a frequent choice. Closure with a running suture is more rapid and often produces a tighter closure than do interrupted sutures. Use of towel clips to approximate skin edges assists in achieving secure galeal closure.

Infiltration of 0.25% Marcaine into the scalp periphery immediately postoperatively may substantially decrease postoperative discomfort. Rapid acting steroids intramuscularly (IM) or orally may also help. Following completion of serial scalp reduction, placement of punch grafts into the scar aids in its camouflage. Bleeding occurring in conjunction with galeal relaxation incisions can be controlled by use of a suction electrocautery or by percutaneous suture ligatures of 4-0 Chromic. Planning of the frontal hairline should be modified if punch grafting is to precede scalp reduction (see Discussion section relative to Figure 6-10).

Complications

Complications of scalp reduction are similar to those of other flap procedures; they include bleeding, hematoma, infection, skin necrosis, scar formation, foreign-body granuloma secondary to buried hair or suture material, hypesthesia, and telogen effluvium ("resting-phase" temporary hair loss).

DISCUSSION

PUNCH GRAFTING

There are several general considerations regarding the advisability of punch grafting. With increasing frequency surgeons are confronted with patients who exhibit early thinning of the hair and request hair transplantation. In general, punch grafting can be considered in such cases if transplanted hair will have a density greater than that already present. Also, early balding makes it more difficult to plan the hairline. The surgeon should remember that the motivation of younger patients with early degrees of baldness is often somewhat tenuous and thus such patients are more likely to discontinue hair replacement surgery prior to achieving the maximum benefit of serial procedures.

Selection of the hairline is another primary consideration. Proper placement of frontal hairline is of prime importance in hair transplantation with punch grafting. As desires of the patient may conflict with the reality and logistics of each individual situation as well as with the aesthetic sense of the surgeon, the plan for replacement of the frontal hairline should be determined by careful communication between surgeon and patient. In terms of the aesthetics of hair replacement, few, if any, factors are as important in the ultimate result as is proper hairline placement. Attempts to correct poorly placed hairlines are difficult and seldom produce good results.

The most anterior point of the U-shaped outline shown in Figure 6-5 corresponds to the midline of the frontal area and the limbs of the U curve posteriorly to meet the temporal fringes just anterior to or above the auricle. The surgeon must also consider that there will be a continuing, gradual rearward movement of the temporal hairline. Areas of temporal recession should rarely, if ever, be incorporated into the hairline, and grafting should never be attempted in or below the partline, as the slightly tufted appearance of the grafts will always show in this area. The hairline should always be as high as possible (Figure 6-5B) and plugs should never be wasted in forming a broad arc that fills in much of the temporal recessions, nor in moving the hairline forward (Figure 6-5A). Surgeons generally advise higher hairline placement than the patient initially requests. Patients can take some solace, however, in the fact that when transplanted hair is combed forward, the hairline will appear $\frac{1}{2}$–$1\frac{1}{2}$ inches more anterior than it actually is.

Fine wispy hairs such as those shown in Figure 6-6 often persist for years after completion of hair transplantation. The surgeon should also point out that a more anterior "youthful" hairline may appear unnatural as the patient ages. Six rows of densely transplanted hair generally suffice to give the frontal illusion of thick, youthful hair. Only three spaced rows need to be transplanted across the bald scalp at each session. Generally, 60–75 4-mm plugs will be required per three-row session in the average patient.

Regarding the selection of donor area Figures 6-7–6-10, close inspection of hair density, coupled with history regarding the extent of eventual balding in both males and females in the family, will yield a reasonable impression of the extent of the possible donor area. Almost all patients can have plugs harvested from the majority of the occiput and posterior parietal areas. The lowermost and extreme lateral occiput may be too thin except for plugs that the surgeon wishes to yield fine delicate hairs, that is, for filler areas.

The size of the punch used for boring recipient holes in punch grafting varies from surgeon to surgeon. Most surgeons prefer 3.5–4.0-mm punch grafts for use in the frontal hairline, although some recommend 5.0-mm plugs. Since the recipient sites expand somewhat following removal of the bald plug, recipient holes should be made with a punch approximately 0.5 mm smaller than that punch selected for harvesting donor plugs.

The occiput is usually chosen as the initial donor area. It is beneficial to harvest plugs on one side of the midline or other during each session so that the patient has at least one part of the posterior scalp that is not tender and on which to sleep.

The surgeon must choose between a strip and block method of harvesting plugs (Figure 6-8). The strip method appears to be more popular among surgeons who transplant larger numbers of grafts per session, as this method allows for easier coverage of the donor sites by adjacent hair. Other surgeons, however, feel that the block method allows a greater number of plugs per square centimeter to be harvested and thus prefer this technique. The block method is the most effective way of conserving the donor area when round punches are used.

It is extremely important that the transplant punch be razor sharp in order to reduce compression of the scalp, which results in loss of viable follicles at the periphery of each plug. Hair yield per plug can be maximized by increasing the rigidity of the donor scalp with generous saline injections.

When using a hand-held punch, the surgeon makes the initial scalp incision vertically. At a point approximately 1 mm deep, the punch is turned parallel to the hair shafts and twisted delicately through the skin. Surgeons who use power punches recommend that the entire incision be made parallel to the hair shafts.

Pressure generally controls bleeding. Injection of additional anesthetic solution or saline containing 1 : 100,000 epinephrine will often stop more troublesome bleeding. Other methods of controlling bleeding include application of powdered thrombin or Surgicel into the donor holes. Control of bleeding can also be achieved by a deep suture of the donor site.

There is some controversy regarding plug size. The most common plug sizes are 4.0–4.5 mm; however, some surgeons utilize 3.0-, 3.5-, and 5-mm plugs. Even smaller plugs are occasionally used for fill-in procedures to enhance the frontal hairline. Studies have shown that the yield of hair per surface area of plug is virtually identical for 3.5–4.5-mm plugs but is diminished when smaller or larger grafts are used. It has also been shown that there is no significant difference in the number of viable hairs in plugs properly harvested with hand punches versus power punches.

The number of grafts used per session varies tremendously from surgeon to surgeon, ranging from as few as 10 to as many as 150 plugs per session. The majority of surgeons perform approximately 50–75 punch grafts per session. This provides for a donor area that is easier to cover with surrounding hair and results in minimal patient discomfort. Many surgeons suggest that the blood supply to the transplanted plugs may be jeopardized if more than 100–150 plugs are transplanted per session.

The time between punch grafting sessions is another factor that varies from surgeon to surgeon. There is general agreement that this time interval should be greater when larger numbers of plugs are transplanted, particularly in the central portion of the scalp.

In grafting the frontal hairline, three rows are constructed per session (Figure 6-14). In order to achieve dense coverage, a minimum of four sessions is required in this area. Separation of the new plugs at each session allows good blood supply and good growth. Note the tight honeycomb gridwork at the front which is formed by this method of plug placement. (Eight rows can be used instead of six.) If the initial transplanatation in the frontal hairline consists of 50–75 plugs, experience has shown that a second session can be safely undertaken in 2–4 weeks. Many surgeons, however, feel that in critical areas such as the frontal hairline and midvertex, it is best to wait 3 months or more following the second and subsequent sessions in order to allow hair growth that will facilitate precise placement and sizing of subsequent punch grafts in spaces between existing grafts to produce maximum hair density. During these intervals, however, transplantation may proceed in other areas of the scalp. Scalp reductions may also be safely undertaken during these waiting periods.

There is controversy regarding bock versus strip methods of plug harvesting (see Figure 6-8). The block method is a more efficient per unit donor area than the strip method yielding 25–30 4.0-mm grafts per square inch of donor scalp (about 1.5 mm between plugs). The strip method, leaving approximately 1 mm of scalp intact between each plug in a row, yields 35–45 4.0-mm grafts from ear to ear across the occiput. About 2–3 mm of scalp are left between each horizontal row.

Although camouflage of the donor area is easier following harvest by the strip method, a "block" measuring 2 × $1\frac{1}{2}$ inches yielding approximately 60 4.0-mm plugs is easily camouflaged if the adjacent hairs are at least 2 inches in length. Whichever method is chosen, spacing between plugs should increase in the lower occipital areas to allow for a better camouflage since hair in this area thins with aging. Also, 4.5–5.0-mm plugs require wider spacing, as they leave larger scars if they remain unsutured.

Suturing of the donor area is also a controversial

issue. Many hair transplant surgeons state that there is no significant difference in the final appearance of the donor site, regardless of whether the donor holes are sutured or left open. Unsutured donor sites generally heal in approximately 2 weeks. Some surgeons feel that suturing increases postoperative pain and also increases the possibility of local inflammation and infection. Although suturing may decrease the incidence of postoperative bleeding, the incidence of this complication is very low, approximately 0.2 percent in patients with unsutured donor sites. Surgeons who perform large numbers of grafts per session or those who harvest plugs using the strip method are more likely to recommend suturing of donor sites.

SCALP FLAPS

General considerations regarding patient selection discussed earlier are applicable to patient selection for flap transposition. A discussion of factors of special importance in flap surgery follows.

The pattern of baldness should be stable, particularly in the fringe area from which the flap is obtained. If further temporal recession occurs following flap transposition, the base of the flap may develop alopecia. Additional parietal recession could be even more troublesome, as the reconstructed frontal hairline might exhibit hair loss. The surgeon must thus proceed with caution in recommending flap surgery in younger patients (early and midtwenties) with frontal recession in whom further hair loss might denude portions of the flap. In such cases it is often wise to defer flap surgery until the status of the fringe area can be predicted with more confidence (i.e., midthirties). In addition, the extent of frontal and central alopecia present at this age is often an important factor in recommending the type most suitable for transposition (i.e., short vs long flaps). Contraindications to flap surgery include the presence of scars or other local donor site factors which may jeopardize the blood supply of the proposed flap.

The following flaps are used for reconstruction of the frontal hairline: the Juri flap, for the entire frontal hairline; the temporoparietal flap, for one-half of the frontal hairline, with a contralateral flap being transposed to complete the reconstruction; and the temporoparietooccipital flap, for reconstruction of approximately three-fourths of the frontal hairline. Occasionally this flap will span the entire hairline.

For determination of the hairline, factors mentioned in regard to punch grafting are applicable to planning the hairline in flap surgery. Conservation is of prime importance in hairline selection, and as a rule of thumb, the distance from the midpoint of the hairline to the glabella is no shorter than that from the columella to the chin (Figure 6-9). In some cases the aesthetic sense of the surgeon will dictate higher placement. As with punch grafting, higher hairline placement conserves donor follicles as the length of the flap required for hairline reconstruction is diminished.

Of utmost aesthetic importance is retention of the natural recession between the junction of the temporal and frontal hairlines (the "temporal gulf"). Blunting of this gulf is a frequent problem following flap surgery and produces an unnatural appearance (Figure 6-18B).

Considerable controversy exists regarding whether flaps or punch grafts yield the best results. The fact that opinion is largely polarized according to the discipline of the transplant surgeon (i.e., dermatologists tend to prefer punch grafting whereas other surgeons are inclined toward the use of flaps) renders absolute judgment regarding this controversy impossible. Both procedures yield excellent results in properly selected patients, and since many candidates for hair replacement surgery can be considered candidates for either procedure, the advantages and disadvantages of each method should be carefully discussed with the patient, allowing patient participation in selection of the technique to be used. (Table 6-1 summarizes the advantages and disadvantages of each technique.)

Regarding the design of short flaps, some surgeons base the leading edge of the flap on the anterior temporal hairline in order to minimize the dog ear of rotation. Flaps based in this position, however, tend to blunt the temporal gulf, creating an unnatural hairline.

Flaps based somewhat more posteriorly (Figure

Table 6-1
Comparison of Punch Grafting and Scalp Flaps

	Punch Grafting	Scalp Flaps
Hair Density	Always Less than Normal	Normal
Direction of Hair Growth	Can be Controlled by Plug Placement to Match Normal Direction in All Areas of Scalp	Predetermined by Orientation of the Flap, i.e., Always Posterior in Hairline in Contrast to Normal Anterior Growth
Time Required for Cosmetic Benefit	Some Improvement in 6–9 Months; Substantial Benefit in 12–18 Months	No Telogen Hair Loss, Resulting in "Instant" Hair
Appearance During Healing Phase	Erythema and Possible Cobblestoning of Plugs, Tufting	Dog Ear for 3–10 Weeks, Erythema of Scar
Magnitude of Procedure	Multiple Small Procedures	Major Surgical Procedure
Number of Sessions Required	6–12	1–2 Plus Minor Revisions
Effect on Future Scalp Reduction	None	Tightening of Scalp May Make Significant Reduction Difficult or Impossible
Complications	Minor, Easily Corrected	Potentially Serious, i.e., Flap Necrosis, Donor Site Alopecia

6-21) can be transposed into the frontal hairline, which maintains the natural temporal frontal recession (gulf) characteristic of the mature male hairline (Figures 6-16 and 6-18A and B). Although a significant dog ear is more likely with such a flap, these dog ears frequently resolve spontaneously. When correction of a dog ear is required, it is generally more satisfactory than attempts to correct blunting of the temporal gulf. A more posteriorly based flap has the additional advantage of including the posterior branch of the superficial temporal artery at its base, thus incurring an extra margin of safety. The dog ear may be decreased by designing the flap base vertically (Figures 6-16 and 6-18A and B).

Although the vast majority of short flaps are viable without delay, necrosis of the distal 0.5–1 cm (or temporary telogen effluvium) occasionally occurs. In order to minimize the incidence of this complication, some surgeons recommend a 1-week delay (incision of the flap without undermining) prior to transposition. As this maneuver divides the total operative time into two shorter segments and probably decreases blood loss and patient discomfort, and additionally probably decreases the small yet finite risk of significant complication in an aesthetic procedure, it merits consideration.

SCALP REDUCTION

The general criteria for patient selection discussed toward the beginning of this chapter are applicable to patient selection for scalp reduction surgery. The amount of bald scalp that can be excised is a function of scalp elasticity which varies from patient to patient. The scalp elasticity appears to correlate better with tissue thickness than adherence of the scalp to calvarium; thus various methods of estimating laxity preoperatively may be misleading, as they are influenced by "adherence" as well as elasticity. "Tightness" of the scalp, therefore, does not necessarily preclude successful scalp reduction surgery. Many surgeons state that scalp elasticity can be substantially increased by serial relaxing incisions in the galea. Serial scalp reductions are generally required to maximize excision of alopecia. Serial procedures are normally performed at the 6-week to 3-month intervals.

The selection of scalp reduction pattern is dependent on the areas of alopecia present in each individual patient, the plan of the surgeon regarding subsequent hair replacement surgery, and the areas of maximum scalp laxity. The specific patterns illustrated in Figures 6-22–6-27 have been advocated.

Following completion of undermining in the scalp reduction procedure, some surgeons recommend serial relaxing incisions in the galea in order to reduce tension. The amount of bald scalp that can be excised varies from patient to patient as well as with the pattern utilized. In an average patient, a strip of scalp 2–4 cm wide can be excised when using the midline longitudinal ellipse (5–6 cm or more is sometimes possible). Some surgeons feel that it is safe to close the scalp under moderate tension when using the midline longitudinal patterns.

There is controversy regarding the timing of scalp reduction in relation to punch grafting. Some surgeons recommend that scalp reduction be performed prior to punch grafting, whereas others state that patient motivation is best maintained if the results of punch grafting in the frontal hairline are discernible prior to the initial scalp reduction. Telogen effluvium is rarely a problem in the grafted area if punch grafting precedes scalp reduction unless the grafted area is placed under excessive tension. If punch grafting is performed prior to scalp reduction, the surgeon must plan the hairline more anteriorly and wider than usual since posteromedial displacement is anticipated for each longitudinal midline reduction that is performed (Figure 6-10).

Timing of scalp reduction in conjunction with flap surgery is another controversial issue. Although scalp reduction may precede or follow punch grafting, most surgeons agree that if flaps are to be utilized to reconstruct the frontal hairline, they should be transposed *prior* to scalp reduction. If reduction precedes flap transposition, closure of the flap donor site may be difficult because of decreased scalp elasticity resulting from the reduction procedure.

The pattern of scalp reduction also varies. The C, J, and U patterns result in transection of many of the neurovascular bundles supplying the central scalp. As the vascularity of the central scalp is impaired, these patterns should be closed without significant tension in order to minimize the incidence of scalp necrosis and scar widening. Hypesthesia of the central scalp is often a problem following use of these patterns. In order to minimize elevation of the frontal hairline when using these patterns, undermining of the anterior flap is avoided, thus limiting the amount of alopecia that can be excised. The T or Y ("Mercedes") patterns create multiple flaps, the tips of which converge under tension at the central closure site. This results in an increased risk of necrosis and scar formation there. The longitudinal median ellipse and paramedian crescenteric patterns allow maximum excision of alopecia while preserving the blood supply to the central scalp.

As the vascular supply of the scalp remains intact, many surgeons state that the skin edges may be closed under moderate tension (following secure galeal approximation), thus further enhancing the extent of alopecia excision. If these patterns are planned prior to punch grafting of the frontal hairline, the hairline should be created more anteriorly and wider than usual as posteromedial displacement is anticipated for each longitudinal midline reduction performed (Figure 6-10). The length of such patterns is determined by the extent and distribution of alopecia, whereas the width of excision is a function of scalp elasticity as well as the experience and skill of the surgeon.

The relative benefit of galeal relaxing incisions is also a debated issue. Many surgeons feel that relaxing incisions in the galea do not add sufficient elasticity to justify the time and risks incurred, whereas others feel that flap advancement and subsequent skin excision is significantly enhanced by these incisions, particularly in patients with reduced scalp laxity. If relaxing incisions are used, they should be placed parallel to the skin edges, since serial incisions are separated by approximately 0.5 cm and extending the full length of the exposed galea. Incisions should extend just through the galeal thickness as evidenced by visualization of subcutaneous fat through the incision. Severing of the many nearby vessels should be avoided.

REFERENCES

1. Alt, T. H.: Scalp Reduction as an Adjunct to Hair Transplantation. *J. Dermatol. Surg. Oncol.*, 12: 401–408, 1980.
2. Ayres, S.: Hair Transplantation. In: Skin Surgery, E. Epstein, and E. Epstein, (Eds.). Thomas, Springfield, 1977.
3. Bosley, L. C., Hope, C. R., Montroy, R. E., et al.: Reduction of Male Pattern Baldness in Multiple Stages. *J. Dermatol. Surg. Oncol.*, 6:6–10, 1980.
4. Elliott, R. A.: Lateral Scalp Flaps for Instant Results in Male Pattern Baldness. *Plast. Reconstr. Surg.*, 60:699–703, 1977.
5. Fleming, R. W. and Mayer, T. G.: Short versus Long Flaps in Treatment of Male Pattern Baldness. *Arch. Otolaryngol.*, 107:403–408, 1981.
6. Juri, J.: Use of Parieto-occipital Flaps in the Surgical Treatment of Baldness. *Plast. Reconstr. Surg.*, 55:456–460, 1975.
7. Kabaker, S. S.: Juri Flap Procedure for the Treatment of Baldness. *Arch. Otolaryngol.*, 105:509–514, 1979.
8. Norwood, O.: Hair Transplant Surgery, Thomas, Springfield, 1973.
9. Norwood, O. T.: Male Pattern Baldness: Classification and Incidence. *Southern Med. J.* 68:1359–1365, 1975.
10. Orentriech, N.: Punch Grafts. In: Aesthetic Plastic Surgery, T. D. Rees (ed.). Saunders, Philadelphia, 1980.
11. Stough, D. B., Cates, J. A., Dean, A. J., Jr.: Updating Reduction and Flap Procedures for Baldness. *Ann. Plast. Surg.* 4:287–295, 1982.
12. Unger, W. P., Baron, R.: Hair Transplantation, Marcel Dekker, New York, 1979.

7
Otoplasty

K. J. Lee
J. N. Hausfeld

TECHNIQUE

The procedure can be performed under local anesthesia using 1% Xylocaine with epinephrine 1 : 100,000 concentration or under general anesthesia in young children. Sufficient hair is shaved around the auricle on both sides before surgery (Figure 7-1). The hair is combed backward and the head is placed in a donut-shaped pillow to stabilize the head and to elevate it away from the operating table so that both ears can be prepped and draped simultaneously. A large 3M tympanoplasty drape is used. Both ears are draped simultaneously. (Under local anesthesia, it is sometimes easier to prep and drape each ear at a time.)

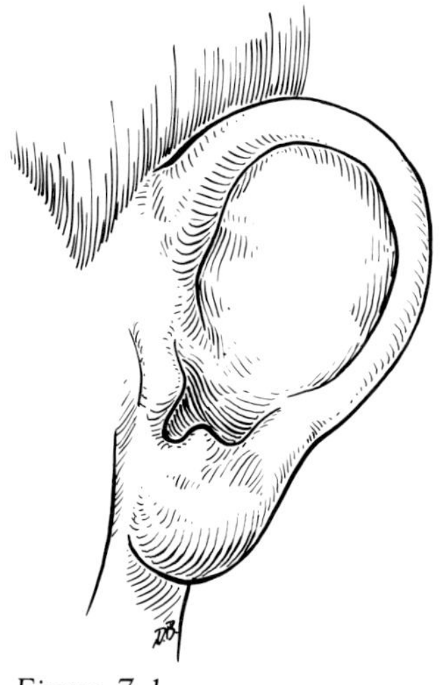

Figure 7-1

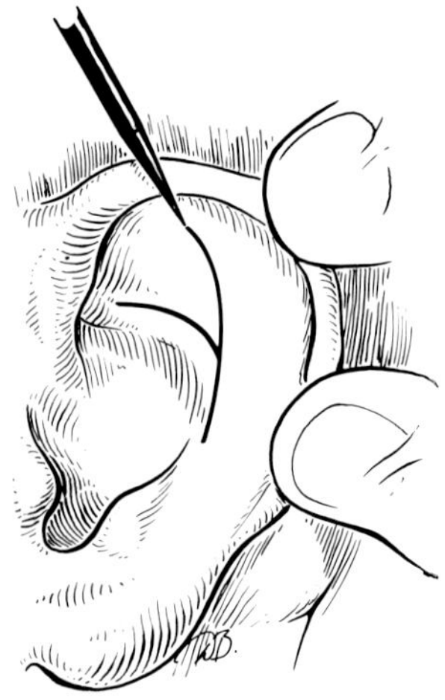

Figure 7-2

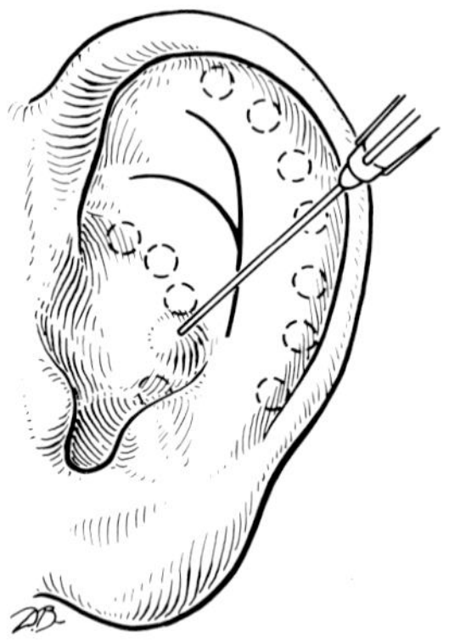

Figure 7-3

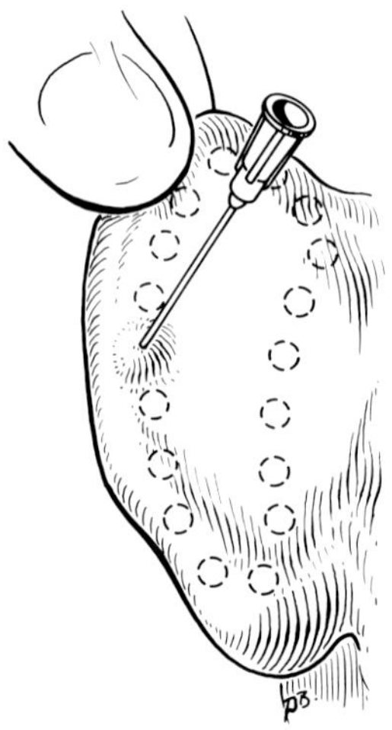

Figure 7-4

There are four aspects to an otoplasty (not all four steps need to be used in every case):

- Step 1. To create the antihelix.
- Step 2. To set back the concha toward the mastoid region. This is needed in a patient with a deeply cupped concha whose concha "bowl" is far away from the mastoid region, resulting in an excessive conchalmastoid angle.
- Step 3. Excision of a crescent of conchal cartilage in those patients with excessively large conchal cartilage.
- Step 4. Partial removal of the caudal helix and extraresection of the postauricular lobule skin inferiorly to correct a protruding lobule.

Depressing the auricle posteriorly outlines the new antihelix (Figure 7-2). The center line of the antihelix as well as the superior and inferior crura can be penciled in with a surgical marker.

The anterior aspect of the auricle is infiltrated with 1% Xylocaine with epinephrine 1 : 100,000 concentration (Figure 7-3). This gives hemostasis and also dissects the skin away from the perichondrium.

The same is done on the posterior aspect of the auricle (Figure 7-4).

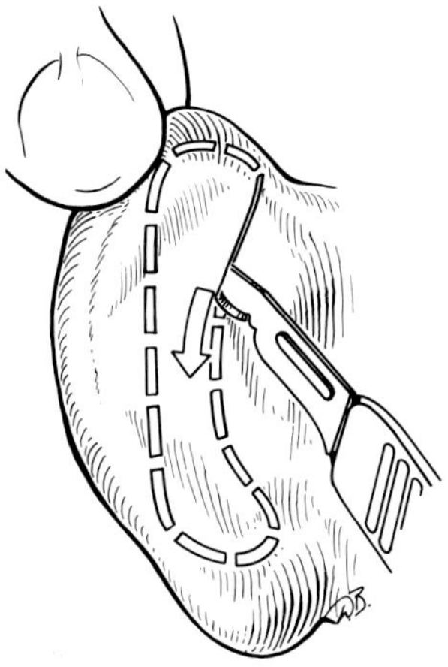

Figure 7-5

A dumbbell-shaped ellipse of skin measuring 0.5–1.5 cm is outlined and excised (Figure 7-5). The skin and subcutaneous tissues are removed, leaving the posterior perichondrium intact. Hemostasis is achieved with cautery. The removal of the dumbbell-shaped skin enables the surgeon to bring back further the superior aspect of the auricle as well as the lobule to avoid a "telephone ear." In the case of excessive protrusion of the lobule on creating a new antihelix, wider excision of skin can be accomplished in the inferior portion of the incision. A W-plasty is helpful.

The skin flaps are raised above the perichondrium anteriorly to the helical rim and posteriorly to the junction of the concha on the mastoid periosteum (Figure 7-6).

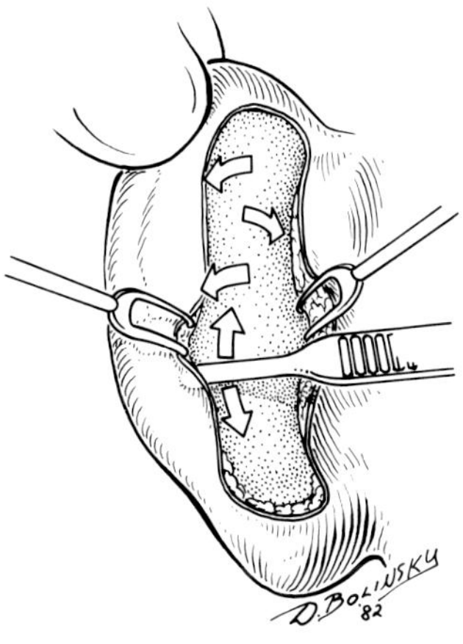

Figure 7-6

Fish-scaling of the posterior layer of perichondrium and full thickness of the cartilage is then done with a No. 15 Bard-Parker blade or a Holmes' cartilage knife (Figure 7-7). The Beaver blade also serves this purpose very well. It is important not to penetrate the anterior auricular skin. The area of fish-scaling should be centered around the centerline of the antihelix and the superior crus. The area of fish-scaling can be extended laterally or medially in order to achieve the desired "break" of the existing cartilage spring. If the cartilage is too thick or resistant to folding, a diamond burr may be used to thin the cartilage after a small section of the perichondrium has been stripped away.

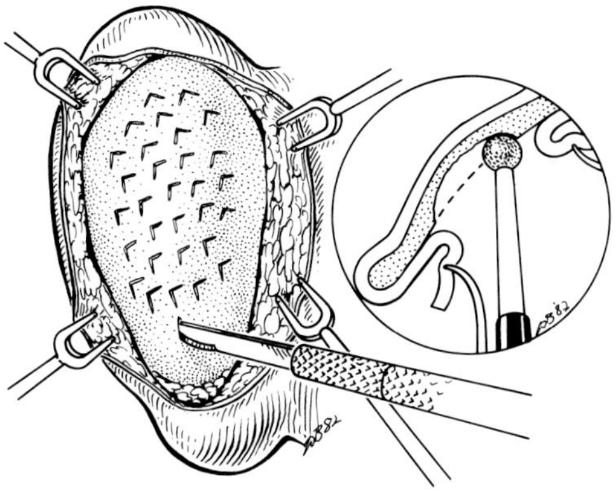

Figure 7-7

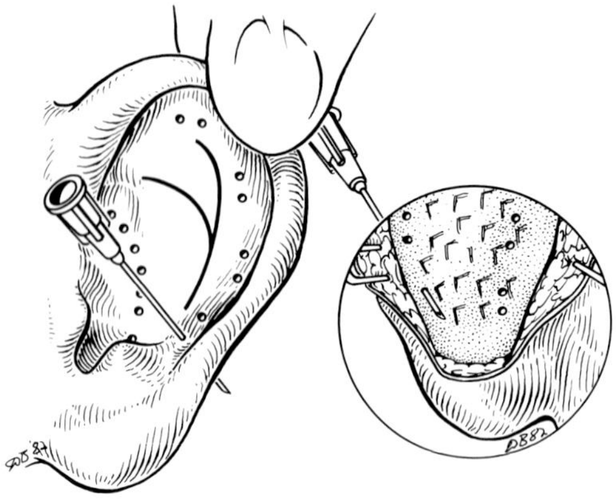

Figure 7-8

The placement of three to five mattress sutures is planned. The position of the proposed mattress sutures is outlined in a radial fashion on the anterior aspect of the ear (Figure 7-8). With the use of a small No. 26 needle, through-and-through punctures are then made on either side of the centerline of the desired antihelical fold. The needle is introduced anteroposteriorly, passing through the anterior auricular skin, anterior perichondrium, cartilage, and posterior perichondrium. The tip of the needle is touched with a cotton applicator soaked with a dye solution prior to withdrawal. On withdrawal of the needle, the desired position for the mattress sutures is stained on the posterior perichondrium. When marking the position for the most superior suture, it is important to place it such that the curve of the newly created antihelix is more in a superoanterior direction rather than in a straight superior direction. This avoids a "pointed ear" appearance.

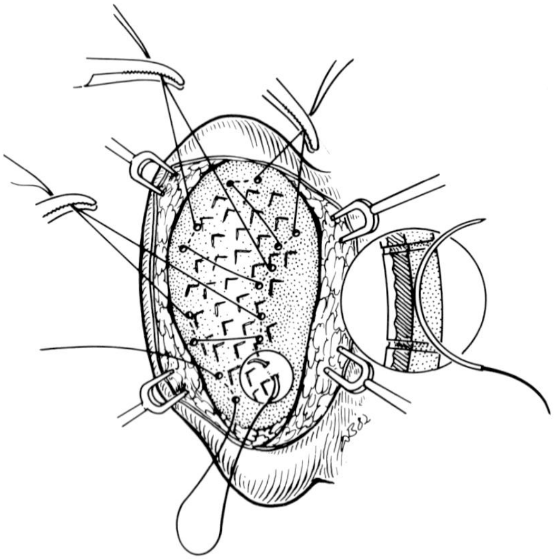

Figure 7-9

Either 4-0 white mersilene, 4-0 clear nylon, or 4-0 white cotton can be used for these mattress sutures. A noncutting needle is preferred in order to avoid damaging the cartilage. As shown in Figure 7-9, the needle pierces the posterior perichondrium, the full thickness of the cartilage, and the anterior perichondrium, avoiding the anterior auricular skin. It is advanced underneath the anterior auricular skin for 5–6 mm and then passed through all the three layers again posteriorly. After this arm of the horizontal mattress suture is completed, the same motion is performed in the opposite direction on the other side of the antihelical fold guided by the correct dye indicator marks. As each mattress suture is placed, each should be temporarily snugged down to show its effect on the antihelix. An improperly placed suture should be removed at this time and replaced. When a mattress suture has been placed correctly, the ends of the suture are temporarily held with a mosquito clamp. It is important not to tie the sutures until all the sutures have been properly placed.

By temporarily snugging down all the sutures, if it is felt that the lobule protrudes, the sutures are loosened and the caudal helix is dissected and partially removed (Figure 7-10). Partial or complete removal of the caudal helix will prevent protrusion of the lobule. When the surgeon is satisfied that the sutures are properly placed, beginning with the most inferior suture, they are tied with four to five square knots. The tension of the sutures vary depending on the deformity and the desired result. The auricle should be adjusted so that it lies 16–18 mm from the skin overlying the mastoid.

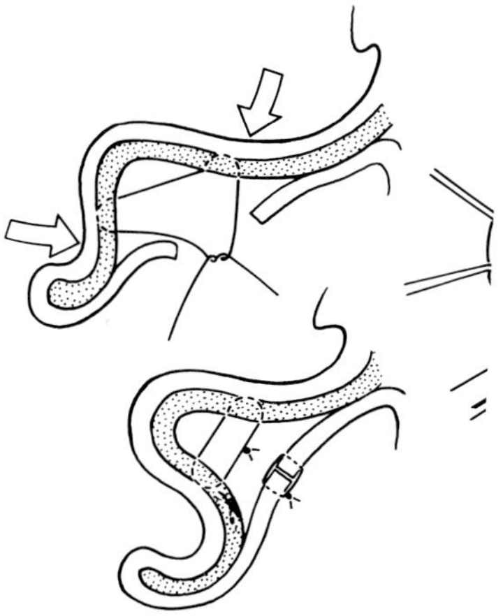

Figure 7-10

Hemostasis should be rechecked at this stage. The skin incision is closed with interrupted 5-0 nylon sutures (Figure 7-11). A rubber drain is not always necessary. Cotton saturated with bacitracin ointment is then carefully packed into the convolutions of the auricle anteriorly and posteriorly. A mastoid-type dressing is applied. The dressing is changed within 48 hours to inspect for hematoma. Then a similar pressure dressing is applied and left on for 7–10 days subsequently. Oral antibiotics are given for the first week postoperatively. An elastic headband is used to splint the ears at night for an additional 4–6 weeks.

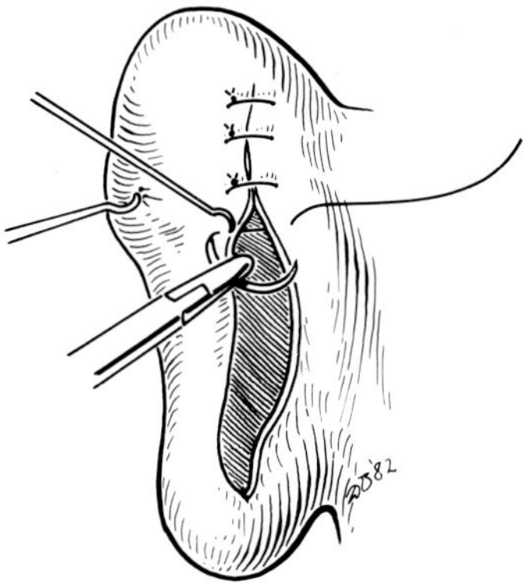

Figure 7-11

ALTERNATIVE TECHNIQUES

In patients who exhibit a deeply cupped concha that is laterally displaced from the mastoid region, resulting in an excessive conchal-mastoid angle, extra stitches of 3-0 clear nylon, 3-0 white mersilene, or 3-0 white cotton in a horizontal mattress fashion can be placed from the mastoid fascia to the periosteum of the concha cup. Three or more of these conchal-mastoid sutures can be placed prior to placing sutures mentioned above to create the antihelix.

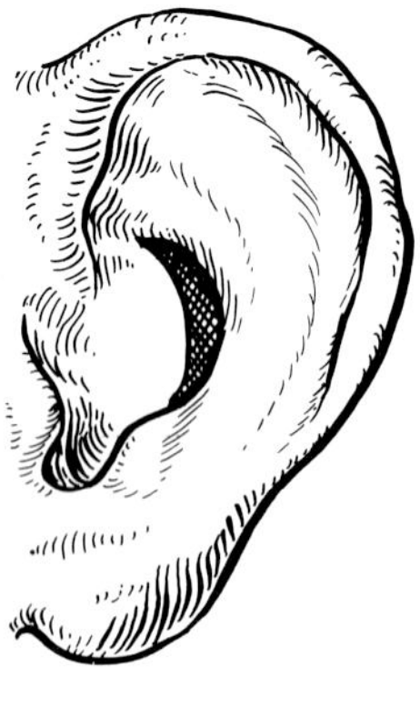

Figure 7-12

In patients who have an excessively large concha cartilage, a crescent of concha cartilage can be removed (Figure 7-12). The crescent of the concha cartilage is to be removed from the area of the concha just anteromedial to the centerline of the antihelix. Whenever cartilage incisions are made, it is important to avoid producing sharp, unnatural edges. This can be minimized by proper cartilage thinning with the diamond burr, as well as meticulous approximation of the cartilage edges.

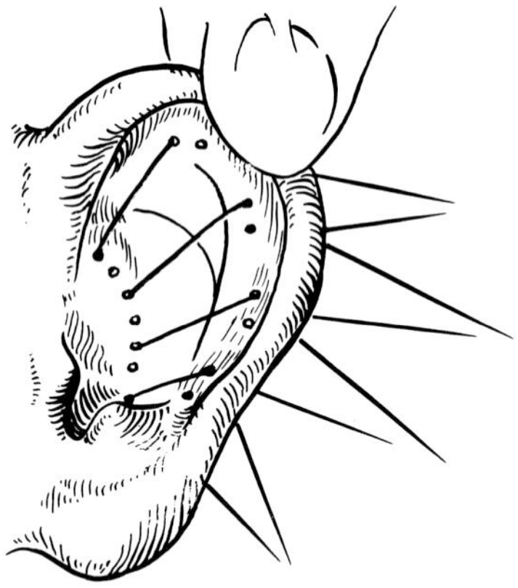

Figure 7-13

Instead of using the No. 26 needle and a dye to mark the posterior perichondrium to guide the placement of sutures, Maniglia *et al.*[1] use temporary 4-0 black silk simple stitches as guides. A straight Keith needle threaded with 4-0 black silk is introduced anteroposteriorly, penetrating the anterior auricular skin, anterior perichondrium, cartilage, and posterior perichondrium (Figure 7-13). The silk is then removed from the needle and, after rethreading, is again introduced anteroposteriorly. The silk marks the position for the 4-0 white mersilene mattress stitches.

REFERENCES

1. Maniglia, A. J., Maniglia, J. J., Witten, B. R.: Otoplasty—An Eclectic Technique. *Laryngoscope* 87: 1359–1368, 1977.
2. Mustardé, J. C.: Correction of Prominent Ears Using Simple Mattress Sutures. *Br. J. Plast. Surg.* 16:170–176, 1963.

8

Ancillary Procedures for Facial Rejuvenation

Frequently the aesthetic result of any facial plastic surgery may be enhanced by local procedures to harmonize the cosmetic result. This chapter covers chemical peeling, dermabrasion, collagen augmentation, skeletal and soft-tissue augmentation, local rhytid excision, and superficial vein cauterization.

CHEMICAL PEEL

The basic formula for chemical peel is 88% phenol, 3 ml; distilled H_2O, 2 ml; Septisol, 8 drops; and croton oil, 4 drops. Storage in a dark bottle will prevent gradual breakdown of the formula. The mixture can be diluted with isopropyl alcohol to make progressively weaker solutions for lighter peels. A more dilute solution will not coagulate the epithelium as readily; weaker solutions are used to feather and blend different areas of the face.

A full face peel is a major operation, necessitating an EKG monitor, intravenous (IV) fluids, and standby oxygen and crash cart. This equipment is necessary in the event that cardiac arrhythmias develop from phenol toxicity. Adequate sedation with a narcotic by weight and supplemented with IV diazepam (Valium) assures patient comfort. The patient's face and hair must be washed the night before and the morning of surgery. Gauze sponges moistened with acetone are used to remove the excess oil from the facial skin. In order to remove the oil uniformly, the face is wiped frequently. When a scraping sound is present as the sponge wipes the face, the formula may be applied to the face. Uneven peeling may result from an unequal removal of the facial oil.

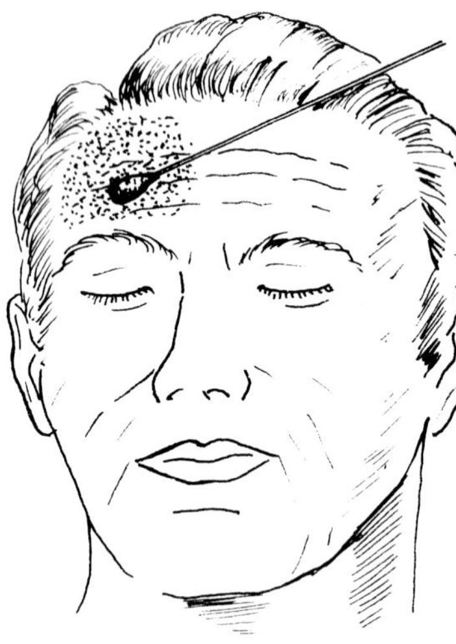

Figure 8-1

The peel solution is applied in segments to the face on Q-tips rolled moderately dry on the edge of the medicine glass (Figure 8-1). The Q-tip reduces the amount of chemical applied, thereby prolonging the procedure and also allowing the solution to penetrate the fine rhytids of the face. Rubbing and reapplying the moistened Q-tips to the same area will increase the depth of the peel. Taping the peeled areas will increase the depth of the peeling by preventing evaporation of the formula. A full face peel should be done in segments (forehead, cheek, circumoral), leaving an adequate amount of time between each facial unit to prevent phenol toxicity. A 1–1.5-hour period is required for a full face peel. During the first 12 hours following application of the solution, the patient will complain of a burning sensation that will require strong oral or intramuscular (IM) analgesics. Vegetable Crisco oil, applied to the face along with cool, moist compresses helps to relieve this discomfort. The patient is instructed to keep a layer of Crisco on the treated areas. After the crusts fall off at 5–8 days, a water-based makeup may be used.

Regional chemical peeling to correct circumoral rhytids, dark circles under the eyes, and glabellar or lateral canthal folds are not as formidable a procedure as a full face peel but require the same technique and postoperative management.

Complications of chemical peeling are best avoided by knowing the contraindications. Chemical peeling is not recommended for male patients; use in the neck region; for patients who have heart, liver, or kidney disorder or diabetes mellitus; or for persons who have deep pores (they will be accentuated by a peel), dark complexion and/or dark eyes, are taking birth control pills, or refuse to wear makeup. Minor complications and irritations from chemical peeling usually resolve with time and patient reassurance. These include erythema (may take 6 months to resolve), sun sensitivity, milia, bleached skin, and persistent burning that is exacerbated in the first few months by sun exposure and exercise.

DERMABRASION

The removal of the epidermis and part or all of the dermis by an abrasive wheel or brush is indicated primarily for acne scars, superficial traumatic and operative facial scars, and fine rhytids. All acne scarring is improved with dermabrasion, but the degree of improvement is variable. Discrete, well-defined, punched out craters yield the best results. Deep, poorly defined contractures with involvement of the dermis are less dramatically affected by dermabrasion. Deep ice pick scars with epithelial tracts that extend to the subcutaneous tela resist improvement. Punch excision with or without graft replacement prior to dermabrasion will afford the best postoperative result. Areas of atrophic depression are first elevated with collagen before dermabrasion.

As with chemical peeling, the face may be dermabraded completely or in sections. Because of possible delineation of abraded areas and pigmentary changes, patients with diffuse acne scarring should have full-face dermabrasion with extension into the hairline and just below the border of the mandible. Feathering the edges of a treated area for acne is difficult but may be done when treating isolated small scarred areas. Light dermabrasion of a surgical or traumatic scar to blend it into the surrounding area is easy and readily done. Perioral dermabrasion of the vertical rhytids is done as a facial unit from the nasolabial folds to the submental area.

TECHNIQUE

The patient's face and hair must be washed the night before and the morning of surgery. Male patients are instructed to shave before coming to the office. All patients are instructed to take no aspirin for 2 weeks and no alcohol for 5 days prior to surgery. Active acne must be under control, and if present on the day of surgery, must be brought under control with tetracycline. No birth control pills must be taken for 1 month pre- and 3 months postoperatively.

The patient should be sedated with narcotics by weight 30 minutes before surgery. For the apprehensive patient, IV diazepam (Valium) will reduce the anxiety. Ice packs are placed on the cheeks prior to freezing with Freon-114 (Frigiderm).

The face is divided into approximately 18 sections. Each section of approximately 7 cm^2 (3 $inch^2$) to be frozen is delineated by four gauzes held firmly in place during freezing. Protection of the eyes, nostrils, and lips is important. Two cans of Freon-114 are used simultaneously.

Start some distance from the skin, gradually approaching to within 4–6 inches. The skin is not placed on stretch during the freezing to allow natural ridges and contours to remain on the skin. After approximately 15 seconds, the skin turns white and should be firmly frozen to -30°F. The gauze sponges are removed completely from the operative field, and dermabrasion begins immediately. Freezing last about 15 seconds; the assistant now stretches the skin.

Begin to plane at the periphery of the frozen field since this is the first area to thaw. Plane slightly beyond the peripheral freeze line since this helps to reduce lines of hyperpigmentation. The rotating wheel is kept parallel to the surface of the skin as it is moved in short, rapid, light-pressured, parallel strokes over the frozen patch. The fraise makes contact only when pulling the abrasive wheel toward the operator; never abrade when pushing the wheel away from the operator. After the area is completed and the skin thawed, lay a gauze over the distal half and wipe the new area free of blood. As you progress around the face, the freezing zones are overlapped. The depth of dermabrasions is important. The epidermis is removed first. Small punctate bleeding from the papillary dermis occurs as the skin thaws. Heavy bleeding indicates the level of the pars vascularis.

As the resistance increases on the abrasive wheel as it is pulled toward the surgeon, the deep papillary or reticular dermis has been reached. The surface appears shredded, and dermabrasion is stopped. If small herniations of fat pop through minute holes, the instrument has reached the bottom of the reticular dermis and should be stopped immediately. Planing through the reticular dermis increases the likelihood of scarring postoperatively. Generally, the deeper the dermabrasion, the more likely there will be hypopigmentation, atrophy, and hypertrophic scarring.

Circumoral abrasion must extend carefully onto the vermillion border to prevent a postoperative line around the lips. Placement of a gloved finger and gauze intraorally will provide direct support. Several dressings are available. Operative-site polyurethane sheeting with adhesive that adheres to intact stratum corneum but does not open wounds and allows for the exchange of gases but not fluids is sometimes used. Biobrane, a plastic sheet bonded with collagen fibers that adheres to a wound to decrease pain, promotes healing and controls bacterial contamination. Debrison beads are also used. Telfa pads with or without an antibiotic ointment covered with gauzes and wrapped may be used. The face may be dusted with thymol iodide powder to absorb the serum and form a crust. After 3 days, the crust is softened with cool water followed by an antibiotic ointment. Saran wrap applied to the abraded skin and covered with abdominol dressing (ABD's) is removed in 24 hours. A bland ointment keeps the crust soft.

Postoperatively, IM steroids (Kenalog, 40 mg) will reduce facial edema. Analgesics (codeine, oxycodone) may be supplemented with aspirin or acetaminophen. Elevation of the head reduces oozing and discomfort. A burning sensation lasts for 24–48 hours as the serum dries and forms a crust. The crust will begin to come off in 7–10 days to expose a reddish skin. Once all crusts are off (usually 1 week) water-based makeup may be applied. The patient is instructed to allow 10–14 days before going out in public.

Dermabrasion may introduce a number of complications. Milia is present in 50 percent of patients who have full face dermabrasion. It can be removed early with an acne stylet or iris scissors. Erythema can also result; however, it usually fades quite well in 2 weeks, although it occasionally may last for up to 6 months. It is exacerbated by sensitivity to cosmetics, soaps, perfumes, and sunlight. Acneiform lesions may form as a foreign-body reaction. The affected area should be cleaned for 7–10 days with gentle evacuation and systemic tetracyline administered. Dermatitis (contact, atopic, eczematous, seborrheic) may flare up after 2 weeks and is treated with topical steroid creams. Telangiectasis in the new skin may be lightly electrodesiccated. Hypopigmentation is to be expected because of removal of melanocytes and lack of solar exposure. After 3 months, gradual exposure to sunlight is permitted with the use of sun-blocking agents; full exposure to the sun is allowed at 6 months. Hyperpigmentation related to injurious exposure of sunlight, perfumes, drugs, soaps, and birth control pills may also occur. To bleach the areas involved, 4% hydroquinone sulfate, 15 g, Retin A (tretinoin) 0.1%, 15 g, with or without triamcinolone acetonide 0.1%, 15 g is applied twice daily until the pigment resolves. The rate of hyperpigmentation is 1–5 percent in blond Caucasians and dark Negroes, 30–40 percent in brunette Caucasions and light-brown Negroes, and 80–90 percent in all Orientals. If hyperpigmentation persists, phenol may be used to lighten the patches. Herpes simplex is another possible complication. If it occurs, surgery should be postponed if the infection is active or recent. Vira-A (vidarabine) ointment, Herplex (idoxuridine), applied several times daily will help. Bacterial infections are rare. Hypertrophic scarring may occur; triamcinolone 8 mg/ml by Dermajet or dermal infiltration will reduce the deformity. Hypertrophy is considered to be due to secondary infection over areas of bony prominence with too deep dermabrasions and excessive facial manipulation.

COLLAGEN AUGMENTATION

Since medical-grade silicone has not been approved by the U.S. Food and Drug Administration (FDA) for general use, the development and approval of bovine collagen has given us a tool that greatly increases the armamentarium of the aesthetic surgeon. Depressed scars of acne, trauma, surgery, chicken pox, and the rhytids of the face not corrected with other procedures are particularly amenable to intradermal augmentation. The patient must be cautioned that multiple treatments will be required to gradually fill in the defect as 80 percent of the material is a liquid and will be absorbed.

TECHNIQUE

The patient should be skin-tested 4 weeks before treatment. A 30-gauge needle is inserted directly into the rhytid to achieve a dermal filler; the skin will blanche and a wheal is produced. Multiple direct punctures are made along a rhytid. A depressed scar is approached by inserting the needle at the periphery and advancing it to the depressed scar. Careful, slow injection is necessary. Frequently the material will escape from a skin pore or break through an area of atrophic skin. Stop injection and return to this area 2–4 weeks later.

Complications are rare if the skin test is nonreactive. All complications will resolve in time and are treated symptomatically (antihistamines, steroids, etc.).

FACIAL AUGMENTATION

In selected individuals with flat malar eminences, augmentation with Silastic implants may be efficacious. Congenital or acquired depressed areas of the face may be augmented with alloplastic implants. Free autografts of fat or dermis do absorb. Supramed mesh or carved Silastic blocks may be used by a variety of approaches to augment the forehead, orbital rim, or malar areas. Implantation of several sheets of Supramed mesh in the abdomen for 9–12 weeks to allow fibrous tissue ingrowth greatly reduces the likelihood of its later being rejected. The allograft material is then harvested, trimmed, and placed in the specific area to be augmented. Slight underestimation of the size of the implant necessary to fill out the defect will prevent revision surgery to reduce excess bulk once it has been implanted.

For malar augmentation, preformed Silastic implants are commercially available (Figure 8-2).

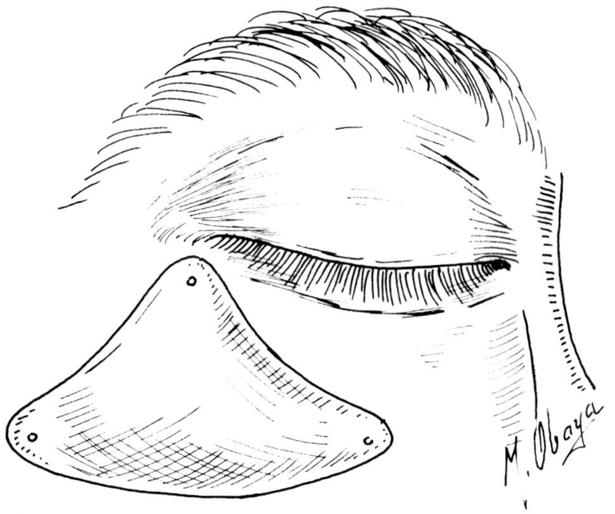

Figure 8-2

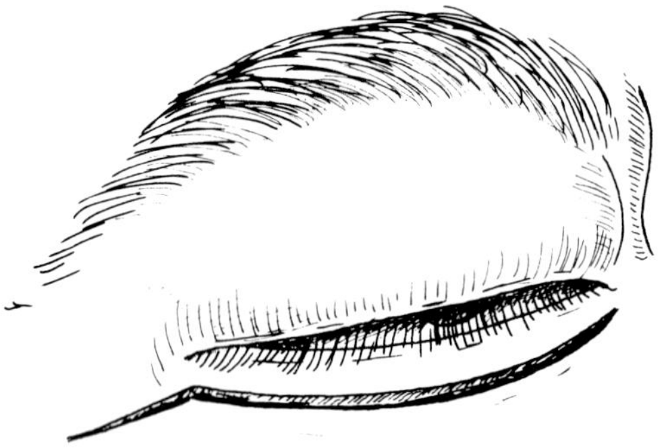

The malar eminence is approached through a lower lid blepharoplasty incision or intraorally. A subciliary incision is made (Figure 8-3).

Figure 8-3

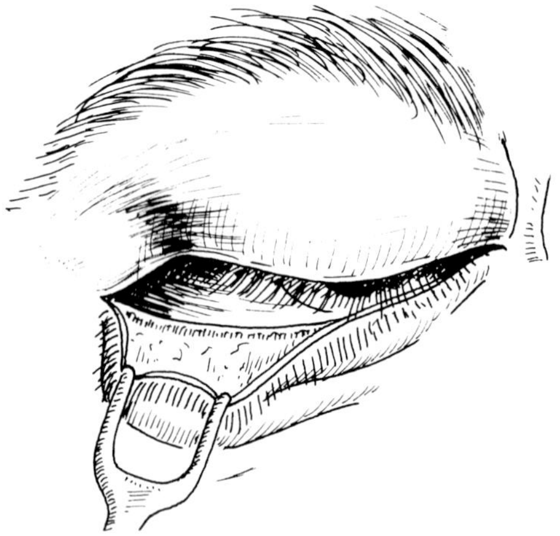

The skin muscle flap is retracted (Figure 8-4) and a pocket is created to accept the implant.

Figure 8-4

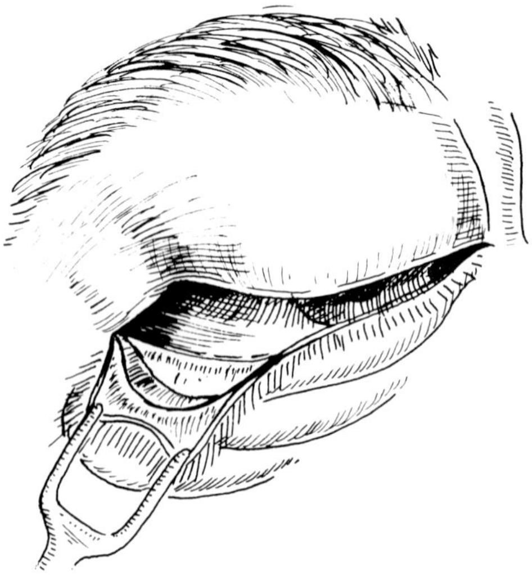

An incision is made in the periosteum (Figure 8-5).

Figure 8-5

Figure 8-6 shows the subperiosteal dissection.

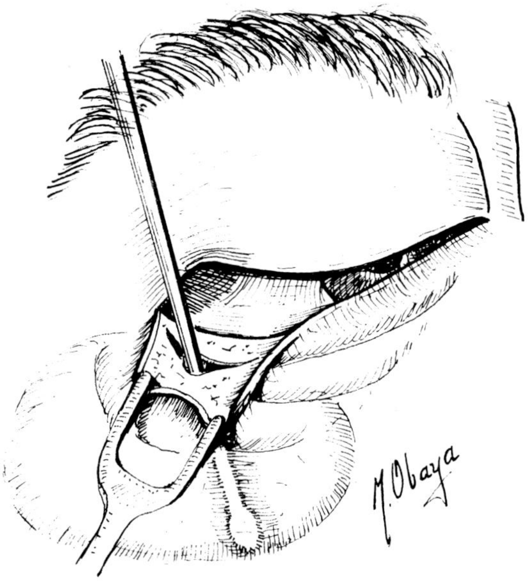

Figure 8-6

After the implant is dipped in an antibiotic solution, it is placed in the pocket (Figure 8-7) and the wound is closed.

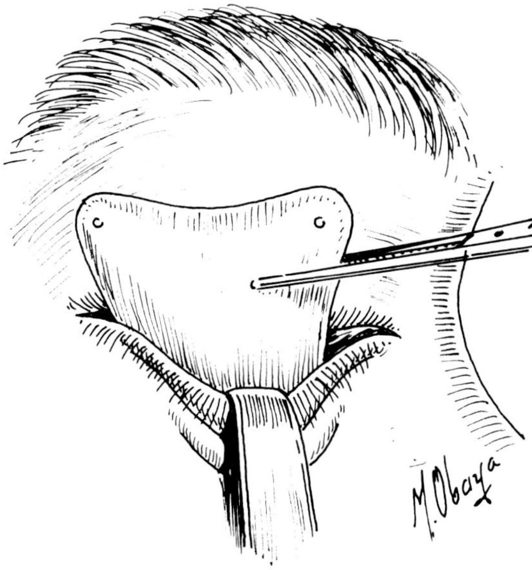

Figure 8-7

SEGMENTAL RHYTID EXCISION

Frequently the patient desires a local area treated without other facial surgery. Local excision of the specific area (glabellar lines, nasolabial folds, etc.) will suffice if the patient is willing to accept a scar in place of a rhytid.

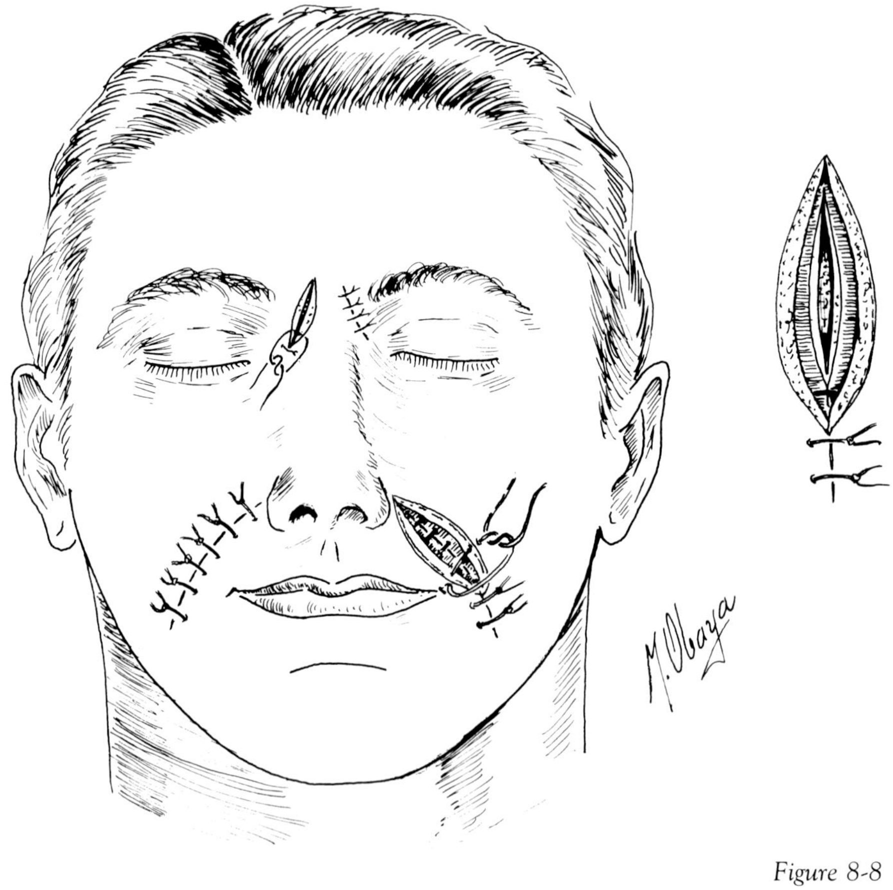

Figure 8-8

The area to be excised is marked, infiltrated, and locally excised (Figure 8-8). The muscle is sectioned and a piece removed to prevent its recurrence. The edges are then minimally undermined and closed in layers with eversion of the skin edges and subcuticular closure.

SUPERFICIAL FACIAL TELANGIECTASIS REMOVAL

Superficial telangiectasis of the face may be readily removed with microelectrode cauterization. The dilated veins of the bulbous nose or the isolated cutaneous "spider" hemangioma are treated.

As shown in Figure 8-9, the insulated microcautery needle is placed at several points in the feeding vessel if possible, and the vessel is lightly cauterized. Only the tip of the needle carries current, and therefore the skin is not burned. It may be necessary to "spotweld" several places along the vessel to effectively coagulate it. Two weeks later the small branches may have to be recauterized.

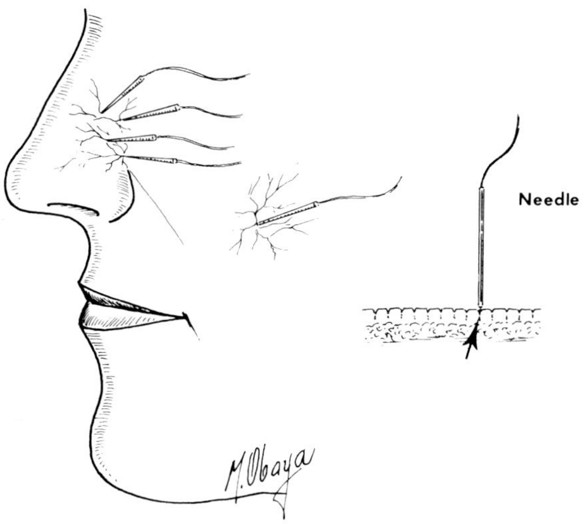

Figure 8-9

DISCUSSION

There is some controversy regarding the value of chemical peel versus dermabrasion. Chemical peeling in the younger patient should rarely be done because of the reduced sun exposure that is necessary for the rest of the patient's life. Chemical peeling is superior for thin, light-colored, dry skin, whereas dermabrasion is better for dark, thick, oily skin. Black patients may be dermabraded safely; they repigment in 5–6 weeks. Dark brown skins do better than do light-skinned patients. All patients who have a chemical peel or dermabrasion should be on antibiotics (erythromycin or tetracycline). Fine rhytids of the aging skin are probably best treated with a chemical peel since the results are smoother, more uniform, and less demarcated and seem to last longer. Because dermabrasion is not as deep, it will not affect the melanocytes as readily as will a chemical peel.

REFERENCES

1. Brennan, H. G.: Augmentation Malarplasty. *Arch. Otolaryngol.*, 108:441–444, 1982.
2. Stegman, S. J.: A Comparative Histologic Study of the Effects of Three Peeling Agents and Dermabrasion on Normal and Sundamaged Skin. *Aesthetic Plast. Surg.*, 6:123–135, 1982.
3. Stegman, S. J. and Tromovitch, T. A.: Implantation of Collagen for Depressed Scars. *Dermatol. Surg. Oncol.*, 6:6, 1980.
4. Straith, R. E., Lawson, J. M., and Hipps, J. C.: Postgraduate Medicine, Vol. 29, No. 2, February 1961. Presented before the 45th Annual Assembly of the Interstate Postgraduate Medical Association at Pittsburgh.
5. Stucker, F.: Autoalloplast. *Arch. Otolaryngol.*, 108: 130–141, 1982.

9

Cervicofacial Liposuction

Douglas D. Dedo
K. J. Lee

Approximately 5 years ago, the French began to employ lipolysis for the removal of unsightly fat and cellulite in the abdomen and legs. The original technique involved injection of saline and enzymes to break the fat down prior to extracting the subcutaneous fat with suction curettage. The French technique has been modified by a group of Americans who observed the French operate. They returned to this country and pioneered the liposuction dissection technique for fat removal. From the success obtained with abdominal, buttock, and thigh sculpturing, smaller cannulas were designed and used to remove the fat in the nasolabial fold, jowl, and neck areas of the head and neck. Although this method of fat removal and sculpturing is in its infancy and extremely new, it is being included in this textbook to present the latest state of the art for facial and neck sculpturing.

A review of the anatomy in Chapter 1 will show that the layer of fat being removed in the neck is the insulating layer of fat just beneath the skin and on top of the platysma muscle. In selected individuals, the deep submental fat pad may be judiciously aspirated to contour the submental area.

For the first time we have an alternative to excision of the nasolabial fold skin that becomes redundant with the passage of time. Prior to fat suction, the only method for improving the fullness of the nasolabial fold was direct excision as presented in Chapter 8.

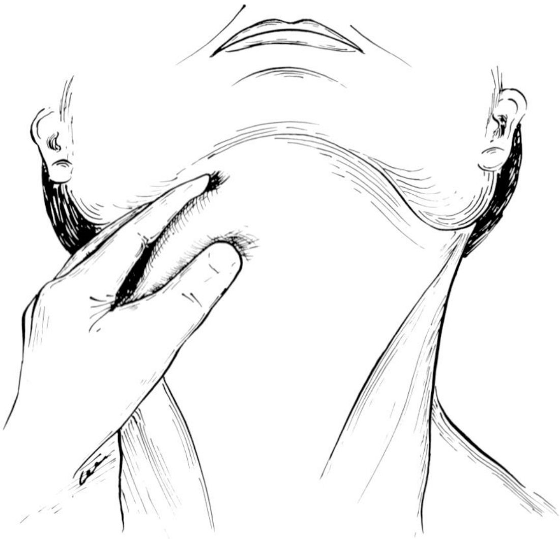

Figure 9-1

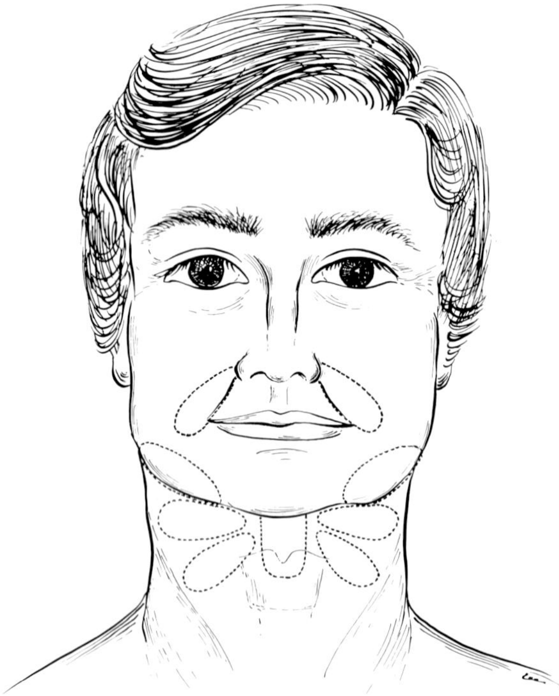

Figure 9-2

OPERATIVE TECHNIQUE

The patient is placed in the sitting position so that the dependent areas of fat collection may be identified. If the patient is placed in the supine position, the nasolabial folds will flatten as well as the jowl and submental areas. The skin is grasped between the thumb and the index finger, and the fat is palpated beneath the skin in the nasolabial fold, submental, submandibular, and jowl. These areas are delineated with methylene blue (Figures 9-1 and 9-2).

To reduce distortion of the subcutaneous fat, the smallest volume of local solution is used. The infraorbital nerves and cervical plexus are blocked with local solution as described in Chapter 1. The areas of undermining are lightly infiltrated with 1% lidocaine (Xylocaine) and 1 : 100,000 or 1 : 200,000 epinephrine (Adrenalin).

The submental collection of fat may be approached through one of three incisions (Figure 9-3). If a chin implant is to be used in the Class V patient with excessive adipose tissue, the incision is made at the first submental crease (Figure 9-3, incision A), approximately 0.5 cm in length. If platysma muscle excision, plication, or flaps are to be made, the incision is placed posterior to the first submental crease as discussed in Chapter 1.

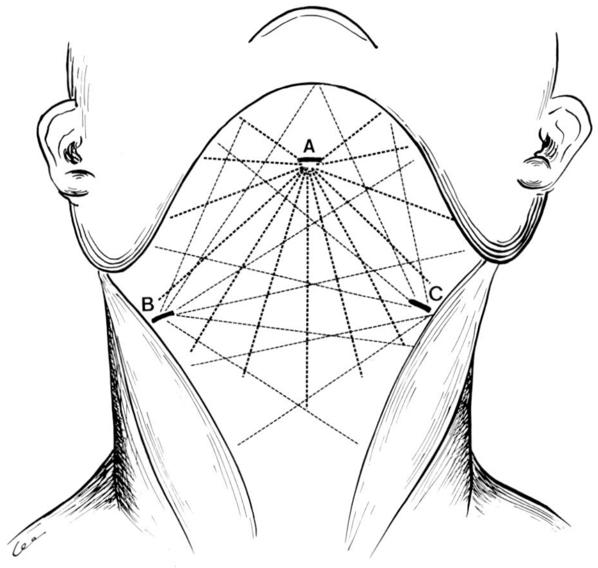

Figure 9-3

Blunt scissors are then introduced into the stab incision and thrust into the fat, down to the level of the platysma muscle (Figure 9-4).

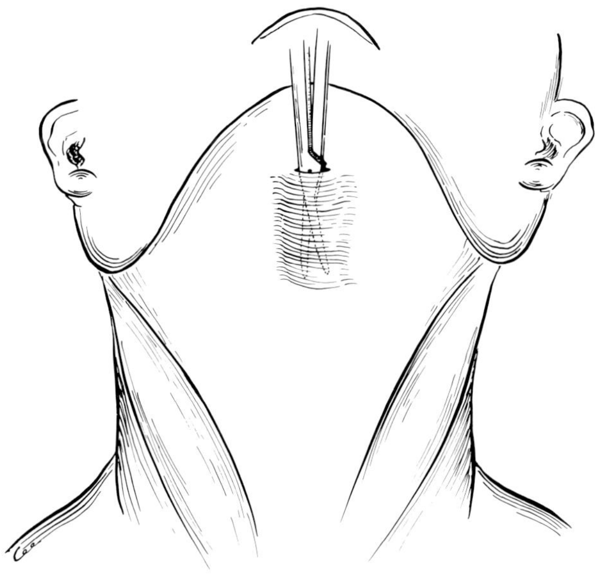
Figure 9-4

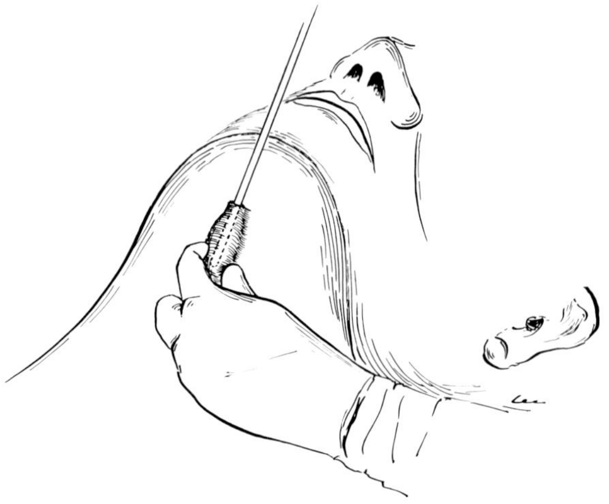

Figure 9-5

The $\frac{3}{16}$-inch suction cannula is inserted with the opening facing away from the skin (Figure 9-5). The skin and subcutaneous fat are pinched between the thumb and the index finger and elevated. The cannula is then pushed bluntly and gently to the limit of the marking of methylene blue and the suction turned on.

Withdrawing and inserting the cannula multiple times, one can squeeze and "milk" the fat into the opening of the cannula as it is gently but firmly withdrawn toward the skin. While introducing the cannula, it is important to advance gently. If resistance is felt, it may be preferable to withdraw and readvance in a slightly different path.

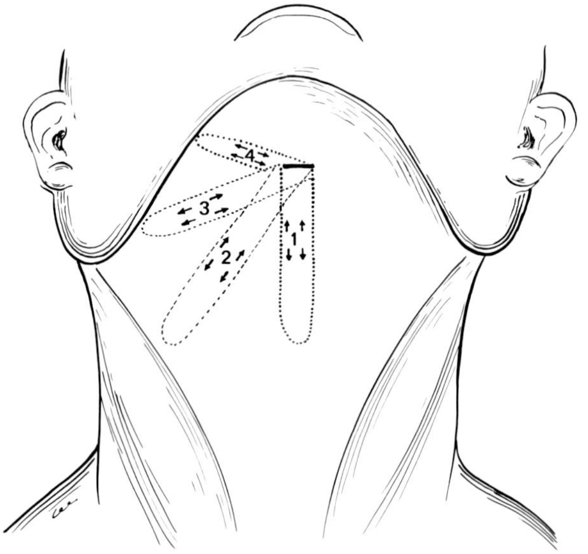

Figure 9-6

It is important to begin deeply and work more superficially. Once the area of fat is removed in the midline, the suction is turned off and the cannula directed approximately 30° to the right and passed down in a deep plane on top of the platysma muscle, and again, by using an in-and-out motion, the cannula is gently but firmly worked toward the surface of the skin as the thumb and index finger squeeze the skin and subcutaneous layer of fat (Figure 9-6). Once this area has been aspirated, the suction is turned off and the cannula is then inserted in a plane in the submandibular area to aspirate and remove this fat. It is possible to remove fat in the jowl area again by pinching it with the thumb and forefinger and pushing the cannula back and forth. Thus, the right half of the neck has been aspirated of its fat by making individual tunnels as illustrated in Figure 9-6 (1–4). The left half of the neck is handled in identical fashion.

The cannula is never swept back and forth to break the septa between the various channels (Figure 9-7). One will find that when an area has been aspirated, if the cannula is moved laterally or sideways, it will touch the septa. The septa carry the blood vessels and should not be disturbed.

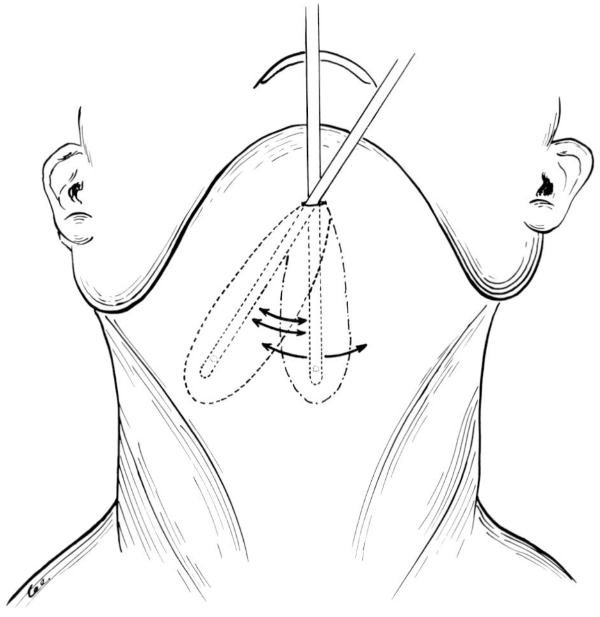

Figure 9-7

The limit of fat suction laterally is the anterior border of the sternocleidomastoid muscle since the muscle itself inserts into the dermis of the skin. Once the entire neck has been aspirated, the suction is turned off and blunt tunnels are made distal to the limit of fat dissection by pushing the $\frac{3}{16}$-inch cannula 1–2 cm beyond the area of fat suction in order to blend and feather the treated areas (Figure 9-8).

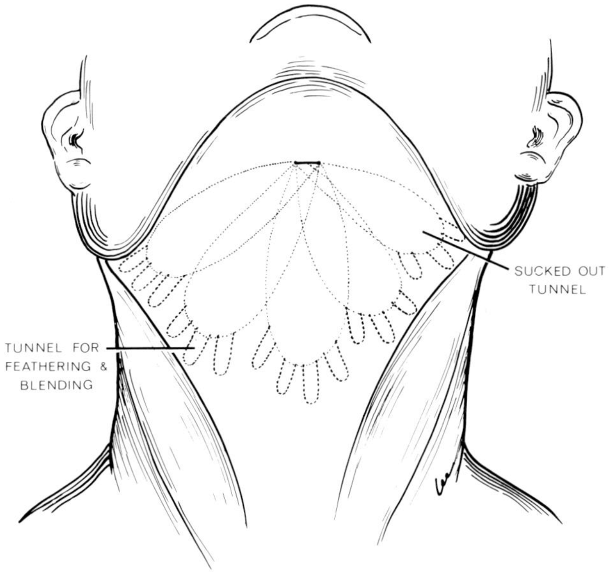

Figure 9-8

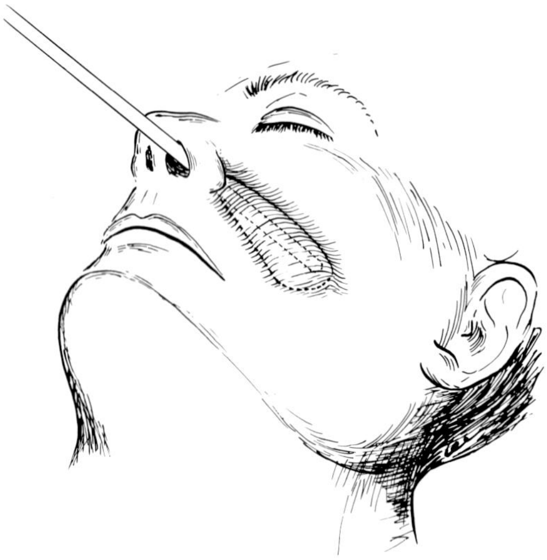

Figure 9-9

For liposuction of the nasolabial folds, the nose is infiltrated with the local solution in the area where stab incisions would be made for lateral osteotomies. A small piece of cotton is placed in the nostril to prevent blood from running down into the pharynx. The nasolabial fold is supplemented with direct local infiltration after the infraorbital nerve block. Scissors are then inserted through the stab wound and spread to the layer of the nasolabial fold. The $\frac{3}{16}$-inch suction cannula is placed into the stab incision, down to the depths of the nasolabial fold inferiorly (Figure 9-9). Again, the opening of the suction cannula *always* faces away from the skin. By gently moving the cannula back and forth and squeezing the nasolabial fold areas, fat is aspirated. Once the fat has been aspirated, the area is feathered with the blunt cannula beyond the area treated, as described previously. The opposite nasolabial fold is treated in an identical fashion. At the end of the procedure, the cotton is withdrawn from the nostrils.

FINESSE

Since liposuction is a new technique, less is better. When fat is removed from the face and neck areas, slightly less should be removed than would be with direct excision. It is a simple procedure, and one can return at a later time and remove irregular collections of fat or remove more fat. Overzealous removal may result in dimpling of the skin and trough formation. The suction cannula must *never* have the opening directed on the facial flaps, as this will cause edema of the dermis and possibly trough formation.

This technique is based a great deal on palpation and feel. The thumb and index finger can literally determine the thickness of the skin flap once the subcutaneous layer of fat has been removed. In order to smooth out the areas of liposuction, it is necessary to tunnel with the blunt cannula the area distal to the site of fat suction in order to allow contraction and a smooth contouring of the overlying flap. Use of a cannula that is too wide in diameter may result in trough formation; a $\frac{3}{16}$-inch cannula is probably the safest and best in the head and neck areas.

COMPLICATIONS

There is continued fat metabolism, necrosis, and contraction of the cervical flaps for several months following fat suctioning. As a result, conservative removal of fat is necessary to allow for the contraction of the cervical skin.

Vertical lines and bands of skin in the submental area have formed but usually resolve gradually over a period of time. If these do not resolve, a secondary facelift procedure may be required in order to redrape the skin posteriorly.

Injudicious fat removal may result in trough formation in the facial areas if the cannula is passed from under the ear lobule to the jowl and the nasolabial fold areas. Placement of the incision inside the nose and the cannula down into the nasolabial fold and jowl areas will prevent this complication. Approaching the jowl fat through the submental area incision will similarly preclude the passage of this cannula under the skin from the lobule. Bleeding, infection, and facial paralysis have not been reported thus far.

DISCUSSION

Regarding the procedure demonstrated in Figure 9-6, some surgeons believe that it is possible to turn the opening of the suction cannula up and remove the globules of fat on the skin flap. This is a controversial issue yet to be resolved; however, the conservative and safest approach is to never turn the opening of the suction on the flap.

While performing the procedure illustrated in Figure 9-8, it is important to repeatedly pinch the skin and feel the thickness of the subcutaneous fat that has been removed. Once the fat has been removed, sweeping the skin up superiorly toward the incision will reveal virtually no bleeding. Because the end of the cannula is blunt, it is almost impossible to perforate major arteries and veins. Since the subcutaneous layer of fat can be readily palpated between the thumb and forefinger, the proper depth of liposuction is maintained, thus preventing injury to major neurovascular bundles. The dissection stays on top of the platysma muscle, and the marginal mandibular branch of the facial nerve will not be injured. Once the area has been contoured by suctioning of the subcutaneous fat, a chin implant is then placed in the routine fashion if clinically indicated.

An alternative incision to the submental stab incision is one placed below the angle of the mandible just in front of the sternocleidomastoid muscle (Figure 9-3, incisions B and C). By placing these incisions bilaterally, one is able to aspirate the fat in the submandibular areas, jowl areas, and midline areas as was done with the submental incision.

An "open" technique for fat suction may be carried out in conjunction with the facelift. Frequently, in the older individual, following fat removal in the neck it will be necessary to perform a concomitant cervicofacial rhytidectomy to correct the laxity of the skin. Following liposuction of the cervical area, less undermining is necessary. Once the preauricular, cervical, and occipital flaps have been elevated, there is readily visualized a layer of fat on top of the subcutaneous musculoaponeurotic system (SMAS). To remove this fat and identify the platysma muscle posteriorly, the cannula is placed on the fat with the opening down and vigorously rubbed with subsequent removal of the fat globules. This open technique may be used at any time during a facelift procedure to contour and sculpture the subcutaneous fat under direct vision.

The amount of suction required for cervical and facial liposuction does not have to be excessive and should not exceed one-half atmosphere of vacuum.

Index

a
b
3 c
4 d
5 e
6 f
7 g
8 h
9 i
8 0 j